Clinical Rheumatology

Clinical Rheumatology

Edited by
MICHAEL MASON, MA, DM, FRCP
and
H. L. F. CURREY, MMed (Cape Town), MRCP
with a Foreword by
SIR HENRY OSMOND-CLARKE, KCVO, CBE, FRCS

PHILADELPHIA, TORONTO
J. B. LIPPINCOTT COMPANY

First published 1970

PITMAN MEDICAL & SCIENTIFIC
PUBLISHING CO LTD
31 Fitzroy Square, London, W1P 6BH

Associated Companies
SIR ISAAC PITMAN AND SONS LTD
Pitman House, Parker Street, Kingsway, London, W.C.2
P.O. Box 6038, Portal Street, Nairobi, Kenya

SIR ISAAC PITMAN (AUST.) PTY LTD
Pitman House, Bouverie Street, Carlton, Victoria 3053, Australia

PITMAN PUBLISHING COMPANY S.A. LTD
P.O. Box 9898, Johannesburg, S. Africa

PITMAN PUBLISHING CORPORATION
6 East 43rd Street, New York, N.Y. 10017, U.S.A.

SIR ISAAC PITMAN (CANADA) LTD
Pitman House, 381–383 Church Street, Toronto, 3, Canada

THE COPP CLARK PUBLISHING COMPANY
517 Wellington Street, Toronto, 2B, Canada

Library of Congress Catalog Card No. 75–133190

SBN: 272 79335 3

Originally published by Pitman Medical & Scientific
Publishing Co. Ltd. under title of
An Introduction to Clinical Rheumatology

Printed by photo-lithography and made in Great Britain at the Pitman Press, Bath

21 2409 11

Contributors

Geoffrey L. Asherson, MA, DM, MRCP, DCH, MC (Path), Head of the Division of Immunology, Clinical Research Centre, Northwick Park, London. (Late Reader in Immunology, The London Hospital Medical College.)

Colin G. Barnes, BSc, MRCP, Physician, Department of Physical Medicine and Rheumatology, The London Hospital.

H. L. F. Currey, MMed (Cape Town), MRCP, Reader in Rheumatology, The London Hospital Medical College. Physician, Department of Physical Medicine and Rheumatology, The London Hospital.

M. A. R. Freeman, MD, FRCS, Orthopaedic Surgeon, The London Hospital. Director, The Biomechanics Unit, Department of Mechanical Engineering, Imperial College of Science and Technology, London.

Graham R. V. Hughes, MRCP, Lecturer in Medicine, The London Hospital Medical College.

Anthony D. M. Jackson, MD, FRCP, DCH, Physician, Children's Department, The London Hospital and The Queen Elizabeth Hospital for Children, London.

J. D. Jessop, MA, MRCPI, MRCP, DPhys Med, Senior Registrar, Department of Physical Medicine and Rheumatology, The London Hospital.

Michael Mason, MA, DM, FRCP, Senior Physician, Department of Physical Medicine and Rheumatology, The London Hospital. Physician in Rheumatic Diseases, King Edward VIIth Hospital for Officers. Civil Consultant in Rheumatology, the Royal Air Force. President, British Association of Physical Medicine and Rheumatology. Hon. Medical Secretary, The Arthritis and Rheumatism Council.

Contents

APPENDIXES

Foreword

Sir Henry Osmond-Clarke, KCVO, CBE, FRCS

Orthopaedic Surgeon to HM The Queen;
Senior Orthopaedic Surgeon, The London Hospital;
Senior Visiting Surgeon, Robert Jones and
Agnes Hunt Orthopaedic Hospital, Oswestry;
Honorary Civilian Consultant in Orthopaedic
Surgery, The Royal Air Force

We are now well into the second half of the twentieth century, a century that has heralded remarkable—often startling—progress in medicine, particularly in the fields of chemical pathology, microbiology, genetics, immunobiology, and therapeutics; the latter, alas, not without iatrogenic hazards. As a result of these advances the management of disease can no longer be undertaken by a single individual, as in previous centuries, when certain surgeons and physicians were regarded, and regarded themselves, as omnipotent! Today, team-work is essential in almost every branch of medicine, and it is particularly true in dealing with arthropathies and other rheumatic diseases. One of the very first hospitals in the United Kingdom to develop a close liaison in research, diagnosis, and treatment of patients suffering from these ailments was The London. It is, therefore, very fitting that the team handling these problems at that hospital should collaborate in producing a book written in clear, comprehensive, and often elegant style, designed primarily, they state, for the medical student. But the authors, under the virile editorship of Mason and Currey, will find it has a much wider appeal, for it is a real vade-mecum for any doctor concerned with these problems.

It seems a long cry, but indeed it is as recently as the thirties of this century, since orthopaedic surgeons attempted to struggle with both the medical and surgical aspects of the sufferer from arthritis. This book well illustrates how far we have advanced, and how much more can nowadays be offered to the community in dealing with a group of diseases causing so much misery and economic havoc.

Preface

In teaching rheumatology to medical students we are often asked to recommend books on the subject suitable for undergraduate reading. We are impressed by the fact that no single work fulfils the requirements of being both readable in its entirety as a general account of the subject, yet sufficiently comprehensive to supply the modest requirements of the student for a book of reference. At present, the student has access only to general medical textbooks in which the rheumatic diseases are often dealt with inadequately; or he must turn to one of the few large textbooks of rheumatology that provide more detail than a student will require for anything but occasional reading in depth.

Hence this volume, written primarily for the medical student, but providing also, it is hoped, an account of the subject that will appeal both to the postgraduate student in general medicine working for higher diplomas, and to the general practitioner. It sets out to introduce the reader to a large and rapidly developing, even an exciting, subject now generally recognised as a 'growing point' of medicine.

The authors are all actively engaged in teaching medical students and (with a single exception) have clinical responsibility for the care of patients suffering from rheumatic disorders. In order to avoid the expression of too many different points of view, or even actual contradictions, sometimes found in multiple-author books, we have restricted the authorship to colleagues from the same teaching hospital. We have worked together at the bedside, in out-patient clinics, and in conference, so that a generally agreed departmental view has matured in the course of many discussions. In certain chapters we have, to a greater extent than is perhaps usual, imposed our own views on our co-authors, when this seemed appropriate, in order to give as authoritative an account as possible. We hope that this is reflected in a consistency of style and content.

The rheumatologist must constantly act in the closest association with his orthopaedic counterpart. He needs to have a working knowledge of the many orthopaedic conditions that overlap with his, and he must know the growing scope of orthopaedic surgery available to his patient. In the United Kingdom at least, and perhaps especially at The London Hospital, the orthopaedic surgeon and the rheumatologist now have the closest possible collaboration in developing the team management of patients suffering from locomotor disorders. We have, therefore, thought it appropriate to include a chapter on the operative treatment of rheumatic disorders.

In addition, if he is to keep pace with the advancing frontiers of his specialty, the rheumatologist must be familiar with the general principles of immunopathology, chemical pathology, microbiology, and genetics. The availability of excellent textbooks on these subjects has made it unnecessary for us to venture into these areas in excessive detail. However, the central position occupied by immunopathology in so much current thinking about the rheumatic diseases has persuaded us of the need to include, also, a chapter outlining the general principles of this rapidly advancing subject.

In brief, we have tried throughout to concentrate on those aspects of the specialty not already covered adequately for students and we have endeavoured to give a clinically orientated account of the subject always, we hope, with a strictly practical approach.

Finally we should like to pay particular tribute to Mrs Dorothy Boyce who typed the manuscript so patiently and so accurately, and to Mr R. F. Ruddick and other members of The London Hospital Photographic Department for preparing the illustrations with their usual skill. Miss Barbara Watson, a student of The London Hospital School of Physiotherapy, kindly modelled for most of the illustrations in Appendix A. Appendix C is reproduced by kind permission of the Royal College of Physicians of London.

The London Hospital,
Whitechapel, E1
May, 1969

Michael Mason
H. L. F. Currey

1

What is Rheumatology?

Michael Mason and H L F Currey

In many branches of medicine the present classification of diseases has been arrived at by a similar process of evolution. That is, by the recognition, initially, of a late end-stage pathological state, followed by a painstaking unravelling of the various separate diseases that may lead to this common outcome. Thus, for example, chronic nephritis, pulmonary fibrosis, chronic dementia, and liver cirrhosis may each be the end result of a whole variety of pathological processes. The patient study of these conditions illustrates the difficulties of establishing the connection between the early stages of a disease and the final picture, often reached many years later.

In the rheumatic disorders, the major part of the present-day classification of arthritis has been arrived at by a very similar process. Here, a common-end picture is 'chronic polyarthritis' or 'arthritis deformans', represented by a disabled patient with multiple, painful joint deformities. We now know that this clinical picture may be the end result of widely differing disease processes, broadly classifiable as *metabolic*, *degenerative*, and *inflammatory* (plus some relative rarities such as haemophilia).

Failure to distinguish the different diseases that may produce chronic polyarthritis confused medical thinking about the rheumatic disorders up to a surprisingly late date, for it was not until the middle of the nineteenth century that gout was clearly divided off as a separate entity; and not until the end of that century that degenerative joint disease, or osteoarthrosis, was finally separated from the other conditions. (The layman's concepts have, of course, developed even more slowly.)

The group that remained, the *inflammatory arthropathies*, consists of rheumatoid arthritis and a number of related conditions. Sub-division of this large and important group has been evolving over recent years. It now includes rheumatoid arthritis, juvenile rheumatoid arthritis (Still's disease), ankylosing spondylitis, psoriatic arthropathy, Reiter's disease, and colitic arthropathy. These appear to be more or less separate diseases, but they have common clinical and pathological features that make it convenient to group them together. As their aetiology is unknown, they are best referred to, noncommittally, as the *inflammatory arthropathies*. Many types of arthritis are, of course, 'inflammatory', but the term is used here in a more restricted sense. These inflammatory arthropathies are broadly sub-divided on the basis of serological tests for the presence of, so-called, *rheumatoid factor*. Thus, rheumatoid arthritis patients tend to be *sero-positive*, and the others *sero-negative*. Interestingly, this immunological division is paralleled by certain clinical differences. Of course, the process of categorisation is still going on. Still's disease, for example, is not a homogeneous category and is undergoing further sub-division.

The conditions mentioned above, particularly rheumatoid arthritis and degenerative joint disease, together represent one of the most important causes of physical suffering and economic loss from illness in any community. The diagnosis and treatment of these conditions, and the research connected with them, demands a physician trained in general medicine but having a particular interest in diseases affecting the joints. This is the Rheumatologist. His specialty, Rheumatology, embraces those diseases mentioned above, among others, in which disorders of joints are the main pathological feature. His interest and responsibility also overlap with other medical specialties in the care of patients suffering from diseases (such as serum sickness) in which the joints are only one among multiple systems involved and do not necessarily constitute the most important feature.

One group of multiple-system diseases that has become the particular province of the rheumatologist is that which includes systemic lupus erythematosus, progressive systemic sclerosis, polymyositis, dermatomyositis, Sjögren's syndrome, and polyarteritis nodosa. Clinically and pathologically these conditions (and rheumatoid arthritis) sometimes overlap and, although the aetiology of none is yet known, they probably have features of pathogenesis in common. Much current research aims at establishing a causal relationship between the obvious immunological activity apparent in these conditions and the actual damage that occurs to tissues. The evidence of this is now sufficiently strong to have stimulated a trial of non-specific suppression of immune processes as therapy. Thus, the rheumatologist is becoming increasingly interested in immunology.

In another direction, rheumatology overlaps with orthopaedic surgery. Not only does this specialty provide the operative surgical treatment of many rheumatological conditions, but there is a no-man's-land of conditions (e.g. capsulitis of the shoulder) that lend themselves to being managed by either specialty.

Under the present organisation of the National Health Service in the United Kingdom, much rheumatology is practised by physicians designated as consultants in *Physical Medicine*. A word is therefore necessary about the relationship of this specialty to *Rheumatology*. The use of the term 'Physical Medicine' to describe a specialty dates from the period when interest in the locomotor disorders centred around the therapeutic use of electricity, massage, and other *physical* methods. This has passed, but the name persists, and the specialty has evolved into one with wide, but variable, responsibility. Thus, a hospital Department of Physical Medicine may care for patients with rheumatic disorders and 'medical' orthopaedic conditions. It may also provide services in electrodiagnosis and general rehabilitation. In addition, it is usually associated with physiotherapy and occupational therapy services. By contrast, appointments in pure rheumatology tend to be available only at academic institutions. Certainly in Britain, a reorganisation of the structure of these two specialties is urgently needed, and the recommendation of the Royal College of Physicians (as set out in Appendix C) that the postgraduate training of the two specialties should be identical is an important step in the right direction.

2

The Immunology of the Rheumatic Diseases

Geoffrey L Asherson

This brief introduction to the immunology of rheumatic diseases outlines the methods whereby immune responses cause tissue damage, discusses the conditions under which autoimmune responses occur, and also describes the underlying aetiology of certain diseases. Relevant to the subject, but for clarity omitted from this discussion, are the topics: immune tolerance, the classes of immunoglobulin, and the principles behind the various immunological tests used in rheumatology.*

GENERAL CONSIDERATIONS

The mechanisms whereby immunological reactions cause inflammation and tissue damage may be the same whether the antigen is an autoantigen, such as DNA in lupus nephritis, or a foreign antigen such as the malarial antigen in the nephrotic syndrome caused by malaria.

The terms *immunity* and *hypersensitivity* sometimes cause confusion. *Immunity* originally referred to a heightened state of resistance to infection caused by previous exposure to a microorganism. The heightened resistance is usually caused by antibody and/or delayed hypersensitivity, and the word immunity now includes both antibody production and delayed hypersensitivity to any antigen, even when the human is in no sense protected by the immune response. Clearly, death due to anaphylactic shock on injection of penicillin is not an example of heightened resistance to a chemical agent. It is, nevertheless, correctly described as an immune response.

*These are dealt with in:

1. Asherson, G. L. (1967) *British Medical Journal* **iii**, 417 and 479.
2. Holborow, E. J. (1967) *Lancet* **i**, 833, 890, 942, 995, 1049, 1098, 1148, and 1208.
3. Gell, P. G. H. and Coombs, R. R. A. (1968) *Clinical Aspects of Immunology*, 2nd ed. (Oxford: Blackwell).

Hypersensitivity refers to an increased response to an agent caused by previous exposure. Hypersensitivity usually, but not always, carries the sense of a damaging reaction.

There is an important distinction between the two main types of immunological tissue damage. Some tissue damage—anaphylactic hypersensitivity, complement-dependent cytotoxicity, immune complex disease, and the Arthus reaction—is due to circulating antibody or antigen-antibody complexes that can usually be demonstrated in the circulation. Histology shows oedema and sometimes polymorph infiltration. These reactions are called *immediate type hypersensitivity* because a local reaction appears, and is maximal within a few minutes or hours of skin testing. These antibody-mediated reactions should be contrasted with delayed-type hypersensitivity.

Delayed-type hypersensitivity is not due to a circulating antibody but to sensitised lymphoid cells. These reactions are called delayed because the macroscopic lesion first appears about 8 hours after skin testing and is maximal at 24 to 48 hours. Delayed hypersensitivity is one example of cell-mediated immunity. Other examples are contact sensitivity (contact dermatitis), and many cases of transplantation rejection, as well as tumour rejection in experimental animals.

MECHANISMS OF IMMUNOLOGICAL TISSUE DAMAGE

Gell and Coombs described the different tissue-damaging immune responses as Types I to IV. These responses are discussed below.

Anaphylactic Hypersensitivity (Type I). Antibodies are composed of heavy and light chains. The heavy and light chains together form the antibody-combining sites which combine with antigen, while parts of two heavy chains together form the Fc (crystallisable) fragment (Fig. 2.1).

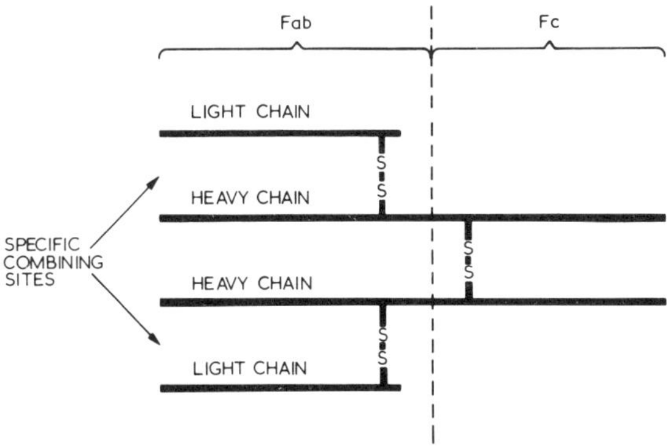

FIGURE 2.1 Diagram of the immunoglobulin G (IgG) molecule

Some antibodies are able to adhere to mast cells and other cells by the Fc fragment (i.e. by a part other than the antibody combining site). When exposed to antigen, these coated cells release histamine, serotonin, and other pharmacologically active materials. This effect is clinically important in asthma, hay fever, and urticaria. When the interaction between antigen and antibody occurs near the capillaries the release of histamine and other pharmacologically active agents may lead to a sudden drop in blood pressure, and even death. This is the anaphylactic shock that sometimes occurs after the injection of foreign serum or penicillin (especially common in patients with a personal or family history of atopy, i.e. asthma, hay fever, or infantile eczema). These reactions can be transferred by injecting serum into a second person and injecting antigen into the same area 24 hours later. A weal and flare occur within a few minutes. This transfer is called the *Prausnitz-Küstner* (P-K) reaction. (The risk of serum hepatitis should be borne in mind before it is performed.) Anaphylactic antibody, at least of the type responsible for hay fever and the P-K reaction, belongs to a class of immunoglobulin (antibody) called IgE. IgE antibody is probably important in preventing the entry of parasites through the skin. It is not known to be important in rheumatic diseases.

Allergic Cytotoxicity—cell damage mediated by antibody plus complement (Type II). Complement is a group of factors normally present in serum, which is capable of causing lysis of red blood cells when these are coated with complement-fixing antibody (i.e. antibody able to combine with complement). Such complement-mediated lysis causes intravascular haemolysis in a few patients with severe autoimmune haemolytic anaemia. (More commonly, antibody causes haemolytic anaemia by facilitating the phagocytosis of red cells by macrophages in the spleen and liver.) This type of cell damage is less important in solid tissues, probably because of poor access of antibody and complement to the cell surface.

Arthus Reaction (Type III). When complement-fixing antibodies combine with antigen they alter serum complement components so as to liberate a factor chemotactic for polymorphs. When antigen is injected into animals containing such antibodies there is local oedema with infiltration by polymorphs, and damage to blood vessels by the enzymes of the polymorphs. This reaction is maximal at about four hours and is called the Arthus reaction. It is seen in patients with aspergillosis who are injected intradermally with fungal extract, and in a few patients with farmer's lung. This may be the mechanism of certain forms of arteritis.

Immune Complex Disease (Type III). Antibody combined with antigen is called an antigen-antibody (or immune) complex. Some of these complexes are soluble and pass through the endothelial lining of blood vessels. They are known to pass through the vascular lining of the glomeruli, and thus give rise to chronic renal disease. This is the mechanism of lupus nephritis. They cause arteritis and endocarditis in experimental animals, but this is not fully documented in man.

Delayed Hypersensitivity (Type IV). Type I to III reactions are all due to antibodies. They are sometimes described as immediate or immediate-type hypersensitivity because the reaction occurs within a few minutes or hours after the injection of antigen. In contrast, delayed hypersensitivity reactions (also known as delayed-type hypersensitivity or cell-mediated immunity) first appear macroscopically at about 8 hours and are maximal at 24 to 48 hours. This reaction, unlike the other reactions, is due to sensitised cells and not to circulating antibody, and can be passively transferred by immune cells. Classical examples are the Mantoux, Frei, and Montenegro reactions of tuberculosis, lymphogranuloma venereum, and leishmaniasis. Delayed hypersensitivity reactions are able to kill cells in solid tissues and are important, at least in experimental animals, in preventing the development of virus-induced tumours, in killing cells that have been altered by virus, and in resisting infection by viruses and certain bacteria such as *M. tuberculosis* and *B. abortus*. Delayed hypersensitivity tissue damage is characterised by infiltration with lymphocytes and macrophages (histiocytes). This mechanism is important in experimental autoimmune diseases such as experimental thyroiditis, orchitis, encephalomyelitis, and adrenalitis; and, by analogy, in human putative autoimmune disease. It is probably an important cause of tissue damage in rheumatoid arthritis. Contact hypersensitivity and transplantation rejection are other examples of cell-mediated immunity.

Three *in vitro* tests correlate with delayed hypersensitivity in the intact animal. They are mentioned here because they are important in clinical research.

Inhibition of Migration of Peritoneal Exudate Cells. Peritoneal exudate cells (a mixture of lymphocytes and macrophages), when packed into a small capillary tube, will normally migrate out of the tube. The addition to the medium of an antigen to which the cells are sensitive inhibits this migration. This inhibition depends on a factor liberated by lymphocytes when they encounter an antigen to which they are sensitised. This test has been applied to the study of lymph node and peripheral blood cells in man.

In vitro Cytotoxic Killing. 'Activated' lymphocytes are able to kill cells *in vitro*. Lymphocytes may be activated either by phytohaemagglutinin – PHA, or by exposure to an antigen to which they are sensitive. Lymphocytes from animals sensitive to foreign cells will kill these cells *in vitro*. Finally, normal lymphocytes will kill cells coated with small amounts of antibody.

Blast Transformation in vitro. Lymphocytes in human peripheral blood will divide *in vitro*. This may be detected by microscopic examination for transformed cells and cells in mitosis. These are characteristically large (blast) cells, hence the term blast transformation. Another technique is to measure the incorporation of radioactive nucleic acid precursors into nucleic acid, using thymidine labelled with ^{14}C or tritium. This is a measure of the formation of new nucleic acid which occurs as a preliminary to cell division.

Human cells will transform *in vitro* in three circumstances:

(*a*) Cells from immune individuals will divide in the presence of antigen. This test is sometimes positive in penicillin allergy. Animal work suggests that blast transformation correlates with a state of delayed hypersensitivity rather than one of antibody production.

(*b*) Cells from normal individuals will divide in the presence of certain substances that are thought to interact with the cell surface. These include phytohaemagglutinin and certain antibodies against human immunoglobulins.

(*c*) Cells from a normal individual will divide in the presence of cells from another individual because of the antigenic difference. This mixed cell transformation is a primary *in vitro* immune response.

These tests are used in clinical medicine. Blast transformation by PHA parallels the ability of a human to manifest delayed hypersensitivity. The latter is characteristically depressed in sarcoidosis, leprosy, and Hodgkin's disease.

AUTOIMMUNE RESPONSES

The histology of the joint in rheumatoid arthritis is compatible with several pathogenic mechanisms: it may reflect, in part, the direct damaging effect of the (unknown) causative agent, which might be a microorganism; it may be due to an immune response against the causative agent; or it may be an autoimmune response triggered by the causative agent.

The conditions under which autoimmune reactions occur are:

1. Exposure to cross-reactive antigens, i.e. antigens similar, but not identical, to the body's own constituents. The classical example is seen in rabbits injected with altered thyroglobulin. *Native* rabbit thyroglobulin injected by itself causes neither autoantibody production nor thyroiditis. However, *chemically altered* rabbit thyroglobulin which is similar, but not identical, to native thyroglobulin causes both autoantibody production and autoimmune thyroiditis.

This mechanism may be important in two diseases:

(*a*) Autoantibody formation sometimes follows tissue damage, as in the postmyocardotomy syndrome. This may be due to exposure to altered autologous antigen.

(*b*) Certain bacteria such as the streptococcus have antigens resembling those occurring in human heart muscle. These may be responsible for the autoantibodies to heart muscle found in rheumatic fever.

However, the occurrence of autoantibodies need not mean that a disease has an autoimmume pathogenesis. This is because not all antibodies cause tissue damage.

2. Injection of animals with homologous organ tissue incorporated into Freund's complete adjuvant. This is a water-in-oil emulsion consisting of the antigen in saline and a mixture of paraffin oil, emulsifier, and tubercle bacilli that looks like mayonnaise. Freund's incomplete adjuvant, which lacks the tubercle bacilli, does not cause autoimmune disease. Freund's complete adjuvant cannot be used in man because of the severe inflammation it causes. There is no clear-cut example of adjuvant-induced disease in man, but the increased levels of autoantibodies in leprosy may be due to the adjuvant effect of this (mycobacterial) organism.

3. Infections, including syphilis and primary atypical pneumonia due to *Mycoplasma pneumoniae*, may be associated with the presence of autoantibodies (the Wasserman antibody and cold haemagglutinin).

Rheumatoid factor is an antibody to human 7S immunoglobulin (IgG). It sometimes reacts with altered human and/or animal immunoglobulin, sometimes with antigens that occur on the immunoglobulins of some but not all people (allotypic determinants), and sometimes with autologous gammaglobulin. Rheumatoid factor is usually, but not always, a high molecular weight antibody (IgM). It can be produced experimentally in animals by immunising them repeatedly with dead bacteria. Under these circumstances, antibodies against the organism are formed. These combine with the bacteria, and the antibody (which is slightly modified by this combination) acts as the immunogen that stimulates the production of antibody to immunoglobulin. A similar mechanism probably explains the occurrence of rheumatoid factor in subacute bacterial endocarditis (in which there is a chronic bacteraemia), and perhaps in rheumatoid arthritis.

UNDERLYING AETIOLOGY OF RHEUMATIC DISEASES

A few pointers to the underlying aetiology of rheumatic diseases are of immunological interest: one example is the spontaneous disease of NZB mice, which is a good model for human systemic lupus erythematosus. These mice develop a Coombs-positive haemolytic anaemia, antibodies to nuclei (antinuclear factor – ANF), and nephritis caused by circulating antigen-antibody complexes. They commonly develop lymphoma. It is reported that this disease can be transmitted by cell-free extracts and is due to a virus. The mechanism whereby this virus infection leads to the production of autoantibodies to red cells and to nuclei, which are the immediate cause of the anaemia and the renal damage, is unknown.

There has been much work on models of rheumatoid arthritis. In this disease, characteristic changes in the joints include the formation of a pannus which contains macrophages and lymphocytes, and the occurrence of plasma cells and lymphoid follicles with germinal centres. Plasma cells produce antibody, and germinal centres occur in lymph nodes exposed to antigenic stimuli. The finding of these two morphological features suggests very strongly that the synovial tissue in rheumatoid arthritis is exposed to antigen to which these various cells are reacting. These findings can be reproduced in experimental animals by producing delayed hypersensitivity to a particulate antigen such as fibrin, and then injecting the antigen into the joint. Agents that damage lysosomes, such as the streptococcal toxin streptolysin-S (not to be confused with streptolysin-O), are also able to cause progressive joint damage, perhaps by rendering joint components immunogenic.

Dermatomyositis in adults often occurs in association with carcinoma. It has been suggested that the tumour shares an antigen with muscle and skin and that this initiates an autoimmune disease. Recently, antibodies against tumour and muscle have been reported in these patients.

Certain drugs such as penicillin may produce an illness resembling systemic lupus erythematosus. This drug is chemically reactive and combines with tissue components. It is likely that delayed hypersensitivity develops towards the drug-tissue complex and that this immune response precipitates the illness.

These are a few examples taken from the field of rheumatology in which there is some insight into underlying aetiology.

3

Rheumatoid Arthritis

Colin G Barnes

Rheumatoid arthritis (RA) in its fully developed form, is a peripheral, symmetrical, inflammatory disease of synovium that leads to destructive changes in the joints, and is associated with the presence of abnormal antibodies (rheumatoid factor) in the blood. Although arthritis is the most frequent and prominent manifestation, it must be remembered that this is a generalised disease involving many systems so that it can be more correctly termed *rheumatoid disease*. Incomplete forms are common, and these, in the clinical situation, may present considerable problems of diagnosis.

EPIDEMIOLOGY

Females are more commonly affected than males in a ratio of 3:1, with a maximum incidence of onset in the fifth decade. However, the age of onset follows a normal distribution curve, and while the peak is indeed in the fifth decade, no age group is exempt from the disease. The prevalence in those populations surveyed (including the United Kingdom) is approximately 3 per cent of the entire population—2·1 per cent in males and 5·2 per cent in females. This increases with age in both sexes reaching 6 per cent in males over 75 years, and 16 per cent in females over 65 years. While rheumatoid arthritis has always been considered to be a disease of temperate and damp climates, there is no definite evidence that this is so, and the more surveys that are performed the more it seems that the disease has a fairly uniform worldwide distribution.

Examination of relatives of rheumatoid patients (or persons with a positive sheep cell agglutination test) reveals a slightly increased incidence of both RA and of positive tests for rheumatoid serum factor. The interpretation of this is not at present clear.

AETIOLOGY

The cause of RA remains unknown. The more carefully the problem is considered, the more does it seem likely that the aetiology or *initiating* factor may have to be considered separately from the pathogenesis, or *perpetuating* factor. It is conceivable that a wide variety of different initiating factors, either infective or traumatic in the widest sense, may initiate a situation evoking an immune reaction within the joint, which then becomes perverted and self perpetuating, perhaps after the initiating factor has ceased to operate.

This, of course, is highly speculative. Despite intensive search and many claims, no infective agent has been definitely incriminated, and neither mechanical trauma nor other insults are consistently involved. In short, no regular set of circumstances has been shown predictably to produce the disease in man.

As for the immune disturbance there is much circumstantial evidence of immune *over-activity*. This includes –

(*a*) The presence of an immunoglobulin – rheumatoid factor – in the serum of rheumatoid patients.
(*b*) The infiltration of the rheumatoid synovium by immunologically competent cells (lymphocytes and plasma cells), some of which can be shown to be actually producing rheumatoid factor.
(*c*) The presence of immune complex particles within cells of the rheumatoid synovial exudate.
(*d*) The finding of lowered complement levels in the fluid of rheumatoid joints.

In terms of current immunological thought a continuing immune disturbance requires the continued presence of an antigenic stimulus. On the one hand, this might be a persisting microbial agent which, while not itself causing tissue damage, nevertheless provides a continuing antigenic stimulus – the resultant immune response producing the tissue damage. Alternatively, the initiating factor might so alter the antigenic specificity of some component of the joint, or itself contain antigenic determinants cross-reacting with some normal joint constituent, that an immune response is mounted against the host's own joint tissue. The latter would be a true 'autoimmune' situation.

It must be repeated that these hypotheses remain at present purely speculative, and are mentioned only to indicate the directions in which thought is moving with regard to RA. The data do not yet justify classifying RA as an 'autoimmune' disease.

One theory concerning the actual local mechanism for the production of synovitis is based on the observation that neutrophil granulocytes within the rheumatoid joint contain visible particles which can be shown to consist of rheumatoid factor forming a complex with IgG immunoglobulins. It is suggested that these complexes act in a manner somewhat similar to the urate crystals in gout (*see* p. 159) to produce rupture of these leucocytes (which have been called 'ragocytes') and release of the contained lysosomal enzymes; these then act as the chemical mediators of the synovitis. Support for this hypothesis comes from the observation that fluid from actively inflamed joints contains free lysosomal enzymes.

PATHOLOGY

NODULES

The one absolutely characteristic pathological finding in RA is the subcutaneous nodule, usually occurring in pressure areas. Such lesions develop in approximately 25 per cent of patients, most commonly on the subcutaneous ulnar border of the forearm (Fig. 3.1). They may also occur

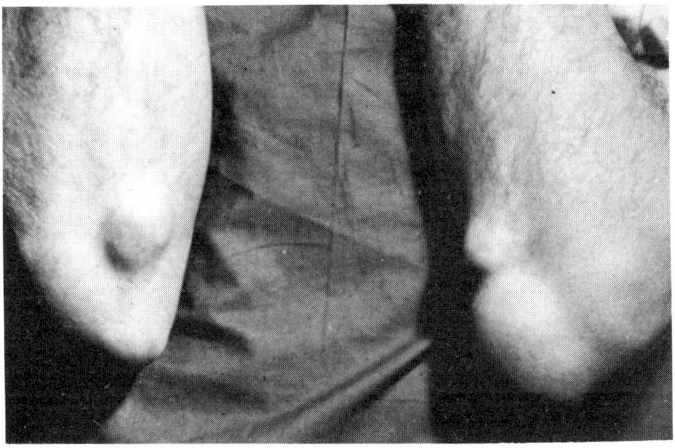

FIGURE 3.1 Rheumatoid nodules on the elbows

in other sites, including the Achilles or other tendons, in the subcutaneous tissue of the fingers, and over the ischial tuberosity.

Macroscopically, a nodule is a non-encapsulated mass, often lobulated and with a central area of necrosis. Histologically, the nodule is a granuloma with three distinct zones: (*a*) central fibrinoid necrosis staining as an amorphous non-cellular material with acidophilic dyes (e.g. eosin); (*b*) a surrounding area of epithelioid cells arranged in a palisade – these are probably macrophages; and (*c*) an outer zone of chronic inflammatory cells – lymphocytes and plasma cells (Fig. 3.2).

SYNOVIUM

Synovitis is the essential change. No synovial tissue is exempt from involvement, hence the lining of tendon sheaths and bursae may be involved in an identical manner. The synovium is oedematous and congested, often appearing as a thick, folded velvety membrane. Synovial pannus (granulation tissue) spreads on to the articular cartilage so that the normally glistening white surface becomes covered with granulation tissue.

Microscopically the synovium is highly vascular and infiltrated with lymphocytes and plasma cells. These inflammatory cells are characteristically clumped together into follicles (Fig. 3.3), some with germinal centres. Immuno-fluorescent methods show that some of the plasma cells contain, and are therefore presumably synthesising, rheumatoid factor.

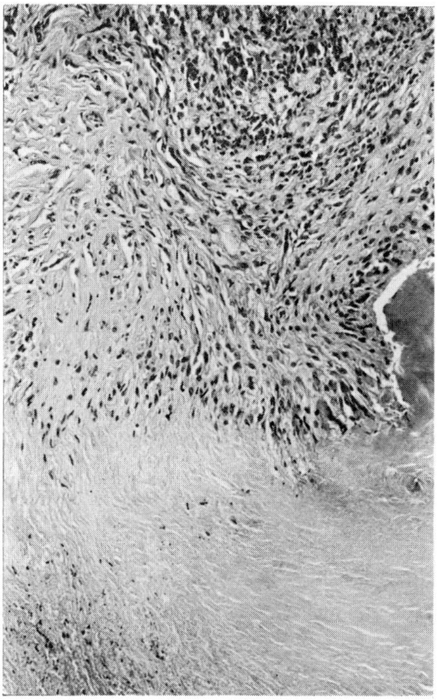

FIGURE 3.2 Section of a rheumatoid nodule (*see* text)

Synovial cells, in health a single layer of cuboid or flattened cells, proliferate into several layers of columnar cells. The synovium takes on a villous form. There is no specific histological feature that can definitely distinguish rheumatoid synovitis from other forms of inflammatory joint disease. Synovial pannus spreading over the articular cartilage produces erosions of its surface, and by breaching the cortex at the cartilage/synovium junction it erodes into the sub-chondral bone (Fig. 3.4). The erosions may become large and cystic. Such changes, together with the loss of cartilage, finally bring about disintegration of the joint surfaces. Erosive changes are usually sufficiently developed to be visualised radiologically (*see* p. 33) within a year of the onset. It has been suggested that the size of erosions are partly dependent on the use to which a joint is put. This is consistent with the hypothesis

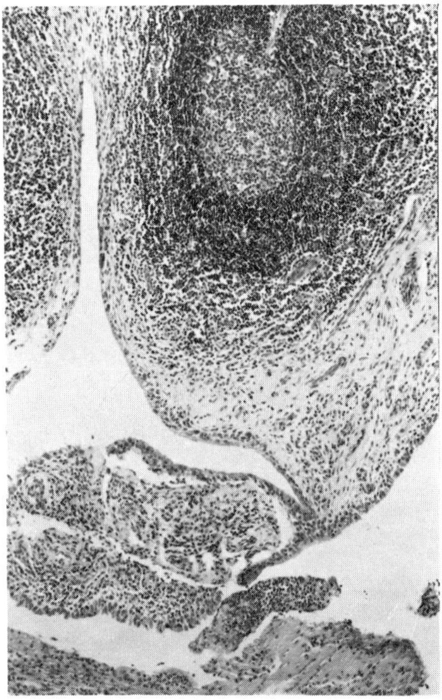

FIGURE 3.3 Section of synovium showing reduplicated synovial cells and aggregation of lymphocytes into a follicle with germinal centre

that there is a 'pumping' action of synovial fluid through the breached cortex, causing distension of subcortical cysts.

ARTERIES

Arteritis occurs in rheumatoid disease. This may conveniently be considered as falling into three categories –

1. Involvement of small end-arteries in the nail folds producing characteristic minute ischaemic areas (Fig. 3.5) which in themselves are usually of no significance.
2. Involvement of small and medium-sized arteries such as the vasa nervorum and digital arteries.
3. Involvement of large arterial trunks, e.g. mesenteric or major limb vessels (*see* Fig. 3.6).

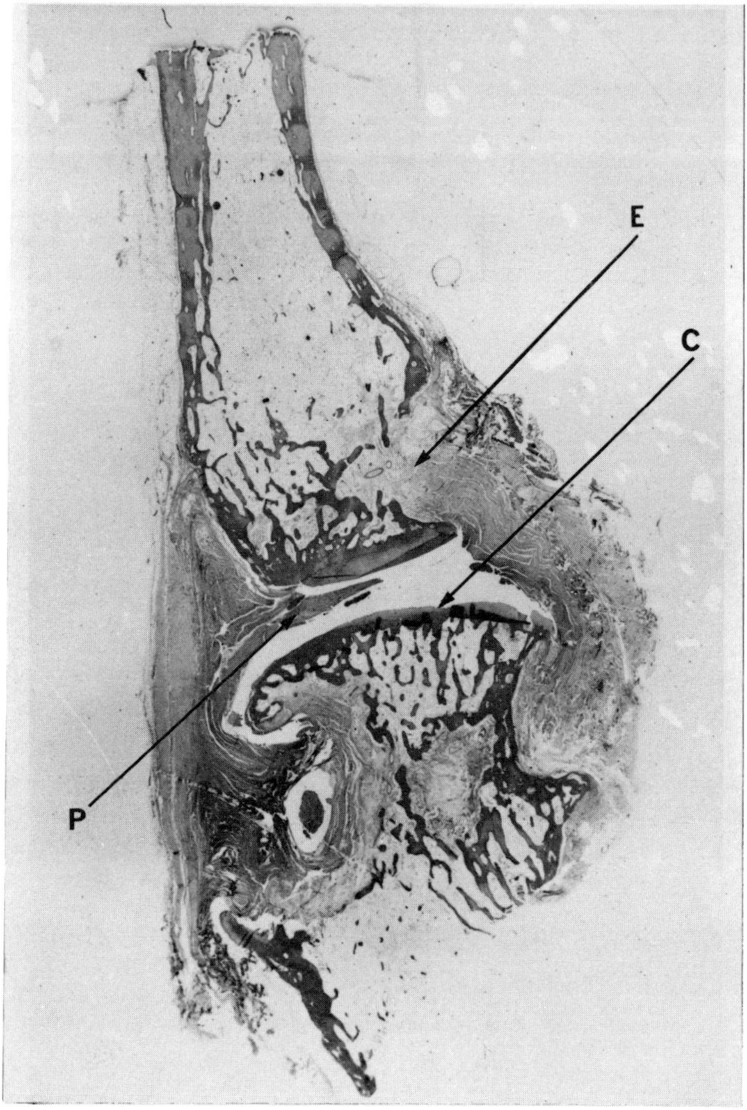

FIGURE 3.4 Section through a metacarpophalangeal joint showing cartilage thinning (C), pannus (P) and erosions (E) (Courtesy Dr J. W. Landells)

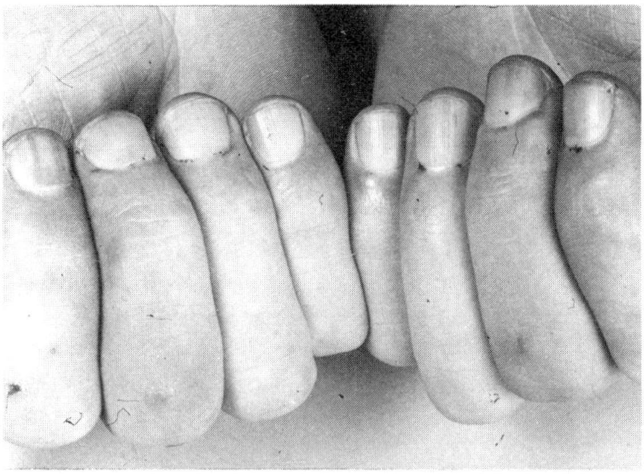

FIGURE 3.5 Arteritic nail-fold lesions

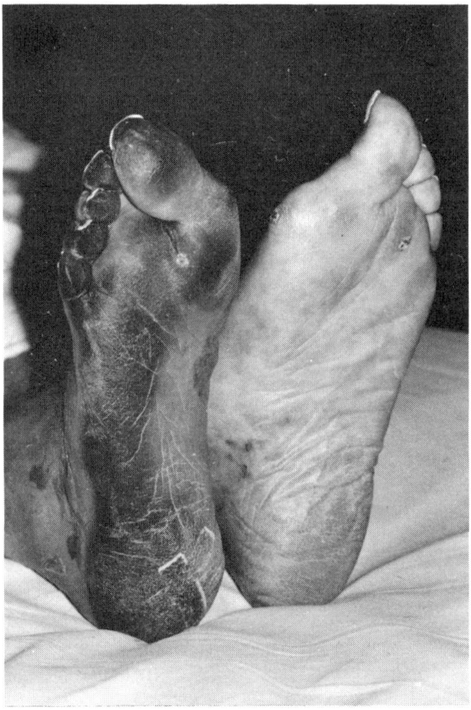

FIGURE 3.6 Peripheral gangrene due to rheumatoid arteritis

The larger the size of vessel affected the more severe is the pattern of arteritis. Thus, the nail-fold lesions result from bland intimal hyperplasia, and the medium-sized arteries show a more active process with fragmentation of the lamina elastica and cellular infiltration. This merges into a picture of gross arterial wall necrosis indistinguishable from polyarteritis nodosa (p. 97).

CLINICAL FEATURES

THE JOINTS

Onset. While rheumatoid disease may present as a generalised systemic illness (*see* below), it usually starts as an inflammatory arthropathy. The onset is very variable and may follow one of three patterns –

1. polyarthritis
2. monarticular arthritis
3. 'palindromic' (episodic) arthritis.

The onset as a *polyarthritis* may be insidious, with joint swelling, pain, and limitation. By contrast, the onset may be an acute polyarthritis which rapidly produces severe pain and disability.

At the onset, RA is not infrequently *monarticular*. The disease may remain confined to one joint for a prolonged period, sometimes years, before becoming polyarticular, or it may remit completely before any other joints are affected.

Initially, the arthritis may be episodic, so-called *palindromic rheumatism*. This is characterised by short-lived episodes of pain with periods of complete remission. Later this often evolves into more obvious RA.

Symptoms. Pain and stiffness are the outstanding complaints, often difficult to separate. In the mildly inflamed joint, pain appears only on movement, whereas with increasing disease activity there is spontaneous pain at rest, too. Perhaps the most characteristic symptom of RA is the severe painful stiffness that is present on waking in the morning and wears off gradually during the day with activity. This *morning stiffness*, recorded as the 'limbering-up time', is the most useful subjective index of rheumatoid activity. This symptom is the hallmark of inflammatory arthropathy. Morning stiffness should last more than half an hour if it is to be accepted as significant.

As joint destruction progresses, the anatomical changes themselves produce increasing functional disability.

Pattern of Joint Involvement. Most commonly affected are the metacarpo-phalangeal, proximal interphalangeal, and the lateral four metatarso-phalangeal joints. Following these come the wrists, knees, shoulders, hips, elbows, ankles, mid-tarsal joints, upper cervical spine, and the

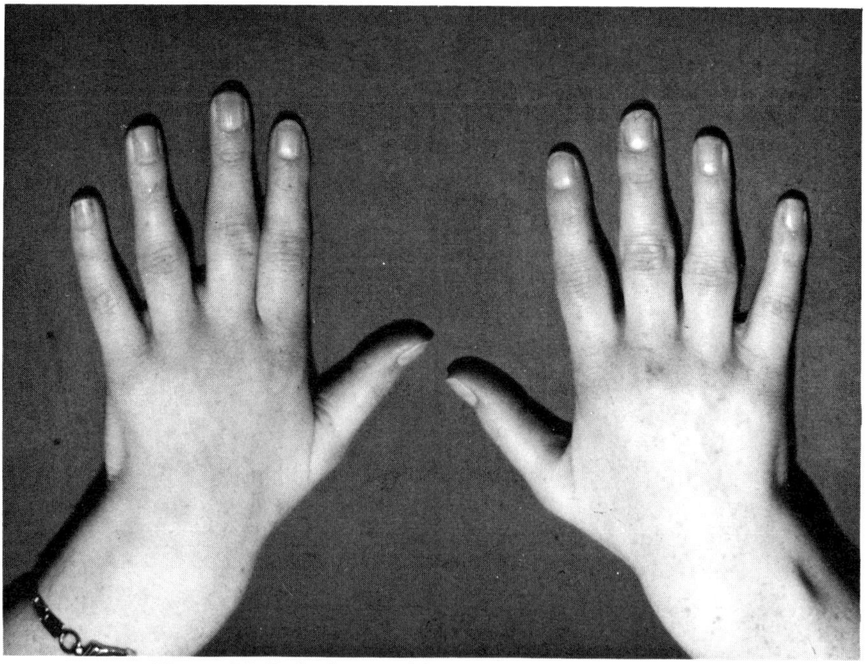

FIGURE 3.7 Early rheumatoid arthritis—spindling of the fingers

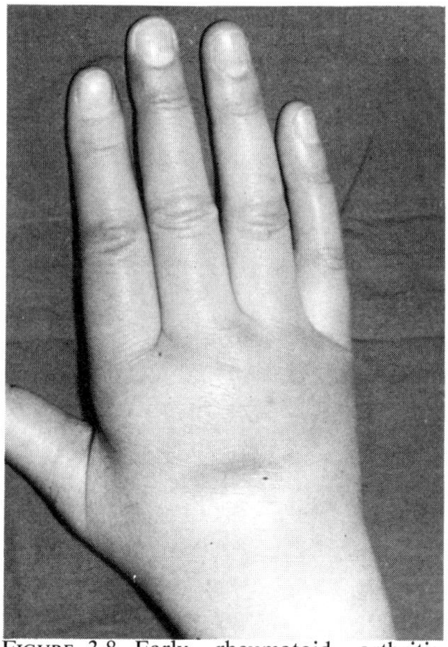

FIGURE 3.8 Early rheumatoid arthritis showing diffuse oedema of the dorsum of the hand

temporo-mandibular joints. Rheumatoid involvement in the cervical spine is usually confined to the Cl-4 segments with the brunt of the inflammatory process falling on the atlanto-axial joint. However, apophyseal joint involvement with subluxation of the upper cervical vertebrae is not uncommon.

Signs. Synovial hypertrophy and effusion produce the typical swelling which, in the fingers, causes a spindle-shaped appearance (Fig. 3.7). In the hands, the swelling is usually confined to the metacarpo-phalangeal and proximal-interphalangeal joints. *Oedema* of the extremities is sometimes a feature of the early stage of the disease (Fig. 3.8). Early synovial swelling of the wrist is highly characteristic and is a valuable sign in distinguishing inflammatory from degenerative joint disease. Synovial swelling of the elbow appears posteriorly on either side of the olecranon, and in the shoulder appears anteriorly. Effusion in the knee joint presents the characteristic horseshoe swelling above and beside the patella. Popliteal swelling and bursal enlargement are common.

Subluxation and Instability. Progressive joint destruction by erosive change leads not only to limitation of movement but, in certain joints, to subluxation. To become subluxed the joints affected must first become unstable. This is usually due to persistent stretching of the joint capsule by effusion, and to ligamentous laxity. The knee, for example, becomes unstable in both the antero-posterior and lateral directions, the latter allowing a valgus or varus deformity to develop. The most common joints to become subluxed are the metacarpo-phalangeal (palmar subluxation) and metatarso-phalangeal joints (dorsal subluxation). Anterior subluxation of the wrist may also occur.

In the cervical spine, atlanto-axial subluxation occurs in about 25 per cent of patients, but only occasionally produces neurological signs from cord compression (*see* p. 25).

Deformity of the hands in RA follows a number of characteristic patterns. *Ulnar deviation* at the metacarpo-phalangeal joint (*see* Fig. 3.9) is common but not pathognomonic of RA, and, surprisingly, by itself produces very little functional disability.

Finger movements at the interphalangeal joints are produced by a number of muscle groups in the forearm and hand; fine movements depend on a delicate balance between the different muscles. Inflammatory, and later destructive, rheumatoid changes may disturb this balance. In practice, one of two characteristic finger deformities may result—

1. *'Swan-neck' deformity* (Fig. 3.10) with hyperextension at the proximal interphalangeal joint and fixed flexion of the terminal interphalangeal joint. The earliest sign of incipient deformity of this type is observed when the patient makes a fist—the interphalangeal joints remain extended until late in the manoeuvre instead of the normal pattern in which the

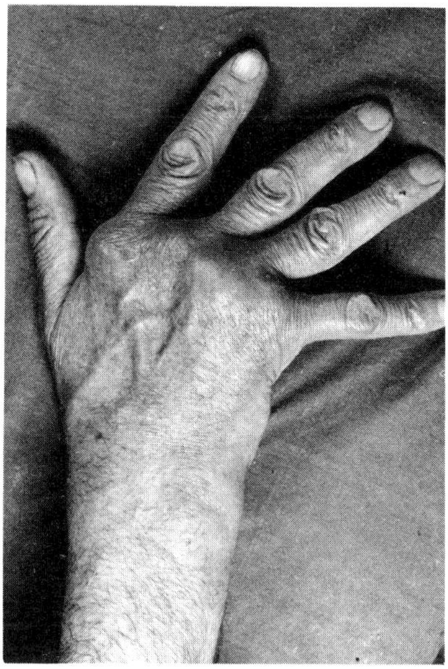

FIGURE 3.9 Subluxation and ulnar deviation of the metacarpophalangeal joints

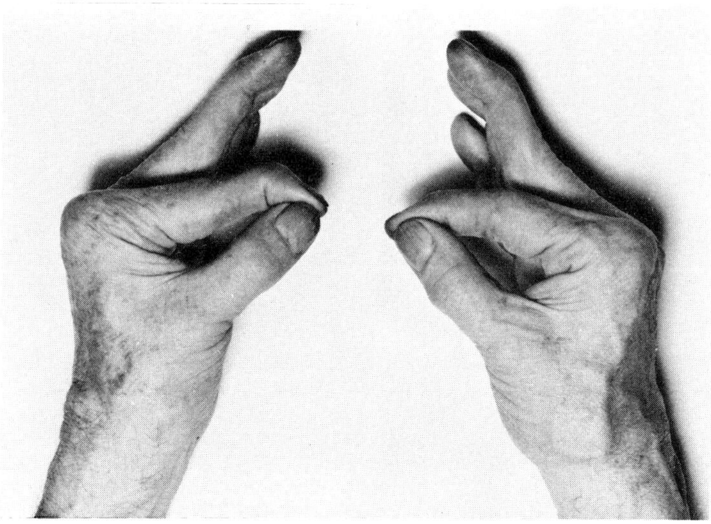

FIGURE 3.10 'Swan-neck' deformities

fingers are rolled up from the distal end. Once a fist can no longer be formed because of inability to overcome hyperextension of the proximal interphalangeal joints the disability becomes severe.

2. *Boutonnière (or button-hole) deformity* is the opposite deformity (Fig. 3.11) and is due to the proximal interphalangeal joint protruding

FIGURE 3.11 Boutonnière deformities

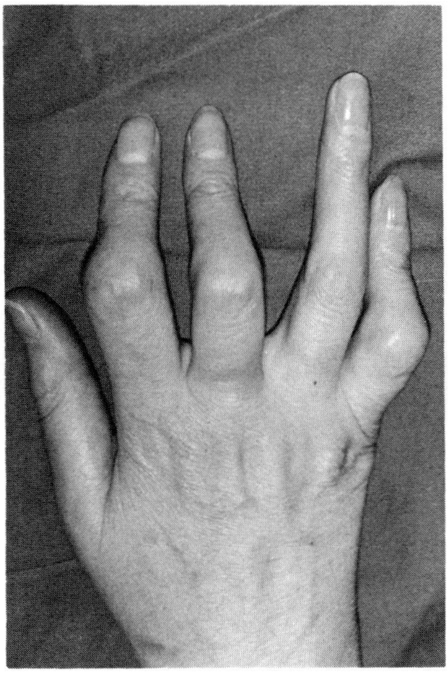

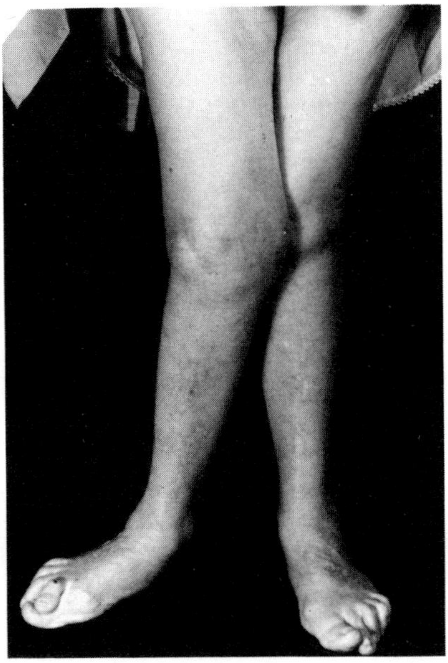

FIGURE 3.12 Flexion and valgus deformity of the knee

through the extensor expansion, the two halves of which slip forwards until, eventually, attempts to extend the joint produce flexion at this joint but extension at the terminal interphalangeal joint.

Outside the hands *flexion deformities* are the most common, e.g. of the knees, hips, and elbows. Such deformities of the knees (Fig. 3.12) and hips are especially important because of the obvious disability they produce. Flexion of the elbow is not so serious a deformity, for if the elbow is badly damaged, and its range severely impaired, then a flexed position is preferable to an extended one, since the former enables the patient to reach his mouth and perform personal toilet.

In the feet and ankles the most common deformities are subluxation of the metatarso-phalangeal joints, with the toes displaced upwards, together with fixed flexion deformities of the interphalangeal joints. This leaves the irritable metatarsal heads exposed to full weight-bearing. Destruction of the mid-tarsal and sub-talar joints leads to a stiff, painful foot. The latter, sometimes together with ankle joint involvement, results in a progressive eversion of the foot with a clumsy gait.

EXTRA-ARTICULAR FEATURES

Fever and Weight Loss. Active RA, being a systemic disease, is accompanied by the usual manifestations of any inflammatory condition. A low grade fever often occurs and may, rarely, precede the arthropathy. Anorexia, weight loss, lethargy, and general malaise are common features, often accompanied by generalised muscle-wasting and weakness. Wasting of the muscles associated with actively inflamed joints may be so marked as to suggest a neuropathic cause to the unwary; and wasting of the intrinsic muscles is part of the characteristic appearance of the rheumatoid hand.

Lymph Node Enlargement. Lymph node enlargement is a common feature of active disease. This involves, particularly, nodes draining actively affected joints; they are discrete, non-tender and moderately enlarged. Histologically they show only non-specific chronic inflammatory changes.

The Subcutaneous Nodule

The nodule occurs in approximately 25 per cent of patients at some time in the course of their disease. It is the only feature that by itself is pathognomonic of RA. It forms a firm non-tender mass varying in size from 2 to 3 millimetres to 2 to 3 centimetres in diameter, usually over a pressure point. The commonest sites, therefore, are over the extensor surface of the ulna at the elbow (*see* Fig. 3.1), then the Achilles tendon, and the ischial tuberosity. In a minority of cases multiple small nodules appear adjacent to the small joints of the fingers and, occasionally, of the feet. Nodules also form in the superficial layers of olecranon bursae.

While rheumatoid nodules are characteristically subcutaneous, they may be intracutaneous, or become adherent to periosteum, and may also occur within tendons. Their size varies from time to time in any one patient and they may completely disappear, only to return later. They are found only in patients with positive tests for serum rheumatoid factor, and their appearance in a patient with negative tests demands biopsy.

Apart from the cosmetic effects and the inconvenience of these firm swellings on pressure areas or on the fingers, the two main disabilities produced are ulceration of the skin overlying the swelling, and pain when the nodules overlie the ischial tuberosities. Under these circumstances they can be excised.

Tendons and Bursae

Tendons (running in synovial sheaths) and bursae are frequently affected by inflammatory changes in common with the synovial membrane of the joints. Bursae, usually the olecranon, become distended by effusions. When tendon sheaths are involved, swelling may be visible and palpable. Extensor and flexor digitorum sheaths are most commonly affected in the hands, thus producing swelling in the palm and of the flexor surfaces of the fingers, and dorsal sheath swellings overlying the wrist and back of the hand. These may be painful, especially on movement.

Nodule formation within the tendons themselves produces palpable swelling and 'triggering' if the flexors of the fingers are affected. Thus, a tenosynovitis, for example of the finger flexors, may produce either palpable tendon nodules and triggering, or palpable crepitus.

Rupture of tendons may occur, especially in the hands. This may be due to nodule formation in the tendon with subsequent softening. Attrition rupture may also occur where the finger extensors course over a roughened, eroded, distal end of the ulna.

Arteries

Arterial involvement (*see* pp. 15–18) occurs only in the strongly seropositive case, usually in those patients with the nodular form of the disease. This may take the form of small nail-fold lesions which appear as brownish-red necrotic areas around the nails, each being 1 to 2 millimetres in diameter. Such lesions are often the first warning that the disease is assuming a more sinister character. Occlusion of medium-sized arteries produces necrotic skin lesions and ulceration, usually on the legs, and by involvement of the vasa nervorum causes the clinical manifestations of 'mononeuritis multiplex' (p. 25).

In the more severe form of arteritis, inflammatory changes occur in the walls of larger vessels leading to peripheral gangrene (*see* Fig. 3.6), mesenteric occlusion, or cerebrovascular accident. The clinical features of this degree of arterial involvement are indistinguishable from polyarteritis nodosa (Chapter 20).

Spinal Cord Compression

This may occur because of external pressure caused by subluxation of the cervical vertebrae. Posterior shift of the odontoid peg (p. 20) or subluxation of the upper cervical vertebrae can, rarely, produce long-tract neurological signs. While this is usually of insidious onset it may be precipitated by trauma to the neck. This complication can be corrected by surgical fusion.

Peripheral Neuropathy

This appears principally in patients with nodular sero-positive erosive RA. Nail-fold arteritic lesions are seen in about one-third of the patients with such a neuropathy. There is no clear-cut evidence that the progression, or improvement, of the neurological lesions is influenced by changes in corticosteroid therapy. Three types of neuropathy are encountered—

Mononeuritis multiplex is the descriptive term given to the clinical picture of ischaemic interruption of peripheral nerves due to occlusive arteriopathy as seen also in polyarteritis nodosa; for example, there may be both motor and sensory features of a median and a lateral popliteal nerve lesion in the same patient. While the asymmetrical single nerve involvement may be obvious in the early stages, these may later summate to produce a polyneuritis which, superficially, can appear so symmetrical as to suggest a metabolic pathogenesis. A carefully taken history should, however, reveal the irregular progress of the neurological deficit.

Symmetrical peripheral neuropathy also occurs in RA, and is of two types. It may be a purely sensory neuropathy of the fingers and/or toes, which carries a relatively good prognosis. Alternatively, there is a more severe form in which sensory and motor signs occur, often in all four limbs. This may be difficult to distinguish from the mononeuritis multiplex described above: it carries a grave prognosis since it tends to accompany widespread and florid arteritis.

Entrapment neuropathies usually occur in one of three sites: compression of the median nerve at the wrist (*carpal tunnel syndrome*), the ulnar nerve at the elbow, or the posterior tibial nerve behind the medial malleolus (*tarsal tunnel syndrome*), occurring in this order of frequency.

About two-thirds of patients with RA develop a carpal tunnel syndrome at some stage, although frequently only with mild compression of the median nerve. However, in a hand that is already the site of an inflammatory arthropathy the superimposition of a neurological lesion may have a profound effect on function. Although wasting of the thenar muscles is an important sign of carpal tunnel syndrome, the significance of it is easily overlooked because it is wrongly ascribed to the joint disease.

Deformities of the elbow may cause pressure on the ulnar nerve as it passes behind the medial epicondyle of the humerus, producing a neurological deficit in the distribution of this nerve.

The tarsal tunnel syndrome is analogous to the carpal tunnel syndrome. It occurs much less frequently.

Lungs and Pleura

These may be involved in rheumatoid disease, and where other causes have been excluded the term *rheumatoid lung* is sometimes used in a broad generic sense. Patients with RA have a higher incidence of previous chest disease than the general population. The significance of this is unknown. It must not be confused with what may be specific rheumatoid lesions occurring during the course of the disease.

Pleural effusion is seen in a small proportion of patients, almost invariably men. It is usually unilateral and its identity as a rheumatoid lesion depends on pleural biopsy or the exclusion of other possible causes. The fluid is sterile, contains lymphocytes and, interestingly, for reasons not explained, has a very low glucose content (less than 20 mg per cent). Unlike most of the extra-articular lesions of rheumatoid disease the effusion may occur early in the course of the disease.

Diffuse interstitial fibrosis is a syndrome that may occur either in isolation or in association with a variety of general disorders, of which RA is one. Whether this should be regarded, therefore, as a specific rheumatoid lesion, or merely as an indication that rheumatoid subjects have an increased liability to pulmonary diseases generally, is not clear. It is associated with sero-positive disease. Clinically, there is progressive dyspnoea, and radiography shows diffuse fine reticular shadowing. Diffusion capacity is reduced.

Rheumatoid nodules, often isolated, may appear within the lung parenchyma and are usually found incidentally on routine chest radiography. Diagnosis may be made only by exclusion or by biopsy (when the characteristic histology is seen). Investigation to exclude the presence of tuberculosis or carcinoma is obligatory. Pulmonary rheumatoid nodules may vary in size and number, and disappear in weeks or months. Occasionally, cavitation occurs due to central necrosis of the nodule. In general, these lesions occur only in the presence of sero-positive erosive nodular disease, although on rare occasions a pulmonary opacity has been investigated in a chest clinic, and found to be a rheumatoid nodule, the arthritis developing later.

Pneumoconiosis and rheumatoid disease occurring in the same patient produce distinctive changes in the lung. Radiologically, a fine reticular shadowing is present throughout the lung fields, and large opacities, frequently becoming confluent, form in the periphery (Caplan's syndrome). Histologically, these nodules are identical to those seen in silicosis, although much larger. This phenomenon perhaps reflects a tendency for any inflammatory process to assume a more florid form if it occurs in the lung of a rheumatoid subject.

The Eye

Contrary to what has been stated in the past, uveitis (iritis) is not a feature of adult rheumatoid disease (it is, of course, well recognised in Still's disease and ankylosing spondylitis). The commonest lesion is keratoconjunctivitis sicca due to reduced lachrymal gland secretions constituting part of Sjögren's syndrome (*see* Chapter 10).

Another typical rheumatoid lesion of the eye is *scleritis* (or *sclerokeratitis*), an inflammatory lesion of the sclera, characterised by nodular infiltration with plasma cells and lymphocytes, with areas of necrosis. Clinically, this produces areas of scleral injection, the bluish colour of the choroid being visible through the thin sclera (Fig. 3.13). Actual nodules

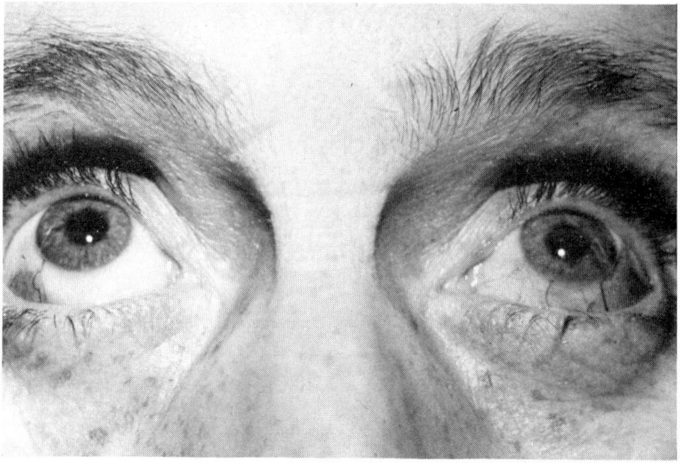

FIGURE 3.13 Longstanding bilateral scleritis with the dark colour of the choroid appearing through the thinned sclera (Courtesy Dr J. White)

may appear in these areas. The presence of scleritis signifies severe disease and a bad prognosis. An important sequel is *scleromalacia perforans*, where the necrotic process is sufficient to produce a breach in the sclera with herniation of uveal tissue.

Skin

In advanced disease the skin becomes atrophic, appearing thin and shiny. This is usually most obvious on the fingers and shins. Ulceration of the skin of the lower leg also occurs spontaneously. It is frequently due to an end-arteritis (p. 15) producing local necrosis. In longstanding disease palmar erythema is common.

The Heart

Cardiac involvement is rarely diagnosed in life. However, at post mortem examination several lesions may be seen. Rheumatoid nodules may be found in the endocardium, myocardium, or pericardium. The incidence of these lesions is uncertain but is probably of the order of 10 per cent.

Pericarditis is found in approximately 40 per cent of patients coming to post mortem study. By contrast, pericarditis is rarely recognised in life although both effusion and constriction have been reported.

Anaemia

Some degree of anaemia almost invariably accompanies RA of any severity. The causes are usually multiple and their precise analysis often difficult. The important causes can be considered under four headings –

1. Iron deficiency.
2. 'Anaemia of chronic inflammation'.
3. Megaloblastic anaemia.
4. Hypersplenism.

1. *Iron deficiency* is common. It is usually secondary to insidious gastro-intestinal bleeding produced by analgesics. (It has been suggested that a significant blood loss may even occur into inflamed joints.)

2. *'Anaemia of chronic inflammation'* occurs with active disease. A haemoglobin of about 11 G per cent is common, but it is occasionally more severe. This anaemia is normochromic or mildly hypochromic, and although the plasma iron is low it differs from the iron deficiency anaemia described above in that the total iron-binding capacity is also well below normal limits. Free iron is generally reduced or absent in the bone marrow. It has been suggested that this represents a defect of iron metabolism due to the rheumatoid disease. Occasionally, an improvement in the haemoglobin level can be achieved by giving iron by injection.

3. *Megaloblastic Anaemia.* Anaemia with a mild megaloblastic picture occurs in about 20 per cent of rheumatoid patients. Folate

measurements yield conflicting results, which do not exclude the possibility that there is a folate deficiency in some of these patients. The prevalence of true pernicious anaemia is the same as that of the general population.

4. *Hypersplenism.* Anaemia may form part of Felty's syndrome.

FELTY'S SYNDROME

Felty's syndrome is defined as the association of RA, splenomegaly, and neutropenia. It usually occurs late in the disease. Ninety per cent of patients have strongly positive tests for serum rheumatoid factor and erosive change, together with positive tests for anti-nuclear factor (ANF) or LE cells. Interestingly, when the fluorescent ANF test is carried out using human peripheral blood as substrate, the anti-nuclear factor can be shown to have a particular affinity for the nuclei of neutrophil polymorphonuclear leucocytes. Splenic enlargement ranges from mild to extreme. The leucopenia affects particularly the neutrophil series (below 2,000/mm^3) and may progress to complete agranulocytosis. Infections are predictably common and there is a failure to respond with a neutrophil leucocytosis. Other features include weight loss, generalised lymph node enlargement, skin pigmentation, and leg ulceration.

Although the granulocyte series is most commonly affected there may also be thrombocytopenia and haemolytic anaemia. Radioactive chromium studies may reveal sequestration of red cells in the spleen. In a sense, the haematological abnormality may be regarded as a special type of hypersplenism. Neither the lymph nodes nor the spleen show specific changes.

The natural history of Felty's syndrome is variable and unpredictable. Occasionally, spontaneous remissions occur. Corticosteroid therapy may induce a remission but this usually requires an unacceptably high dosage for a prolonged period. Splenectomy is sometimes, but not regularly, followed by temporary, or even permanent remission. This operation is therefore limited to those patients in whom depletion of one or other formed element in the blood has reached a critical stage, as judged by recurring infections, haemorrhage, or haemolytic anaemia requiring repeated blood transfusions.

Myopathy

This may occasionally complicate RA, and is fully discussed later, in Chapter 8. It is sufficient here to draw attention to the need, if possible, to differentiate between a primary rheumatoid myopathy and the somewhat similar condition occurring as a side effect of corticosteroid therapy, triamcinolone being a particular offender in this respect.

SPECIAL INVESTIGATIONS

ERYTHROCYTE SEDIMENTATION RATE

Determination of the erythrocyte sedimentation rate (ESR) by the Westergren method is an indispensable investigation in RA. It reflects inflammatory activity. Thus, it may be normal when the disease is in remission, yet rise to over 100 mm/hour during a very active phase. There is, however, considerable variation between individuals, and a normal ESR does not invariably exclude disease activity.

TESTS FOR RHEUMATOID FACTOR

Rheumatoid factor is an IgM type of immunoglobulin found in the serum of approximately 80 per cent of patients with RA. It is an antibody to altered (IgG) gamma globulin (i.e. an 'anti-antibody' or 'anti-globulin') and is detected by adding the patient's serum to an inert marker (sheep red cells or Latex particles) coated with rabbit or human IgG. The various tests are described in Appendix B (p. 315).

Rheumatoid factor is not specific for RA. It is present in the serum of about 5 per cent of normal subjects, and may appear during the course of a variety of chronic diseases, notably bacterial endocarditis and hepatitis. Nevertheless, it remains an outstandingly valuable test in the diagnosis and classification of inflammatory joint disease. It forms the basis for separating the 'sero-negative inflammatory arthropathies' from RA. This is discussed in Chapter 5.

Tests for rheumatoid factor generally become positive early in the course of the disease, and then remain positive. However, some otherwise typical cases never have positive tests, and in others the tests may become negative at a late stage of RA. In general, there is a positive correlation between the titre of rheumatoid factor and both the severity of arthritis and the liability to develop systemic manifestations. Relatives of patients with RA show an increased incidence of positive tests for rheumatoid factor.

ANTINUCLEAR AND LE CELL TESTS

Positive tests for antinuclear factor and LE cells occur in approximately 20 per cent of rheumatoid patients. This finding is limited to those patients who have rheumatoid factor in the serum, and erosive joint change on X-ray. It is more common among those showing systemic features.

The serological overlap between RA and systemic lupus erythematosus is more impressive than the clinical overlap. In practice, the two conditions can generally be distinguished, and intermediate forms are unusual. In an otherwise typical case of RA, the discovery of a positive anti-nuclear factor or LE cell test does not make the diagnosis less secure. It does, however, indicate a somewhat worse prognosis, and a greater liability to develop systemic manifestations.

HAEMATOLOGY

Anaemia is common, and is often the result of a number of different factors, which are discussed on p. 28.

Active disease may produce a modest elevation in the white cell count. Both leucocyte and platelet counts may be lowered by drugs (such as gold and phenylbutazone) which can suppress the bone marrow. Felty's syndrome (p. 29) may be associated with a reduction in all formed elements of the blood.

RADIOLOGY

The basic X-rays required for assessment of a patient with any inflammatory arthropathy are:

- a postero-anterior view of both hands on one plate;
- an antero-posterior view of both feet on one plate;
- an antero-posterior view of the pelvis (showing hips, sacro-iliac joints and symphysis pubis).

It is important to restrict radiology of other joints in order to limit radiation exposure. Further radiology should be requested only in order to answer specific questions relevant to a particular joint.

Early Signs. The first radiological signs of rheumatoid arthritis are non-specific and merely reflect the inflammatory process. They consist of widening of the soft tissue shadows surrounding the affected joint, followed by localised osteoporosis of the adjacent bones (Fig. 3.14).

As cartilage is damaged and eroded, the 'joint space', which represents the thickness of the two layers of articular cartilage on adjacent bone ends, becomes narrowed. This narrowing is first seen in the small joints of the hands and carpus but can affect any synovial joint. A useful diagnostic aid depends on the type of joint space narrowing seen in the hip. Thus, in inflammatory arthropathy the joint space of the hip is narrowed more or less evenly around the circumference of the femoral head. Radiologically, therefore, the head of the femur appears to move deeper into the acetabulum in a direction towards the centre of the pelvis. Later, the medial aspect of the acetabulum may bulge into the pelvic cavity, followed by the femoral head. This is known as *protrusio acetabuli* (Fig. 3.15). Degenerative disease of the hip, by contrast, leads to joint space narrowing which is maximal in the weight-bearing zone, that is, the superior surface of the femoral head, so that radiologically the femoral head appears to have moved vertically upwards (*see* Fig. 14.2, p. 214).

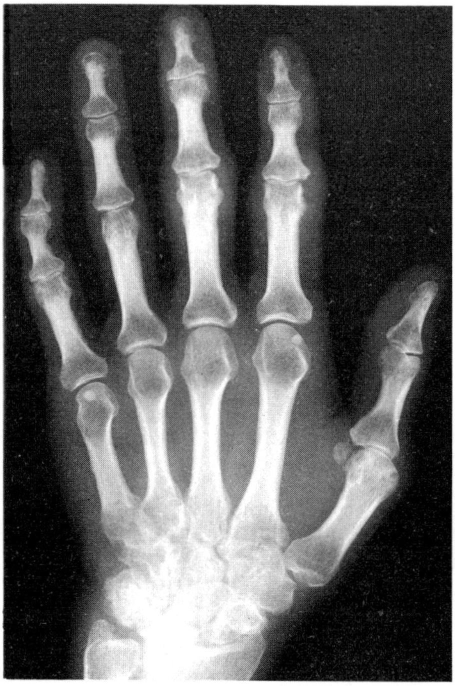

FIGURE 3.14 Radiograph of the hand showing periarticular osteoporosis and loss of joint space in the carpus

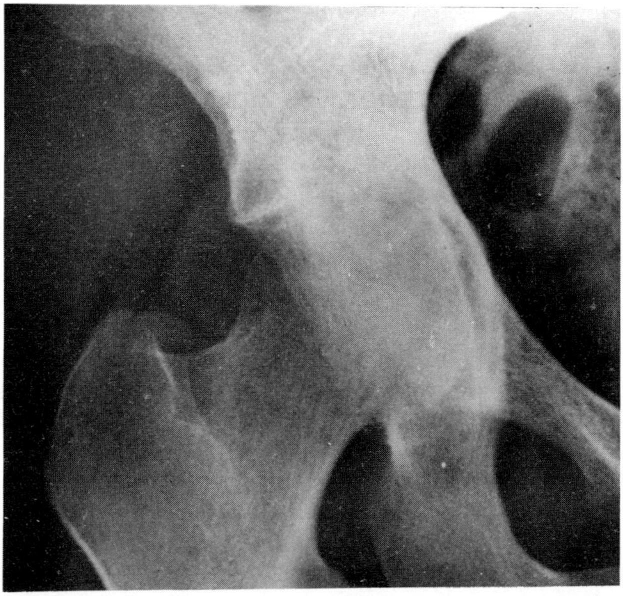

FIGURE 3.15 Rheumatoid arthritis of the hip with loss of joint space and early *protrusio acetabuli*

A faint periosteal reaction may be detected on bones adjacent to affected joints. This is most commonly seen in the hands and feet of younger patients.

Erosions. An erosion is a bone cyst that communicates with the joint cavity through the bony cortex. It is the radiological hallmark of RA. The correct radiographic projection is necessary to demonstrate the breach in the cortical bone outline, without which the lesion is termed a cyst, not an erosion.

Erosions are seen in their most characteristic form in the small joints of the hands and feet (Fig. 3.16). Careful radiological examination of the

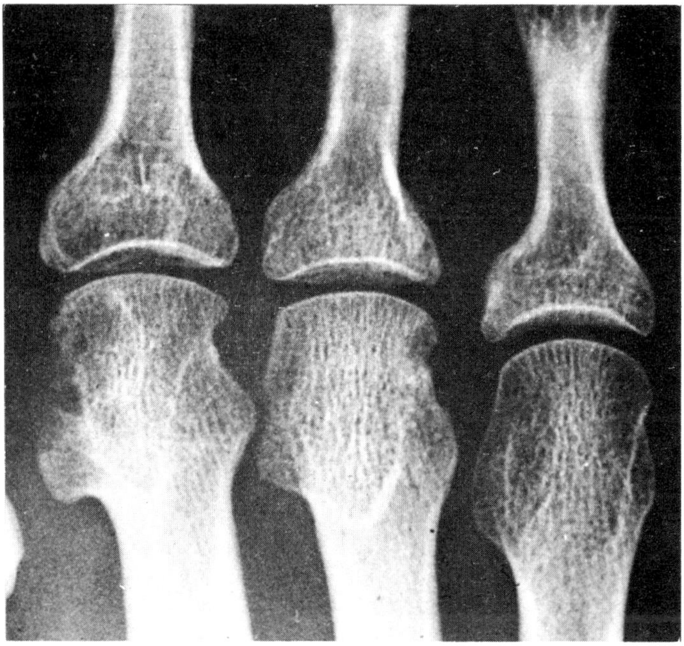

FIGURE 3.16 Erosive change in a metatarsophalangeal joint

(clinically normal) feet in a patient with an otherwise unexplained arthropathy, may sometimes reveal a tell-tale erosion of a metatarso-phalangeal joint (often the 5th). In the hands, erosive changes are most common in the metacarpo-phalangeal and proximal interphalangeal joints. Carpal erosions are not uncommon, and the ulnar styloid process is a frequent site. In the feet it is the metatarso-phalangeal joints that particularly become eroded. The toes are usually spared (unlike some sero-negative arthropathies; *see* p. 73).

No joint affected by rheumatoid arthritis is exempt from erosive change, and this radiological feature may be seen in the hips, knees, elbows, shoulders, temporomandibular joints, and the odontoid peg as well as in the more common sites mentioned above. However, an erosion in a larger joint is less easily visualised than in the small peripheral joints, because of the greater bone density. It is for this reason that the smaller peripheral joints are the most sensitive areas for observing early erosive changes.

Late changes. Erosive changes may progress to the point where there is collapse of the joint surface with subluxation and malalignment of the joints. Malalignment need not result, even from gross destructive changes, if the 'pen and egg-cup deformity' (Fig. 3.17) develops.

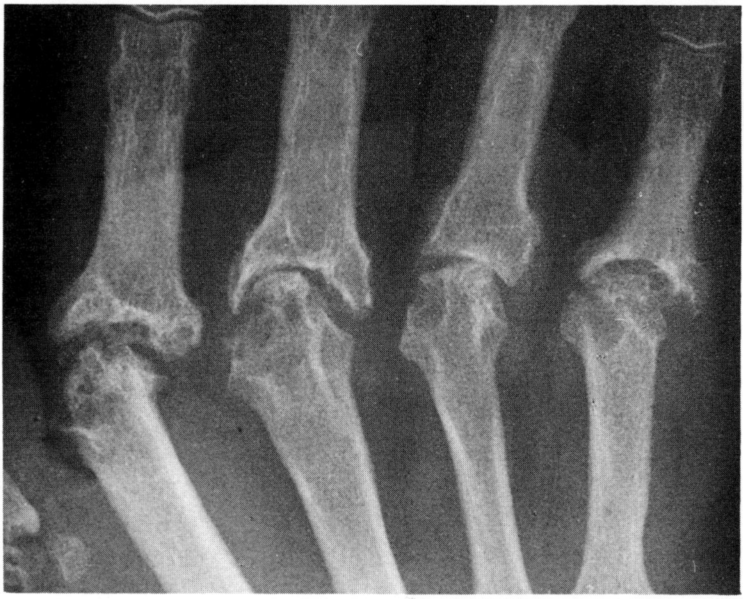

FIGURE 3.17 'Pen and egg-cup' deformity in metacarpophalangeal joints

Gross destruction of the carpus is common, with roughening of the distal ulna. Rarely, gross joint destruction may extend to actual bone resorption and bizarre 'main-en-lorgnette' deformity (*see* Fig. 5.9) more characteristic of psoriatic arthropathy (p. 74).

In the knees, collapse of a tibial plateau may produce either a varus or, more commonly, a valgus deformity (*see* Fig. 3.12). The late stages of hip-joint involvement result in deformity of the femoral head with flattening superiorly and complete loss of joint space. This is due to erosive change both in the femoral head and in the adjacent acetabulum. In some cases the changes of 'avascular necrosis' are superimposed (*see* p. 275), leading to segmental collapse of the upper surface of the femoral head. 'Protrusio acetabuli' is common (Fig. 3.15).

Cervical spine. In contrast to degenerative joint disease, the upper rather than the lower cervical spine is affected by RA. Erosions of the odontoid peg are recognised, but the more significant finding here is forward subluxation of the atlas on the axis. This is considered to be present when a lateral X-ray centred on the odontoid peg, with the neck fully flexed, shows the space between the odontoid peg and the anterior arch of the atlas to exceed 4 mm (Fig. 3.18).

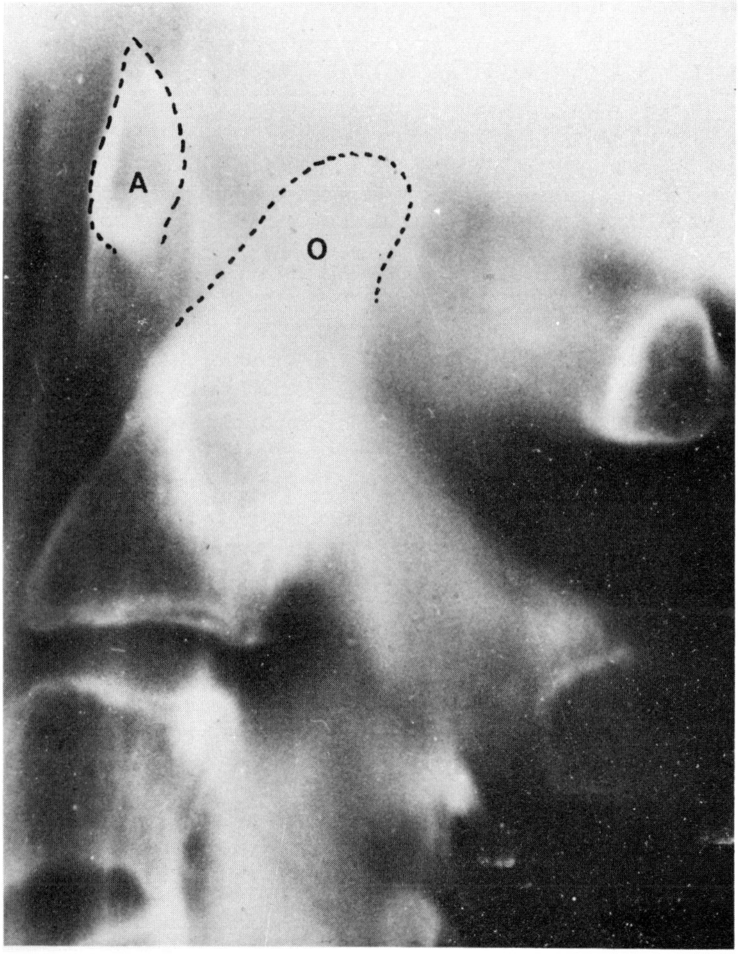

FIGURE 3.18 Radiograph of the cervical spine in flexion showing atlanto-axial subluxation, i.e. abnormal separation between the odontoid peg (O) and the anterior arch of the atlas (A)

Subluxation may also occur in the C2-C5 segments, producing a step-shaped pattern in flexion, with vertebrae tending to slip forwards on those below.

DIAGNOSIS

The only finding pathognomonic of RA is the (histologically proven) subcutaneous nodule. For the rest, the diagnosis depends on the statistical probability of the various clinical and laboratory findings occurring together either as a result of RA, or by chance.

In an attempt to standardise the diagnosis of RA, the American Rheumatism Association in 1958 drew up the following *diagnostic criteria*:

AMERICAN RHEUMATISM ASSOCIATION CRITERIA FOR THE DIAGNOSIS OF RHEUMATOID ARTHRITIS (1958).

Classical Rheumatoid Arthritis

This diagnosis requires seven of the following criteria. In criteria 1 to 5 the joint signs or symptoms must be continuous for at least six weeks.

1. Morning stiffness.
2. Pain on motion or tenderness in at least one joint (observed by a physician).
3. Swelling (soft tissue thickening or fluid – not bony overgrowth alone) in at least one joint (observed by a physician).
4. Swelling (observed by a physician) of at least one other joint (any interval free of joint symptoms between the two joint involvements may not be more than 3 months).
5. Symmetrical joint swelling (observed by a physician) with simultaneous involvement of the same joint on both sides of the body (bilateral involvement of mid-phalangeal, metacarpophalangeal, or metatarso-phalangeal joints is acceptable without absolute symmetry). Terminal phalangeal joint involvement will not satisfy this criterion.
6. Subcutaneous nodules (observed by a physician) over bony prominences, on extensor surfaces, or in juxta-articular regions.
7. X-ray changes typical of rheumatoid arthritis (which must include at least bony decalcification localised to or greatest around the involved joints and not just degenerative changes) – degenerative changes do not exclude patients from any group classified as rheumatoid arthritis.
8. Positive agglutination test – demonstration of the 'rheumatoid factor' by any method that, in two laboratories, has been posi-

tive in not more than 5 per cent of normal controls; or positive streptococcal agglutination tests.

9. Poor mucin precipitate from synovial fluid (with shreds and cloudy solution).
10. Characteristic histological changes in synovial membrane with three or more of the following: marked villous hypertrophy; proliferation of superficial synovial cells often with palisading; marked infiltration of chronic inflammatory cells (lymphocytes or plasma cells predominating) with tendency to form 'lymphoid nodules'; deposition of compact fibrin, either on surface or interstitially; foci of cell necrosis.
11. Characteristic histological changes in nodules showing granulomatous foci with central zones of cell necrosis, surrounded by proliferated fixed cells, and peripheral fibrosis and chronic inflammatory cell infiltration, predominantly perivascular.

Definite rheumatoid arthritis. This diagnosis requires five of the above criteria. In criteria 1 to 5 the joint signs or symptoms must be continuous for at least six weeks.

Probable rheumatoid arthritis. This diagnosis requires three of the above criteria. In at least one of the criteria 1 to 5 the joint signs or symptoms must be continuous for at least six weeks.

Possible rheumatoid arthritis. This diagnosis requires two of the following criteria and the total duration of joint symptoms must be at least three weeks.

1. Morning stiffness.
2. Tenderness or pain on motion (observed by a physician) with history of recurrence or persistence for three weeks.
3. History or observation of joint swelling.
4. Subcutaneous nodules (observed by a physician).
5. Raised erythrocyte sedimentation rate or C-reactive protein.
6. Iritis.*

To these criteria are added a series of 20 specific exclusions from the diagnosis, e.g. the typical rash of disseminated lupus erythematosus, histological evidence of 'peri-arteritis nodosa', 'definite scleroderma', tophi, etc.

These criteria are included here because they are internationally recognised. Although they continue to be used, they are now out of date, particularly because they do not take into account current views about the

*Iritis is no longer regarded as being a feature of adult rheumatoid arthritis (*see* p. 27).

sero-negative group of arthropathies. The first five criteria for example do no more than indicate the presence of an inflammatory arthropathy of any type, although they would, according to this system, enable one to make a diagnosis of 'definite rheumatoid arthritis'. While it is true that the criteria for 'classical RA' (7 criteria) are beyond criticism, the *ARA criteria* are of little value in reaching a diagnosis when an incomplete pattern of clinical features is present—*and this is very common.*

In practice, the essential features are pain and swelling of several joints, with morning stiffness, continuing for at least a few weeks. The pattern of joint involvement is important in that RA commonly affects peripheral small joints symmetrically (with the exception of the terminal interphalangeal joints of the fingers, and the interphalangeal joints of the toes). Firm diagnosis then depends on finding positive serological tests for rheumatoid factor, perhaps subcutaneous nodules, and erosive changes on X-ray. Negative tests for rheumatoid factor demand very careful exclusion of all the sero-negative arthropathies (*see* Chapter 5). It must be realised that in the early phases of the disease it may be possible to diagnose only 'inflammatory polyarthropathy—type uncertain' although statistically RA may be the most likely possibility. The subsequent course of the disease is likely to make possible a more precise diagnosis.

DIFFERENTIAL DIAGNOSIS

When RA presents as a symmetrical small-joint polyarthritis, the correct presumptive diagnosis is usually clear. Difficulty arises when the presentation is atypical. Thus, a *monarticular* presentation may require synovial biopsy to exclude conditions such as tuberculosis. It should be added, however, that biopsy of the early rheumatoid joint usually reveals rather non-specific changes. In the elderly, RA may present with features of *polymyalgia rheumatica* (*see* Chapter 7, p. 105). Rarely, the presenting feature may be *extra-articular*, usually pulmonary; so tests for rheumatoid factor are worth performing in any patient with unexplained pulmonary or pleural lesions. An onset as *palindromic rheumatism* (*see* p. 18) is confusing until the typical pattern of attacks is established, then a reasonably confident diagnosis of the underlying rheumatoid nature of the disease can be made.

The differential diagnosis of an inflammatory polyarthropathy in a patient who is sero-negative is discussed on p. 90. The systemic 'connective tissue disorders', systemic lupus erythematosus, dermatomyositis, and progressive systemic sclerosis, may all produce polyarthritis which is, however, non-erosive. Rarely, the symmetrical polyarthritis of RA may to some extent be mimicked by gout, pyrophosphate arthropathy, or sarcoidosis.

COMPLICATIONS

Neuropathy, scleritis, nodule formation, Felty's and Sjögren's syndromes, tendon ruptures, lung and pericardial involvement are all considered to be part of the rheumatoid process itself. Amyloidosis and superadded septic arthritis may, however, be regarded as *complications*.

Amyloidosis. In rheumatoid subjects coming to autopsy, between 20 and 25 per cent show evidence of amyloidosis, although this is frequently of very mild degree. The incidence of amyloidosis producing clinical manifestations is very much lower, and occurs only in patients with longstanding active disease. The occurrence of amyloidosis is more closely related to the duration of disease and its activity than to the age or sex of the patient. The most common presentation of amyloidosis is the incidental finding of albuminuria. This may progress to a nephrotic syndrome, and is likely to lead eventually to renal failure, and death. Other findings may be hepato-splenomegaly and, occasionally, intestinal malabsorption. While it has been suggested that amyloid deposits may regress if the disease is controlled, there is little histological evidence to support this view. The diagnosis is established by histology. In a patient with obvious renal or hepatic pathology suspected of being amyloidosis, then biopsy of kidney or liver respectively is appropriate. Where these are contra-indicated, or there is no firm lead as to which site may be involved, then both rectal and gingival biopsies are very simple to perform, and both are adequate screening tests. The Congo red test is seldom indicated.

Septic Arthritis. Very rarely, septic arthritis may develop in a rheumatoid joint. This is commoner in patients on corticosteroid drugs (when the signs may be masked) but not limited to them. The diagnosis must always be considered when an undue exacerbation occurs in a rheumatoid joint, particularly if accompanied by general signs of infection. Immediate diagnostic aspiration is the only safe course (*see* Chapter 12).

PROGNOSIS

Natural History. It is difficult, if not impossible, to predict reliably the course that rheumatoid disease will follow in the individual patient. It is a disease characterised by spontaneous exacerbations and remissions. The popular belief that the diagnosis of RA is a 'passport to a wheelchair' is a fallacy. In the United Kingdom, of those developing definite RA (of sufficient severity to bring them to hospital) the following approximate generalisations can be made –

(*a*) 20% – Short-lived activity of joint disease which 'remits' without significant residua.

(*b*) 25% – Joint disease which remits to leave only mild or moderate residua.

(*c*) 45%—Persistent activity of arthritis punctuated by exacerbations and remissions leading to progressive deformity of variable degree.
(*d*) 10%—Severe inflammatory disease leading to complete disability so that the patient becomes restricted to a bed or wheelchair life.

The prognosis for males generally is significantly better than for females. But it is also true that the most severe forms of the disease are seen in men. An oversimplified generalisation is that if the severity of the disease is regarded as a spectrum ranging from the very mild to the most severe, then men group largely at the mild end of the spectrum with a few at the very severe end, whereas women form the bulk of the patients in the centre.

Rheumatoid arthritis (unlike systemic lupus erythematosus) usually goes into remission during pregnancy. After delivery, the arthritis relapses, and there is no indication that pregnancy itself influences the long-term course of RA.

Assessment of Prognosis. There are no certain indicators of the course that rheumatoid disease will take, but the following features to some extent correlate with a *less* favourable prognosis—

(*a*) Insidious onset of the disease.
(*b*) Persistent active disease without remission beyond one year.
(*c*) Positive tests for rheumatoid serum factor within the first year.
(*d*) Early appearance of radiological erosions.
(*e*) Early appearance of nodules.

The longer that active, progressive disease continues, the worse the outlook becomes. The appearance of extra-articular manifestations such as arteritis, neuropathy, or eye lesions, carries a particularly poor prognosis.

Causes of Death. While rheumatoid disease may produce complete crippling of the patient, death directly attributable to the disease is uncommon. Death may result from the effect of arteritis (p. 15), amyloidosis (p. 39), atlanto-axial subluxation (p. 25), and the leucopenia of Felty's syndrome (p. 29).

Death may, of course, result also from the complications of treatment. Analgesics may cause gastro-intestinal bleeding (salicylates, phenylbutazone, indomethacin), renal damage (phenacetin), and blood dyscrasias (phenylbutazone). Gold salts are known to cause bone marrow suppression, nephropathy, and exfoliative dermatitis. Corticosteroid therapy carries an appreciable mortality risk from peptic ulceration, infection, and inability to respond to stress.

TREATMENT

Treatment of RA must be a combined effort between physician, surgeon, physiotherapist, occupational therapist, and instrument maker, and long-term planning is essential. Both the patient and her relatives will need a careful explanation about the disease and the planning of treatment. The least that a rheumatoid patient deserves is a sympathetic physician with time to discuss the many and varied problems RA introduces into her life. The key to the successful management of the patient is the ability to grasp her confidence at the first consultation. Failure to establish a satisfactory doctor/patient relationship is perhaps the main reason why patients turn to practitioners of unethical medicine and quack remedies. Explanatory handbooks for patients of the type issued in the United Kingdom by the Arthritis and Rheumatism Council* can be very valuable in this context.

In a disease for which there is no specific cure, treatment aims at improving the lot of the patient by a comprehensive approach to the disease, the patient, and her life. Broadly, therapy can be planned under two headings –

Modification of the patient	*Modification of the environment*
Rest	Appliances
Physiotherapy	Housing adjustment
Drugs	Occupational adjustment
Surgical operations	Transport

GENERAL TREATMENT

Rest

While it is generally agreed that rest is of value, the exact manner in which it should be applied is controversial. In the presence of very actively inflamed joints it seems reasonable to prescribe rest. In a non-specific way this appears to reduce inflammatory activity, and the rheumatoid patient admitted to hospital will often show improvement without any other change in treatment. However, there is little to support the view that rest in itself produces any long-term benefit, or modifies the disease process.

Splints. The prolonged immobilisation of rheumatoid joints in plaster of Paris splints is not recommended. Splints should be reserved for specific functions –

*Obtainable without charge on application to the Secretary, Arthritis and Rheumatism Council, Faraday House, 8/10 Charing Cross Road, London W.C.2.

(*a*) Maintenance of joints in the correct position while the patient is at rest, e.g. 'back slab' plaster of Paris or plastic splints for the knees, worn at night to prevent flexion deformities.

(*b*) For the correction of deformity, e.g. fixed flexion of the knees; serial splints, each one being a little straighter than its predecessor, are applied. Such splints should also be worn while the patient is weight-bearing.

(*c*) To stabilise a painful joint such as the wrist, so that activity can continue without pain. Below-knee calipers for stabilisation of the painful ankle or subtalar joint may produce great symptomatic relief and enable the patient to walk more comfortably.

(*d*) To relieve entrapment of the median nerve at the wrist by immobilising splints worn at night.

(*e*) Stabilisation of unstable joints may be attempted with plastic splints or calipers. In non-weightbearing joints such as an elbow, plastic splints may be very effective, but weight-bearing joints usually require calipers. Fixed valgus or varus deformity of the knee presents a problem that cannot satisfactorily be solved by splints.

Physiotherapy

Physical methods of treatment are an invaluable adjunct in the treatment of RA. However, before any treatment is ordered, a specific aim must be defined, and treatment must be adapted to the individual's requirements (and, of course, in a changing disease, this must be kept constantly under review). Outpatient care of rheumatoid subjects encourages the prescription of token physiotherapy in the department. It is important to remember that a few minutes of planned exercise, short of fatigue, several times a day, is more rational than half an hour's treatment with a physiotherapist, to the point of fatigue, two or three times a week. The physiotherapist's function is far more one of supervision, instruction, and encouragement, and for this purpose she is invaluable.

Such physiotherapy falls into three categories –

1. The maintenance of joint movement and the prevention or correction of deformity. Active joint movement may be increased by remedial exercises, and where the movement is painful this can often be facilitated by exercising in a deep pool. The early correction of flexion deformities of the knees and hips is of particular importance.
2. The strengthening of muscle groups by remedial exercises. As an example, quadriceps muscle weakness due to immobility or secondary to painful involvement of the knees must be corrected.

3. Walking re-education, especially instruction in the use of appropriate aids such as walking sticks or crutches.

As already emphasised, it is essential that the patient should be taught and encouraged to perform her own physiotherapy at home. The development of flexed knees, for example, is not infrequently due to the failure of the physician to instruct the patient about the importance of maintaining a correct posture, or failure to forbid the use of pillows under the knees in bed.

Various forms of electrotherapy, and sources of local heat (e.g. wax baths) have had their vogue in the past. These have very limited application in the modern treatment of RA. Two might be mentioned. First, in the painful and limited joint, local application of heat (by any convenient method) may produce sufficient temporary relief to enable the patient to perform remedial exercises more effectively. The heat itself has no remedial property.

Secondly, faradic stimulation may be used to re-educate a patient to contract weak muscles. This is purely a method of demonstrating to the patient a contraction that he must then be encouraged to carry out for himself. Once the patient can voluntarily produce a contraction, then faradism is of no further use, and active strengthening exercises are performed under the guidance and encouragement of the physiotherapist.

Occupational Therapy

This must not be considered solely as a method of producing time-filling diversions for a bored patient. It may indeed be of great value to an immobilised patient, but occupational therapy has far more important functions. These include –

1. Aid and instruction to patients in performing normal personal and household activities within the functional limits imposed by their disability. This may involve the use of trick movements, or the provision of household appliances adapted to the patient's requirements, gadgets to enable her to dress herself, or modified equipment such as typewriters, telephones etc.
2. Re-training in the performance of simple manoeuvres hindered by the arthritis. With careful planning, this can be designed to strengthen weak muscles or mobilise stiff joints.
3. Assessment of patients for employment where their previous occupation has had to be abandoned (resettlement).

Resettlement. A patient who is becoming progressively more disabled is likely to find increasing difficulty in performing his normal daily activities. In some cases his occupation may be obviously unsuitable (e.g. heavy labouring), and it is better to explore the possibility of his changing to a more suitable job (with industrial re-training if necessary) before he loses his original work through disability. Modifications to the home—the kitchen layout, the step at the front door, the position of the bath—should be considered before the existing arrangements make it impossible for the patient to manage. Simple procedures such as the fitting of handrails over the bath, the conversion of a single steep step into two shallower ones, make life much easier for the disabled patient. In some cases, change of accommodation has to be considered and, again, this should be thought of early rather than late.

This combined approach to making the patient's life more comfortable and convenient aims, above all, at maintaining his or her independence.

DRUG TREATMENT

Analgesics

Pain relief forms a major part of the treatment of RA, and virtually all patients benefit from a regular background of medication with an effective analgesic. The more useful analgesics are listed below. *They do not influence the basic pathological process.*

Salicylates. These remain the mainstay of symptomatic treatment and should always be used as the drug of first choice. Appreciable pain relief is usually achieved, but large doses are necessary, and until the patient has been persuaded to take 4 G of aspirin a day regularly it cannot be regarded as ineffective. Actual reduction in joint swelling (regarded as an 'anti-inflammatory' effect) has been shown to occur when doses greater than 3 G a day are taken.

Dyspepsia, with or without peptic ulceration, is a troublesome side effect, but it can sometimes be avoided by the use of soluble or enteric coated preparations or aloxiprin. A major disadvantage of all salicylate preparations is their tendency to cause gastro-intestinal blood loss. Apart from the obvious haemorrhages that may occur from acute gastric erosions or chronic peptic ulcers, salicylates tend to produce an insidious and steady blood loss into the gut. This can be detected and measured only by radio-isotope studies. The blood loss usually amounts to a few millilitres daily—enough, in many people, to produce a chronic iron deficiency anaemia. The possibility of this type of blood loss has constantly to be remembered when reviewing the haemoglobin level of patients taking salicylates. Once a patient proves to be a 'salicylate bleeder', all salicylate preparations should be discontinued.

Paracetamol. This is a milder analgesic than aspirin, which is nevertheless valuable because of its almost complete lack of toxic effects. Thus, it can be used in patients intolerant of salicylates. Doses up to 6 G daily may be used. Phenacetin is converted *in vivo* to paracetamol but, at the moment, there is no evidence to link paracetamol with the renal damage thought to result from chronic phenacetin ingestion.

Codeine. Codeine, and its derivative dihydrocodeine, suffer from the drawback of causing constipation and, sometimes, nausea. However, they are occasionally useful as alternative analgesics. Many proprietary salicylate preparations contain small quantities of codeine. Care must be taken to see that such compound tablets do not also contain *phenacetin*, the chronic ingestion of which is thought to predispose to renal damage (particularly papillary necrosis).

Phenylbutazone and Oxyphenbutazone. These analgesics also have anti-inflammatory properties. In a minority of patients they prove somewhat more effective than salicylates. Their major toxic effects are gastro-intestinal disturbances and bone marrow suppression. Bone marrow suppression is a rare but serious complication that occurs in two situations: first, acute granulopenia or agranulocytosis appearing soon after treatment is started, suggesting a hypersensitivity reaction; secondly, aplastic anaemia leading to pancytopenia may occur after prolonged treatment, and in susceptible individuals seems to be a dose-related effect. Gastric intolerance occurs in approximately 25 per cent of patients treated with either phenylbutazone or oxyphenbutazone, although there is not complete overlap between the patients affected by these two preparations.

The dose of phenylbutazone should not exceed 300 mg daily, and since it may be mildly cumulative, treatment on six days a week is sometimes recommended. On this regimen, haematological side effects during long-term treatment are rare, and most of the reported cases have been on larger doses. Nevertheless, blood counts should be performed *before starting* the drug and at least every three months thereafter.

Indomethacin. Indomethacin is a newer analgesic, also with mild anti-inflammatory properties. Some patients find it more effective than salicylates. Toxic effects occur in one-third of patients and consist of a characteristic headache, dizziness, visual disturbance, mental confusion, and gastro-intestinal disturbances. The usual dosage is 75 to 100 mg/day in divided doses.

Indomethacin is also available as 100 mg suppositories, and if administered last thing at night these may considerably reduce morning stiffness.

Other Analgesics. The fenamates (mefenamic and flufenamic acid) and dextrapropoxyphene, while occasionally useful, have not proved to have any real advantage over aspirin or phenylbutazone.

Gold and Chloroquine Compounds

Both gold salts and chloroquine compounds are thought to achieve something more than the analgesics mentioned above. Their use is based on the hope that they suppress the disease process in some more fundamental way and may actually influence favourably the long-term course of the disease. The evidence for the efficacy of these drugs is sufficiently strong for their use to be routine in most rheumatology units. But it must be admitted that this is also a reflection of the absence of any really satisfactory drug for this disease.

One or other of these drugs is usually started once a firm diagnosis of definite, progressive RA is made. Neither drug has any analgesic action, so analgesic drug therapy is required concurrently.

Gold Salts. The mode of action of gold is unknown. It does not suppress immune responses, but it has been shown both to stabilise lysosomal membranes and to inhibit the activity of lysosomal enzymes. If lysosomes are concerned in rheumatoid inflammation then this may be relevant.

The evidence for the efficacy of gold in RA comes from a controlled trial conducted in 1961. This showed that 1,000 mg of sodium aurothiomalate (Myocrisin – of which 50 per cent is metallic gold) given as weekly injections of 50 mg for 20 weeks, produced significant improvement in the recipients compared to controls, which was maintained for 18 months, but which disappeared by 2½ years. X-rays showed no significant differences.

It is now felt that if gold is effective it should be continued indefinitely, rather than being given as a 'course'. The plan of administration has to allow for gold salts being cumulative. A typical regimen is to give weekly intramuscular injections of sodium aurothiomalate, starting with test-doses of 10 and 20 mg, then 50 mg weekly until a total of 500 mg has been administered. This is about the 'load' needed to produce a clinical response. If the response is encouraging, the injections are continued at the rate of 50 mg every second week until an overall total of 1,000 mg is reached, when the frequency is reduced again to 50 mg every fourth week. This is then continued indefinitely on the theory that this rate of administration is of the same order of magnitude as the renal excretion at this stage. Newer methods of measuring gold in biological materials should in future provide a method of controlling the dose of gold.

The administration of gold salts may be associated with a number of serious toxic reactions –

1. *Albuminuria.* Rarely, this may develop into a full nephrotic syndrome.
2. *Skin rash* preceded by pruritus and sometimes eosinophilia. This is an eczematous eruption which may become generalised exfoliative dermatitis.
3. *Bone marrow suppression.* This may present as an isolated thrombocytopenia, or granulopenia, and progress to complete marrow aplasia.

4. *Stomatitis*, *gastro-intestinal haemorrhage*, and *diarrhoea*.
5. *An acute allergic reaction* following the initial injection. Although very rare, this imposes the necessity for small test doses at the start of treatment.

In view of these potentially serious reactions every injection must be preceded by an enquiry about pruritus or skin rash, and examination of the urine for albumin. Full blood counts, including platelet counts, must be performed at least monthly (when weekly injections are being given), and three monthly (if monthly injections are given). Exfoliative dermatitis is exceedingly rare if injections are stopped at the first sign of skin toxicity, and any skin rash that does occur will usually respond to local or, if necessary, systemic, corticosteroid preparations. Similarly, serious bone marrow suppression is rare if blood counts are carried out regularly and treatment stopped at the first sign of any bone marrow suppression. Permanent renal damage does not occur if no further gold is given after the first appearance of albuminuria.

The chelating agent *dimercaprol* (British Anti-Lewisite or 'BAL') is capable of producing relatively rapid elimination of gold from the body, and has been recommended as a treatment for gold toxicity. Its value is limited.

Chloroquine Compounds. The mode of action of chloroquine preparations is unknown. Like gold, no response is seen until some time after starting treatment. Both *chloroquine* and *hydroxychloroquine* are used, generally in doses of between 200 and 400 mg daily. Toxic effects include skin eruptions, hair depigmentation, and corneal deposits, all of which are reversed by stopping the drug. However, these drugs may also cause *retinal damage*, with serious loss of vision which is irreversible and which may continue to progress after the drug is stopped. Retinopathy is probably dose-related but neither the arbitrary limitation of the course of the drug to, for example, one or two years, nor frequent ophthalmalogical surveillance have proved a complete safeguard against this very grave complication. For this reason antimalarial therapy is now usually reserved for patients who are unable to tolerate gold salts.

Corticosteroid Preparations

Adrenal corticosteroid drugs, or 'steroids', are the only preparations that will predictably suppress rheumatoid activity. Unfortunately, the relatively high doses necessary to achieve suppression, and the continued administration required to maintain this, produce so many serious side effects that this form of treatment now finds application only in a small proportion of patients with RA. Generally, the use of steroids is limited to cases of severe, progressive disease not controlled by any other methods, and the objective is usually long-term, partial suppression with the minimum possible dosage. Analgesics and other forms of therapy are continued simultaneously.

The use of steroid drugs is so much conditioned by their side effects that these are listed below. They are, of course, the same as the features of Cushing's disease.

Osteoporosis leading to vertebral collapse or other fractures.
Peptic ulceration, with dyspepsia, perforation or haemorrhage.
Liability to infection, particularly tuberculosis and skin sepsis.
Salt retention leading to hypertension, oedema and 'moonface'.
Skin atrophy and bruising which, like the osteoporosis, is due to collagen protein breakdown.
Pituitary-adrenal axis suppression, with (potentially fatal) inability to respond normally to stress. This may persist for many months after stopping the drug, and requires steroid supplementation during periods of stress, such as surgical operations.
Decreased glucose tolerance, with transient glycosuria or diabetes.
Other side effects, including hypertrichosis, myopathy, hypokalaemia, cataract, avascular necrosis of the femoral head, and psychotic changes. Stunting of growth in children is discussed in Chapter 4.

A variety of natural and synthetic corticosteroid preparations is available. Compared with cortisol, the more potent synthetic preparations provide greater anti-inflammatory effect relative to their salt-retaining action, and experience suggests that the two most generally satisfactory preparations are *prednisone* and *prednisolone*. Dyspepsia may be slightly reduced by using a soluble form (e.g. Prednesol) or enteric-coated pills. Prednisolone tablets of both 5 and 1 mg are available. The latter are useful for the fine adjustment of dosage.

Corticotrophin (ACTH) and Synacthen provide alternative forms of therapy. Advantages claimed for them are a lower incidence of gastric side-effects and less difficulty in stopping treatment (because the adrenal medulla is hypertrophic rather than atrophic). Against this must be set the need for daily injections and greater salt retention than occurs with prednisolone. Policies vary, but on the whole prednisolone is used very much more widely than ACTH.

Doses are kept to the minimum that will produce adequate relief. Prednisolone 10 mg daily is about average, and above this dosage level the incidence of serious toxicity rises sharply. One very disappointing aspect of corticosteroid therapy is the way in which the same dose that in the first few days of therapy produces apparently miraculous improvement, later seems to achieve much less, despite increasing evidence of side effects. Such an effect may be greatly exaggerated when therapy is initiated by unnecessarily large doses—the 'steroid honeymoon'. Controlled long-term studies to determine the manner in which prednisolone alters the natural history of RA are very difficult to perform, but the one thing that corticosteroid drugs do seem to achieve is a reduction in the number of new radiological erosions appearing.

In some senses, prednisolone is almost a 'habit forming drug' for the rheumatoid patient. Even in subjects whose disease is poorly controlled by prednisolone, withdrawal of the drug can precipitate a very severe flare-up of the arthritis and considerable constitutional disturbance. This can be avoided only by reducing the dose very gradually (for example by reducing the daily dose by 1 mg once a month). Patients on corticosteroid drugs or ACTH should carry *steroid cards* recording dosage and other details.

From what has been said it should be clear that a decision to start a rheumatoid patient on prednisolone is never undertaken lightly. In general, the drug is reserved for patients whose pain and stiffness remain intolerable despite vigorous non-hormonal treatment. Obviously, each patient is an individual problem. The following considerations may influence the decision—

1. Intolerable morning stiffness can sometimes be controlled by a small dose (prednisolone 5 mg) taken last thing at night.
2. Very acute disease with systemic features may rarely be an indication for using larger, suppressive doses for a limited period. This is exceptional; normally the dose should be limited by the knowledge that it will have to be continued for years. Short-term therapeutic advantage may be bought only at the price of disaster in the long run.
3. RA in the elderly can be a pathetically distressing disease. They have less to lose from steroid therapy.
4. Functional disability in RA is due both to inflammation (reflected by the ESR and morning stiffness) and to mechanical (anatomical) derangement. Only the former can be influenced by steroids.
5. No patient should be allowed to become bedridden without corticosteroid therapy being considered.
6. In the relentlessly progressive case in which it is clear that steroids are likely to be needed at some stage, it is not always wise to put off the decision until the last possible moment. There are situations where it may be better to take advantage of the functional improvement offered by prednisolone at a somewhat earlier stage. Examples are the mother with young children to bring up, or the bread-winner faced with reduction in his earning capacity.

Local Corticosteroid Injections. Intra-articular corticosteroid injections are used to suppress local inflammation. The effect is usually transient, lasting for a few hours to, at the most, several weeks, so the purpose of the injection is to tide the patient over an acute exacerbation in a particular joint – a *temporary* solution to a local problem. Insoluble preparations are used; for example, hydrocortisone acetate (100 mg) for a knee joint. Meticulous antiseptic precautions are essential.

It has been suggested that many repeated injections may themselves damage a joint. In practice, this form of treatment is not sufficiently popular for this hazard to arise.

Occasionally, it is helpful to inject small volumes of a corticosteroid suspension into an inflamed tendon sheath, bursa, or 'triggering' tendon.

'Immunosuppressive' Agents

The cytotoxic and antimetabolic groups of drugs (developed originally for the treatment of cancer) have been shown capable of suppressing immune responses, and they have been used successfully to prevent the immune rejection of transplanted organs.

If immune mechanisms play a role in the pathogenesis of RA, then these drugs would appear to offer a logical approach to the treatment of rheumatoid disease. This form of therapy is being tested, and the reports so far are encouraging. Of course, these drugs may suppress the bone marrow, and this form of therapy requires very careful supervision. Of the drugs currently available, most interest centres round azathioprine, cyclophosphamide, and chlorambucil.

At present it would seem wise to regard the use of these drugs as still requiring assessment, and to limit their use to specialised centres.

Haematinics

Haematinics, especially iron, are frequently needed as part of the treatment of rheumatoid disease. Hypochromic anaemia may result from gastrointestinal blood loss due to the use of analgesics, especially aspirin, and requires treatment with iron. The normochromic anaemia associated with active disease (p. 28) may respond to parenterally administered iron preparations. Rarely, folic acid is required for the treatment of an associated megaloblastic anaemia, but only after full investigation.

SURGERY

The role of orthopaedic surgery in the management of patients with RA is dealt with fully in Chapter 16. It is only necessary to say here that, as a rule, a particular operation can be no more than an incident (albeit often a critical one) in the treatment programme of an individual patient. It is also important to appreciate that there is a strict limit to the number of operations that can be sustained by the patient at one time, or even over a period. Thus, the choice of operation, and its timing, is a matter requiring the most careful consideration. Clearly the usual formal arrangement whereby the patient is referred from one end of the hospital to the other (often literally) for a simple 'yes' or 'no' verdict on a particular operation is usually quite inadequate. There are many factors concerning the patient, the disease, and the environment that have to be carefully considered and discussed. The individual joint in question is never the whole problem.

In this situation experience shows that a good environment for discussing these questions and taking decisions is the *combined clinic* and the *combined ward round*, in which the rheumatologist and the orthopaedic surgeon see the patient together. This enables the particular problem to be reviewed against the whole background of long-term treatment and management. Such consultations inevitably lead to cross-fertilisation of ideas, and a common policy gradually develops, undergoing constant modification, all to the patient's advantage. This approach also leads to the creation of mutual understanding of the kind that facilitates communication, so that even outside the (somewhat time-consuming) combined clinic, referrals in both directions become more effective.

This combined approach to the care of the rheumatoid patient leads to the development of a collaboration between rheumatologist and orthopaedic surgeon to the point where the traditional sharp division between the two disciplines begins to blur. There would seem much to be gained, and little lost, if a similar interlocking of departments gradually follows.

4

Still's Disease

Colin G Barnes

In 1897, Dr George Frederick Still of King's College Hospital described a chronic inflammatory polyarthropathy in children, which was accompanied by systemic manifestations. Subsequently this syndrome became known as 'juvenile rheumatoid arthritis', but as this term implies a more exact identity with the adult disease than is now thought to exist, it seems preferable tc retain the eponym of Still's disease to describe any inflammatory arthropathy occurring in children. The Medical Research Council's Rheumatism Unit (Taplow) defines Still's disease as a chronic polyarthritis affecting children under the age of 15 years, lasting for three months or longer, and affecting more than four joints. This definition probably includes more than one pathological entity (*see* below).

AETIOLOGY

The aetiology remains unknown. Biochemical abnormalities have not been identified, nor has any infective agent been isolated. There is some evidence that hereditary factors may be operative. In relatives of patients with Still's disease there is a significantly increased incidence of arthropathy, either alkylosing spondylitis in male relatives, or a peripheral erosive arthropathy in female relatives.

Just as in the case of adult rheumatoid arthritis, it is suggested that an altered state of immunity exists, although whether this could be the basic abnormality in Still's disease remains unknown. The evidence for such an immune disturbance is the finding of plasma cell and lymphocytic infiltrations in the inflamed synovium, elevation of plasma immunoglobulin levels, and the propensity to develop amyloidosis.

CLINICAL FEATURES

The peak age of onset is between two and four years, with a second smaller peak at about the time of puberty. The female to male ratio is approximately 3:2. The presenting features may be entirely confined to the joints or may be an acute systemic illness.

ARTHRITIS

When the condition presents as an arthritis this may initially be monarticular, involving commonly a knee, with pain, swelling and limitation of movement. Other joints subsequently become affected, although the timing and pattern of further joint involvement is very variable. Alternatively, a widespread acute polyarthritis involving predominantly the peripheral and medium sized joints may be present from the onset.

While no joint may escape involvement, the knees, the small joints of the hands and feet, and the wrists are most frequently affected. Early involvement of the hips and cervical spine is not uncommon. Painless

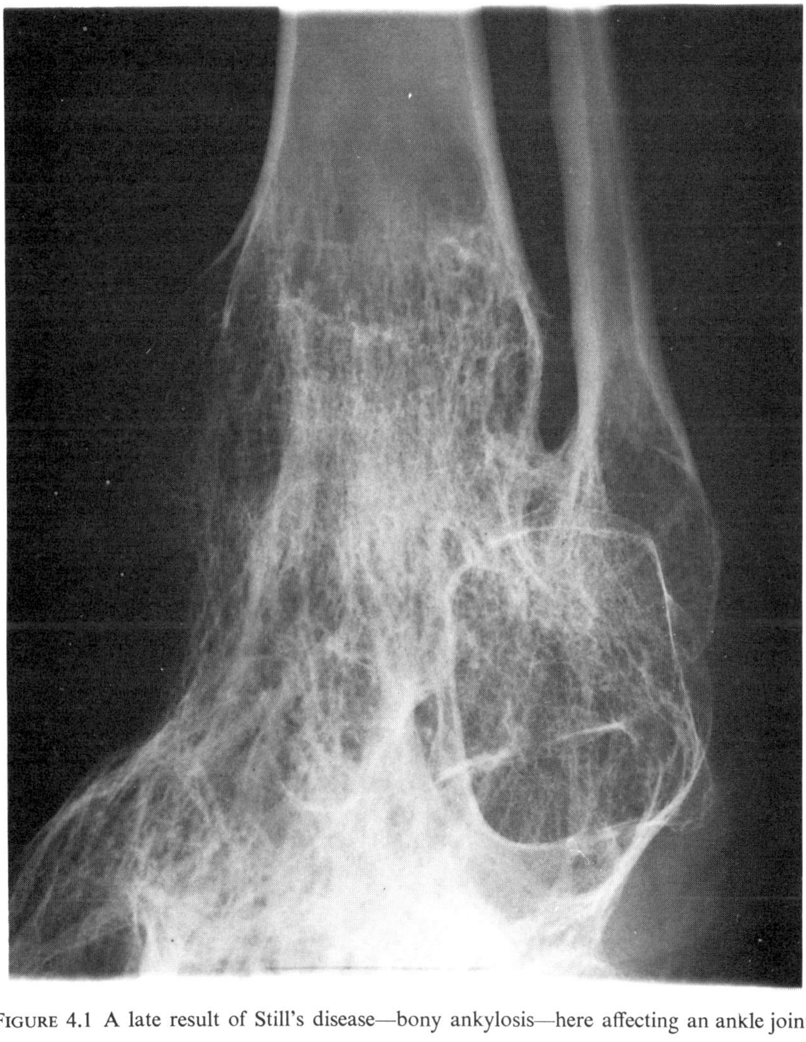

FIGURE 4.1 A late result of Still's disease—bony ankylosis—here affecting an ankle joint

effusions occur although more commonly the swollen joints are warm, tender, painful, and limited. The swelling consists of synovial hypertrophy with effusion.

Sequelae. Destructive joint changes are the usual outcome of continued severe arthritis. These occur rapidly in the older child, but develop much more slowly in the younger patient. Joint cartilage is destroyed and this may be followed by peri-articular bone reabsorption. Bony ankylosis (Fig. 4.1) is another important late result of Still's disease and is much more common than in adult rheumatoid arthritis. This is of serious functional significance when a hip, knee or elbow is affected. In the large weight-bearing joints ankylosis with flexion deformity is of particularly serious consequence.

In the cervical spine the development of vertebrae may be arrested, so that in later life some vertebrae radiologically appear to be normally shaped but smaller than their neighbours. This failure of development is frequently associated with fusion of adjacent vertebral bodies. In addition, bony fusion of apophyseal joints may also occur, resulting in permanent stiffness.

The presence of an inflammatory arthritis adjacent to the epiphysis of a growing bone inevitably brings about disturbances of development. Paradoxically, this may be either retardation or acceleration of growth, either generally or locally. Arrest of growth may occur not only in the cervical spine but also around the hip joint, leading to failure of development of the femoral head, in the region of the wrist and the metacarpals, and characteristically in the jaw. The latter produces the typically receding chin so characteristic of the adult who suffered from Still's disease in childhood, sometimes permitting an instant diagnosis as the patient walks into the consulting room.

General stunting of growth is not uncommon. However, periostitis may cause new bone formation leading to a widening of bones, especially the phalanges, and an actual increase in the length of individual bones may even occur.

EXTRA-ARTICULAR MANIFESTATIONS

During the active phases of the illness, these children characteristically exhibit *fever*, *lymphadenopathy*, and a *rash*. The lymphadenopathy affects mainly the axillary and epitrochlear glands, and the rash is typically a dusky pink maculopapular eruption, the distribution of which varies from day to day, or even from hour to hour. The trunk and limbs may both be affected.

In active disease *anaemia* is present. This is normochromic and normocytic; presumably associated with the active inflammatory process, and is not caused by deficiency of iron, vitamin B 12, or folate. A polymorphonuclear *leucocytosis*, which may exceed 25,000 per cubic millimetre, occurs frequently. *Splenomegaly* is found in a small proportion of cases but the enlargement is usually modest and in itself is thought not to predispose to any haematological disturbance (c.f. Felty's syndrome in the adult, p. 29).

The two most serious systemic manifestations are *iridocyclitis* and cardiac involvement. Iridocyclitis is reported to occur in about 8 per cent of patients and may lead to blindness. This presents either as acute pain and redness of the eyes, or it may be insidious and chronic. *Pericarditis* may occur in active phases of the disease.

Amyloidosis occurs in about 3·5 per cent of cases at variable intervals from the onset of the disease.

SPECIAL INVESTIGATIONS

RHEUMATOID FACTOR

It is usually accepted that standard tests for rheumatoid factor (Latex and sheep cell agglutination tests) are negative in Still's disease. This is certainly true in younger children. In the older (teenage) child, however, there is an increasing incidence of positive tests, indicating that the condition may become identified with adult rheumatoid arthritis when it begins in the older child. An overall incidence of 13 per cent positive reactions is quoted.

RADIOLOGY

Early Features. At the onset, and early in the development of the arthritis, there are no radiological abnormalities to be seen in the bones, but soft shadows around inflamed joints indicate the soft tissue swellings apparent clinically.

Periostitis, indicated by new bone formation and widening of some bones, especially the phalanges, appears early, and is progressive.

The earliest change in or around the joints themselves is a localised or peri-articular osteoporosis. This is followed by narrowing of the joint space, representing loss of cartilage. Erosive change is rare at this stage.

Late Features. Progressive loss of joint space may proceed to complete destruction of the articulation and subsequent bony ankylosis. This is seen particularly in the knees, hips, carpus, and elbows. When bony ankylosis is complete, trabeculae can be seen to cross the site of the former joint space (Fig. 4.1). A 'ghost' of a joint line may sometimes still be apparent.

Later in the disease residual changes may be seen in the cervical vertebrae, with hypoplasia of the vertebral bodies, ankylosis of the apophyseal joints, and sometimes atlanto-axial separation. In the latter case, a lateral view of the cervical spine taken in a fully flexed position shows an increased gap between the posterior surface of the anterior arch of the atlas and the anterior surface of the odontoid peg, representing laxity or even separation of the transverse ligament of the atlas.

Radiological signs of sacro-iliitis are present in about one quarter of these patients, males being more commonly affected than females. The difficulty of interpreting sacro-iliac radiographs in the young are discussed in the section on ankylosing spondylitis (p. 66).

OTHER INVESTIGATIONS

In active phases of the disease the erythrocyte sedimentation rate is accelerated and reflects the severity of the inflammatory process. Plasma proteins show a rise in globulin levels, usually due to an increase in the gamma components. Tests for antinuclear factor are negative.

As has been mentioned above, a normochromic, normocytic anaemia, and polymorphonuclear leucocytosis, the latter often reaching very high values, accompany active disease.

NATURAL HISTORY

It must be emphasised that the term 'Still's disease' is only used to describe an inflammatory polyarthropathy occurring in children ('inflammatory' being used in the restricted sense defined in Chapter 1; it excludes conditions such as rheumatic fever and allergic purpura). No specific investigations are available to make a more precise diagnosis, and it is evident that this diagnostic category includes a number of different diseases. This is suggested by the natural history of Still's disease. At least some cases appear to be examples of adult inflammatory arthropathies occurring in childhood. Perhaps all are.

It would seem a useful, but probably over-simplified, view of the natural history of the disease to divide the cases into three broad categories. The first is the young child with an inflammatory polyarthropathy who, on long-term follow-up, continues to have negative tests for serum rheumatoid factor. The disease in the majority of these patients becomes quiescent within seven to ten years. A minority progress to severe articular incapacity. A second group consists of those patients in whom the condition first appears after the age of ten years, and who develop positive tests for serum rheumatoid factor. In general, the arthritis in these cases tends to behave more like the adult form of rheumatoid arthritis, apart from beginning at an earlier age. The third group consists of a minority of patients, usually boys, in whom the disease progresses to a state indistinguishable from ankylosing spondylitis.

The prognosis is difficult to assess in any individual case. However, the figures obtained from the follow-up of large numbers of patients at

Taplow indicate that in over half the patients the arthritis becomes quiescent, or 'burnt out', leaving negligible or only mild joint residua and excellent functional capacity. It seems as if permanent damage is less severe in those children in whom the disease started at a very young age.

In a minority of cases there is persistent activity of the inflammatory process leading to progressive joint damage and functional incapacity. This is especially true when major weight-bearing joints, such as the hips and knees, are affected.

Iridocyclitis and pericarditis are the leading non-articular causes of morbidity. The former, before the advent of corticosteroid therapy, was a significant cause of blindness; happily this can now largely be avoided. Pericarditis may rarely lead to constriction requiring pericardectomy.

The development of amyloidosis may lead to renal failure and hypertension, carrying a very poor prognosis. At Taplow the incidence of this complication is about 3·5 per cent. Occasionally, improvement in the manifestations of amyloidosis has been recorded with effective treatment or clinical remission of the disease.

DIFFERENTIAL DIAGNOSIS

Rheumatic fever, while uncommon in the United Kingdom, remains the principal condition to be differentiated. However, the flitting nature of the arthritis in rheumatic fever and the more chronic nature of Still's disease usually enables a correct diagnosis to be reached, even in the absence of the characteristic skin or cardiac manifestations of these two conditions. The significance of a preceding sore throat and of estimations for ASO titre are discussed under rheumatic fever (p. 199).

Virus infections, such as rubella or mumps, may cause a polyarthritis which is usually acute but short-lived.

The *systemic connective tissue disorders* seen in adults may also present in childhood. These include systemic lupus erythematosus, dermatomyositis, and polyarteritis nodosa. Psoriatic arthropathy may also start in childhood.

Acute leukaemia may present with joint pain and swelling. In practice, some difficulty may occur in those cases of Still's disease having a marked leucocytosis. However, bone marrow examination should clarify the diagnosis.

Joint infections, particularly tuberculosis, have to be excluded, especially when the arthritis is monarticular. In this situation, examination and culture of synovial fluid and, if necessary, synovial biopsy are essential.

TREATMENT

GENERAL

The treatment of Still's disease is dominated by the special problems of the age group to which these patients belong. Thus, while periods of rest and activity must be carefully co-ordinated, the education of the child must be continued and an environment created in which the child can be happy and can mature even through prolonged periods of hospitalisation may be required.

At home, in special schools, and in hospitals, the combined care of physicians, orthopaedic surgeons, ophthalmic surgeons, physiotherapists, and teachers is necessary, together with the appropriate provision of splints, walking aids and, occasionally, wheel chairs. It is thus vital to appreciate that the correct handling of these children is a matter of team-work.

During acute phases of the illness, rest is an essential element of treatment, both for the systemic manifestations of the disease and also for the arthritis. Wherever possible, however, the patient should be kept mobile and ambulant, and complete bed rest should be avoided except when it is necessary for severe generalised illness, with fever or active involvement of weight-bearing joints. Prevention of flexion deformities, especially of the knees and hips is critical. Thus, during periods of rest the position of the patient must be controlled to maintain correct alignment of joints, which can most easily be achieved by light-weight splinting. Where flexion deformities have already occurred, these must be corrected by physiotherapy and serial splinting. Physiotherapy should be continued at all times to maintain joint movement and muscle strength. Hydrotherapy in a warm pool is usually the most useful form of physical treatment.

DRUGS

Analgesics. Salicylates are the best symptomatic form of treatment. In maximum tolerated doses they are both analgesic and anti-inflammatory. To achieve the most effective dosage the plasma salicylate level should be monitored. The oral dose may then be increased until a plasma salicylate level of 25 to 30 mg/100 ml is obtained, or until side effects develop.

If salicylates are not tolerated then other analgesics may be used, as in adult rheumatoid arthritis (p. 44). It has been shown that children treated early in the disease with salicylates alone fare no worse than those treated with corticosteroids.

Gold. Treatment with repeated injections of gold salts has been shown to be of value in rheumatoid arthritis (p. 46). While formal trials of this method of treatment have not been performed in Still's disease it is, nevertheless, considered to be useful in suppressing disease activity in some cases.

Much smaller doses of gold are given than in adults. Thus, after appropriately small test doses, 0·3–0·5 mg Myocrisin/kg body weight is given weekly by intramuscular injection for twenty weeks, then the same dose is continued monthly. This necessitates the same urine testing, enquiries for rashes, and repeated blood counts as in adults (p. 46). Antimalarial preparations are occasionally used in children intolerant of gold salts.

Corticosteroids. Corticosteroids undoubtedly suppress the inflammatory activity of this disease. The one absolute indication for corticosteroids is iridocyclitis, to prevent blindness.

Rarely is corticosteroid treatment required for the joint manifestations alone, and only occasionally for the suppression of systemic manifestations of the disease.

Those patients who are treated with corticosteroid drugs develop features of Cushing's syndrome with obesity, moonface, osteoporosis, and vertebral collapse. Bacterial infection is more common. Probably the main drawback of long-term corticosteroid treatment in children is interference with growth hormone action, leading to stunted growth. Whether this effect is less marked with ACTH is not yet known. For this reason, if corticosteroids are prescribed, it is mandatory to titrate down the dose meticulously to the minimum that just controls that aspect of the disease for which the drug was given.

SURGERY

Orthopaedic surgical procedures are largely confined to reconstructive techniques in the late stages of the disease. Arthroplasty of the hips is probably the most common procedure. The place of synovectomy, particularly of the knees, has not yet been established.

5

Sero-Negative Arthropathy

Michael Mason

In Chapter 3, attention was drawn to the great importance of the finding in 1940, by Waaler, and again in 1948, by Rose, of the gamma-M immunoglobulin known as rheumatoid serum factor (RSF). This discovery made possible a division of inflammatory arthropathies into two main groups; those in which RSF is present, and those in which it is absent. In general we have, therefore, two types of inflammatory arthropathy: (i) rheumatoid arthritis in which RSF is characteristically present, and (ii) polyarthritis in which RSF is regularly absent throughout the natural history of the disease. (Still's disease may include examples of both types occurring in childhood.) The second group comprises a number of apparently quite separate diseases. Unfortunately, in practice, the distinction may not be quite so simple. The following factors must be considered—

1. *The technique used for identifying RSF*. The reader will find a brief account of the tests for RSF in Appendix B. As with all such tests, alteration of sensitivity may affect specificity, with a tendency for increasing sensitivity to be associated with loss of specificity. Similarly, any increase in specificity may be at the price of loss of sensitivity. Thus, while the test using human globulin on particles of polystyrene (*latex test*) may be slightly more sensitive than that using sheep cells sensitised with rabbit globulin (*sheep cell agglutination test—SCAT*), the latter is the more specific for rheumatoid arthritis.

2. *The absence of positive tests for RSF does not necessarily invalidate a diagnosis of rheumatoid arthritis*. Tests for RSF, by whatever technique used, are not always positive in what appears to be undoubted rheumatoid arthritis by present criteria. Such patients may go through the whole natural history of the disease without this factor ever being identified. Usually, however, sero-negative rheumatoid arthritis is less severe, and other systemic complications such as arteritis and neuropathy are unlikely to develop. Some 25 per cent of any group of patients with rheumatoid arthritis will have negative tests throughout their disease.

3. 'False positive' tests for RSF may occur in other diseases. These include systemic lupus erythematosus, progressive systemic sclerosis, and dermatomyositis, when some 30 per cent of patients will have a positive test. The test may also be positive in the dysproteinaemias, in subacute bacterial endocarditis, hepatocellular disease, chronic pulmonary tuberculosis, and leprosy. In addition, epidemiological studies of the general population show that some 4 per cent of the 'healthy' population have positive tests, with a tendency for these to be found more frequently in the older age groups.

Subject to these limitations of our present techniques, we can define a group of arthropathies in which there is a polyarthritis resembling rheumatoid arthritis but with a different pattern of joint involvement, pursuing a different clinical course, often associated with characteristic multi-system involvement, and in which repeated tests for rheumatoid factor are consistently found to be negative. It is useful and convenient to give these arthropathies separate identities, but it must be recognised that so long as the aetiology remains unknown this separateness is not proven, and in practice very considerable overlap may be found, blurring the edges of these different categories to the extent that a precise diagnosis may not always be possible.

Ankylosing Spondylitis

Definition

Ankylosing spondylitis is an erosive arthropathy with a marked tendency to bony ankylosis, and with a strong predilection for the sacro-iliac joints and the spine. The limb joints are less frequently affected and there is a tendency for the proximal joints to be involved first. The disease characteristically develops in males in the third decade, although females may be similarly affected. A pre-pubertal onset is well recognised, and this may then be diagnosed as Still's disease. The term 'rheumatoid spondylitis' is confusing and should be avoided, and eponymous titles such as Marie-Strumpell's or Von Bechterew's disease are of historical interest only.

CLINICAL DESCRIPTION AND PHYSICAL SIGNS

The disease is commonest in men, the first symptom usually developing in the third decade. Women are affected more than was at one time appreciated, and the sex incidence is of the order of 5 males to 1 female.

Onset. In 75 per cent of cases the initial symptom is low backache which may extend to buttocks and thighs. Characteristically, this is associated with morning stiffness and a 'limbering-up time' of a few minutes to several hours. Backache and stiffness may waken the patient in the early morning. The onset is usually very insidious and the early symptoms may be intermittent, with prolonged periods of remission. Rarely, the onset is acute, resembling a lumbar disc protrusion, and when this is precipitated by trauma the diagnosis is likely to be missed. However, sensory symptoms of a nerve root lesion—paraesthesiae—are absent, and a careful clinical examination should provide the diagnosis. Occasionally, the patient presents with backache and stiffness higher up the spine, in the dorsal or cervical region. This is due to the initial symptoms being trivial and overlooked since there will always be evidence of sacro-iliac and lumbar spine involvement. There is a small group of patients, about 10 per cent, in which the onset is in a peripheral joint, nearly always in the lower limb, such as the hip, knee or in the foot; occasionally, a 'painful heel syndrome'—plantar fasciitis or Achilles tendinitis—may be the first symptom. In this situation it may not be possible to make the diagnosis for some time. Another 10 per cent of patients develop their first symptom before puberty. Where there is, as seems more frequent in this age group, an onset in a peripheral joint, this may be one form of Still's disease, and only prolonged follow-up into adult life will reveal the more precise diagnosis. Finally, an attack of iritis may bring the patient under medical supervision for the first time, and reveal the diagnosis. Screening of all patients with non-granulomatous anterior uveitis for ankylosing spondylitis is now standard practice.

Physical Signs. Physical examination of the spine is critical in making the diagnosis. The patient must be stripped. In the advanced case, loss of movement amounting to ankylosis of all segments, spreading from below upwards with a tendency to fixation in forward flexion is characteristic; but it is in the early stages that the eliciting of signs may require practice and skill. There is diminution of movement of the lumbar spine in all directions, most easily recognised in lateral flexion. This is associated with loss of the lumbar curve when standing erect and an inability to obliterate the lumbar lordosis in full flexion (Fig. 5.1). Mobile hip joints can compensate for considerable loss of lumbar spine flexion (judged by the patient's ability to touch the floor with the finger tips). At this stage the sacro-iliac joints may be irritable, and forced movement of the sacrum on the pelvis may reproduce the patient's pain. This is most easily done by laying the patient on his face, placing the hand on the sacrum and pressing hard downwards (*see* Fig. A6, p. 298). In the early stages of the disease this will produce pain in the sacro-iliac joint region, which is an important sign. In the later stages, when ankylosis has taken place, this sign will, of course, become negative. In the dorsal spine the presence of spondylitis will be revealed by two signs: (i) *loss of rotation.* The patient should be seated in order to fix the pelvis, and the arms folded across the chest (*see* Fig. A5, p. 297). Rotation can then

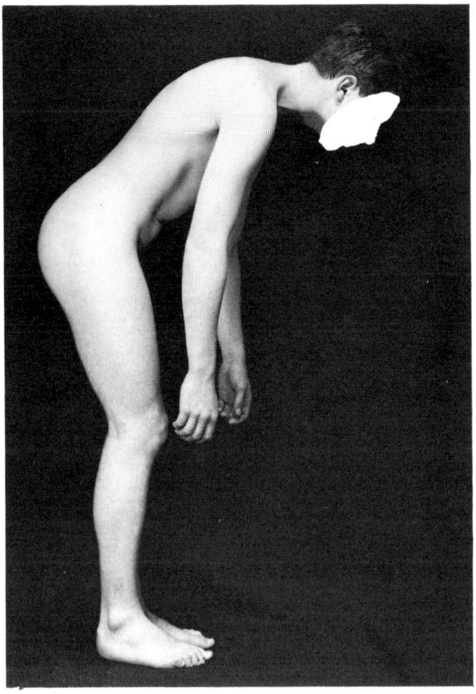

FIGURE 5.1 A patient with ankylosing spondylitis flexing his spine as far as possible. Note the inability to obliterate the lumbar lordosis

be observed and measured. (ii) *Involvement of the costovertebral joints.* When the disease reaches the dorsal spine these joints are invariably affected and a reduction in the respiratory excursion results. A finding of a chest expansion of less than 5 cm in an otherwise apparently fit individual without chest disease is an important physical sign. By the time the cervical spine is affected the diagnosis is usually obvious, hence examination here is less important from a diagnostic standpoint. Loss of range, however, does indicate the extent of the spondylitis and is valuable in following the progress of the disease.

The most important peripheral joints to be affected are the hips since involvement of these leads to critical loss of function. Careful examination of the hip is essential, therefore, with accurate recording of the range of movement (*see* Appendix A, p. 306). When other peripheral joints are affected the signs are those of an inflammatory arthropathy, and are non-specific. Limitation of range of movement is common. The characteristic pattern of joint involvement is for the proximal joints to be affected first, but where the peripheral joints are affected (sometimes initially) the interphalangeal joint of the big toe is often involved, and as we have already observed, the painful heel syndrome is also common.

Occasionally, symptoms may arise from involvement of the manubrio-sternal joint; and arthritis of the symphysis pubis may certainly produce radiological changes, although this is seldom recognised clinically. Nodules are always absent. With active disease the erythrocyte sedimentation rate is likely to be elevated, but this is variable.

COMPLICATIONS AND ASSOCIATED FEATURES

Multi-system involvement is less common in ankylosing spondylitis than in rheumatoid arthritis. However, the following systems may be affected–

1. Ocular,
2. Cardiovascular,
3. Gastro-intestinal,

and when symptoms in these systems predominate there may be difficulty in diagnosis. Occasionally, however, involvement of these systems may give the clue to the diagnosis of an otherwise obscure sero-negative arthropathy.

1. *The eyes.* Iritis (non-granulomatous anterior uveitis) occurs in up to 40 per cent of cases of ankylosing spondylitis at some stage in the disease. It is commoner in the more severe cases, and in those with peripheral joint involvement, but it may be an outstanding feature of mild disease and may, indeed, be the presenting symptom. Routine screening of all patients with iritis will often reveal a mild ankylosing spondylitis which may be symptomless, or with such mild symptoms that the backache has been accepted as of trivial origin and part of some occupational stress. The attacks are usually self-limiting, and with prompt treatment permanent loss of vision is rare.

2. *Cardiovascular System.* The aorta and heart may be affected in a distinctive manner, giving rise to conduction defects and lone aortic incompetence. These defects result from inflammatory changes which cause distortion and dilation of the aortic valve with thickening of the intima, and sometimes spread along the aorta and may even reach the descending portion. The endocardium can also be affected, and there may be interstitial fibrosis in the myocardium. This complication is rare, although routine ECG examination may identify minor defects of conduction. Complete heart block may occur. Lone aortic incompetence is also rare and probably occurs in no more than one per cent of patients with ankylosing spondylitis. But, seen from another point of view, ankylosing spondylitis is an important cause of lone aortic incompetence and, just as in the case of anterior uveitis, patients with this valvular defect should be screened for ankylosing spondylitis.

3. *Gastro-intestinal Tract.* Ulcerative colitis and regional enteritis are both seen with a significantly increased frequency in patients with ankylosing spondylitis. Conversely, patients with ulcerative colitis have a significantly increased incidence of ankylosing spondylitis. The relationship of these two conditions is not clear but will be discussed further in the section on colitic arthropathy (p. 88).

Amyloid Disease. Secondary amyloidosis is a relatively uncommon complication. The possibility of its existence should be considered, however, in the severe and chronically ill spondylitic with peripheral joint involvement, a high ESR, and proteinuria. Renal function tests will show impairment and the diagnosis may be confirmed by renal biopsy, or more simply and almost as reliably, by rectal biopsy.

NATURAL HISTORY

A much increased index of suspicion for the diagnosis of early and mild examples of this disease, together with studies of the relatives of patients with ankylosing spondylitis, indicates that the natural history of the condition is often benign and self limiting. This may vary from virtually asymptomatic bilateral sacro-iliitis, revealed on routine X-ray examination, or occasional low back pain, accepted as part of the aches and pains of some athletic activity, to complete ankylosis of the whole spine, and rarely even of the peripheral joints. Occasionally, an isolated attack of iritis may draw attention to the diagnosis. It seems likely that the picture of the severe spondylitic with a rigid spine fixed in the flexed position is rare indeed. That this is so is perhaps best illustrated by experience in the Armed Forces where ankylosing spondylitis is most commonly observed (because of the age and sex distribution of the disease, young men in the third decade forming the bulk of the Services). For example, in a recent survey in the Royal Air Force it was found that some 60 per cent of the cases diagnosed were able to continue with a full Service career.

PATHOLOGY OF THE JOINTS

Because the earliest changes occur in spinal joints that are not easily accessible to biopsy, knowledge of the initial pathological changes is scanty. This is, however, an inflammatory arthropathy characterised by the formation of granulation tissue, usually arising at the anterior corners of the vertebrae, which gradually extends into the outer layers of the annulus fibrosus to form the syndesmophytes so well seen radiologically. In synovial joints the synovitis resembles that seen in rheumatoid arthritis but without a tendency to necrosis of the surface layer; similar erosions of the articular cartilage occur. Later, the characteristic tendency to bony ankylosis appears. The joint fluid shows no specific features, though rheumatoid factor is invariably absent. Rheumatoid nodules never occur.

RADIOLOGY

Confirmation of the diagnosis depends on radiography. The specific radiological features of ankylosing spondylitis are, therefore, very important and will be described in some detail. The presence of bilateral sacro-iliitis is essential for the diagnosis, though rarely, in very early cases, it may be necessary to observe the patient for some time until the changes become apparent. The standard views required consist of an antero-posterior radiograph of the pelvis and lumbar spine and a lateral view of the lumbar spine. Special views, e.g. postero-anterior or oblique views of the sacroiliac joints, practically never help, often confuse, and should normally be avoided. Unfortunately, the sacro-iliac joints are very difficult to visualise clearly; this is particularly so in the young, especially before the epiphyses are united, when the sacro-iliac joints normally appear to be fuzzy and blurred, often making useful interpretation impossible. The earliest change, however, is blurring of the lower part of the joint with patchy areas of osteoporosis alternating with sclerosis (Fig. 5.2). When

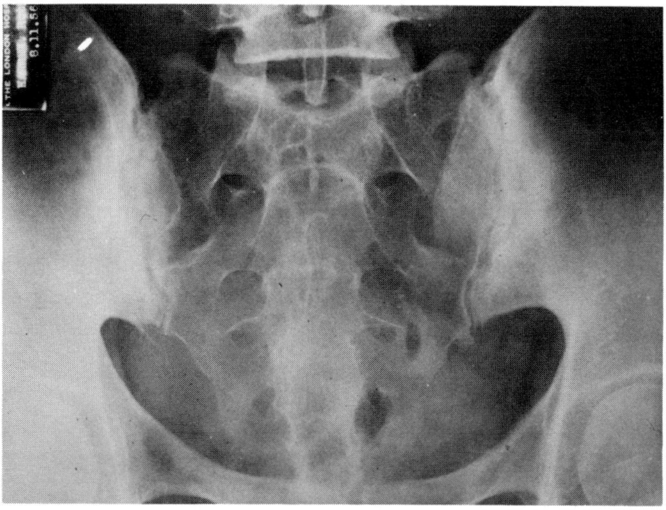

FIGURE 5.2 Bilateral sacro-iliitis with blurring of the sacro-iliac joints due to sclerosis, osteoporosis and erosions

the osteoporosis predominates, the joint may even appear to be widened. If the line of subchondral bone is visible, erosions breaching it may be seen. As the disease progresses, the joint space becomes gradually obliterated until complete bony ankylosis occurs. In the lumbar spine the

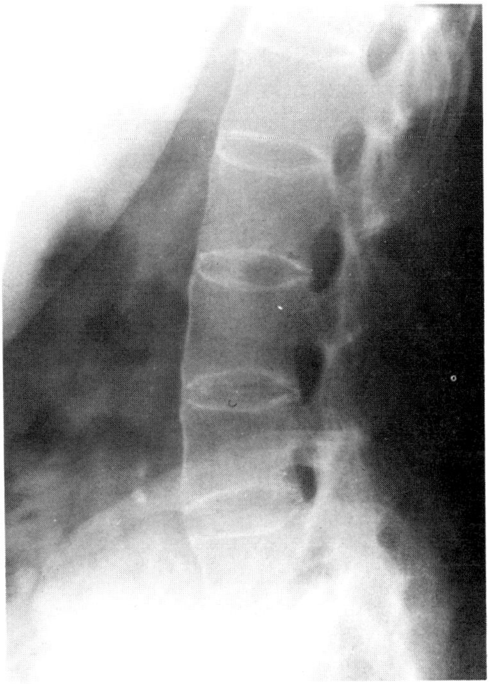

FIGURE 5.3 Lateral radiograph of lumbar spine in ankylosing spondylitis. Anterior calcification can be seen. This leads to ankylosis. The concavity of the front of the vertebral bodies has largely been filled in, giving them a 'squared' appearance

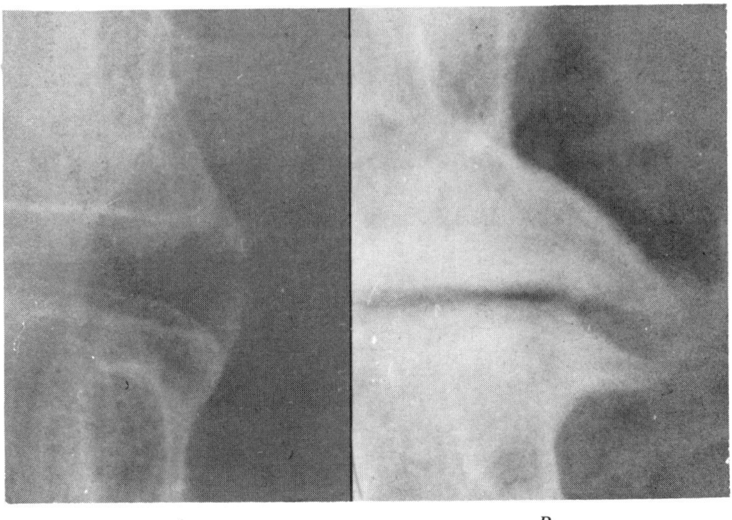

A *B*

FIGURE 5.4 *A* shows a syndesmophyte developing in ankylosing spondylitis. Note that its direction is vertical, while in *B* the osteophyte of spondylosis develops in a horizontal direction vertebral bodies develop a squared appearance, especially seen in the lateral view, with filling in of the anterior concave surface (Fig. 5.3). Small erosions may develop in the upper and lower corners. Sometimes these may be prominent, especially in the lower dorsal spine, and may even suggest a localised infection such as tuberculosis. These changes are followed by calcification in the annulus, forming a *syndesmophyte*. This calcification runs *vertically*, which distinguishes it from the *horizontal* new bone formation (*osteophytes*) of spondylosis (Fig. 5.4), and in the later stages, when the longitudinal ligaments of the spine are affected, gives rise to the so-called 'bamboo spine'. The facetal joints also become affected but they are more difficult to visualise, except in the cervical spine where ankylosis may be obvious (Fig. 5.5). Other characteristic features include

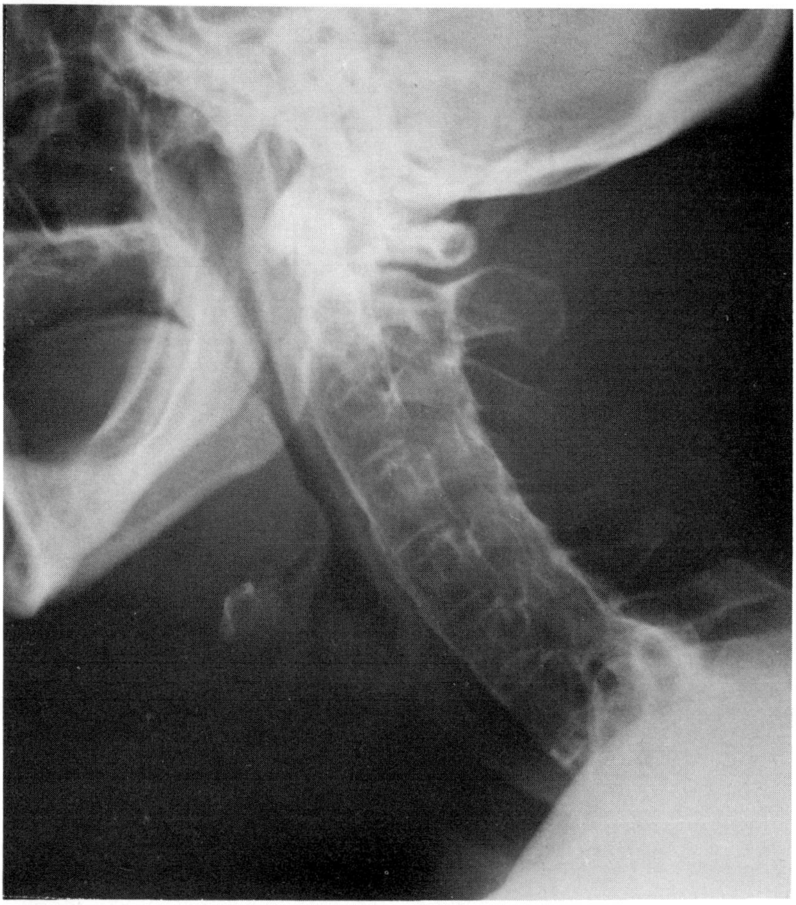

FIGURE 5.5 Advanced ankylosing spondylitis which has reached the cervical spine. This radiograph shows fusion of the vertebral bodies and ankylosis of the facetal joints

erosive changes in the symphysis pubis, which may later ankylose, and a tendency to the formation of periosteal new bone over the ischial tuberosities, often associated with erosions at this site. The costo-vertebral joints are again difficult to visualise but in the ordinary postero-anterior views of

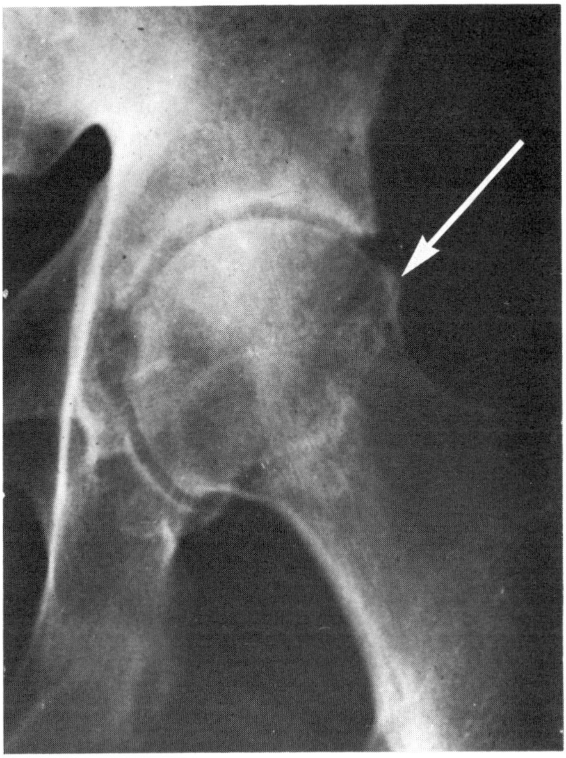

FIGURE 5.6 This radiograph of the hip joint in a patient with ankylosing spondylitis shows early involvement characterised by the development of a 'ruff' at the margin of the joint—best seen on the upper lateral aspect (indicated by the arrow) (*From* Mason, R. M. in *Textbook of Rheumatic Diseases* 1969. Ed. Copeman, W. S. C. Edinburgh: E & S Livingstone)

the chest, or of the cervical spine, the first costo-transverse joint is often well seen, and erosive changes may be recognised here. In the peripheral joints the changes are less specific. Nevertheless, certain features, in the hips and feet particularly, are often helpful. In the hips, a characteristic 'ruff' often develops around the junction of the femoral head and neck (Fig. 5.6). In the feet, the erosive changes are often more localised and associated with less osteoporosis than in rheumatoid arthritis. Involvement of the interphalangeal joint of the big toe is not uncommon in all the sero-negative arthropathies.

AETIOLOGY

Ankylosing spondylitis is a relatively uncommon disease, occurring in less than 0·5 per cent of the male population at risk, but it is much more common among the relatives of patients with ankylosing spondylitis and may be found in about 9 per cent of these. Thus, a *genetic factor* seems to be important, and many families with a high incidence of the disease have been described. Indeed, a careful family history is often of great value in making the diagnosis and, sometimes, in a doubtful case, it is helpful to examine suitable relatives. *Infection* has long been suspected as a possible cause and there is evidence to show that patients with ankylosing spondylitis have a high incidence of chronic prostato-vesiculitis, and prostatic massage will usually produce a purulent smear. This fact, together with the observation that patients with Reiter's disease, ulcerative colitis, and Crohn's disease are all liable to develop spondylitis, lends some support to such a hypothesis. Unfortunately, no organism has ever been regularly identified, and agglutination studies have so far failed to identify any specific antibodies. Recent work has, for example, shown that antibodies to Chlamydia are absent in ankylosing spondylitis (*see* Reiter's disease p. 86). Thus, while the hereditary factor is clearly important, the environmental factor producing the disease remains unidentified.

TREATMENT

Ankylosing spondylitis is one form of inflammatory arthropathy in which rest and immobilisation appear to be downright harmful, leading to rapid loss of mobility and encouraging ankylosis. The whole emphasis in treatment is on active mobilisation, the patient being encouraged to live a normal and reasonably athletic life. Regular breathing exercises to maintain mobility of the thoracic cage are believed to be important, but advice to engage in pleasurable active pursuits such as squash or tennis which cause increased respiratory activity is more likely to be followed. Attention to posture is vital, and aims at ensuring that any ankylosis occurs with the spine in an optimal position. Avoidance of a gross spinal flexion deformity is critical. The patient should have a firm mattress and practise spinal extension exercises. The office worker who bends over his desk all day may be well advised to lie flat on the floor for half an hour on his return from work. Special care is required when the patient develops some intercurrent illness requiring a period in bed. Such a patient merits regular attention from a physiotherapist to keep him mobile. Prolonged bed rest without this precaution may have disastrous results on posture and function.

Analgesics. The proper use of the milder analgesics such as aspirin or its substitutes should not be neglected and will usually keep the patient mobile and comfortable. *Phenylbutazone* or *oxyphenbutazone* seem to have an almost specific effect in ankylosing spondylitis. So excellent is the response in many cases that the administration of these drugs may occasionally be used as a diagnostic test. Small doses are often sufficient, and the daily dose should not exceed 300 mg. Regular blood counts are necessary in view of the possibility of blood dyscrasias being precipitated, but the risk of these should not cause the drugs to be withheld. Gastro-intestinal irritation, and haemorrhage from peptic ulcers are complications that can sometimes be circumvented by using suppositories (250 mg) once or twice daily. On larger doses, some salt and water retention occurs. Whether phenylbutazone has more than a purely analgesic effect is not known. *Indomethacin* may be useful where phenylbutazone is not tolerated, particularly in patients with dyspepsia. This may be administered by mouth or, alternatively, by suppository, 100 mg at night, and in this latter form may be valuable in relieving the characteristic morning stiffness.

Radiotherapy. Deep X-ray therapy will produce palliative relief in over three-quarters of patients with ankylosing spondylitis. However, this relief tends to be transient, lasting no more than twelve months as a rule, and there is no evidence that it has any influence on the natural history considered over a longer term. There is evidence that irradiated patients have up to a tenfold increase in the likelihood of developing leukaemia. For these two reasons irradiation as a method of treatment of ankylosing spondylitis has fallen into disuse in recent years. Nevertheless, deep X-ray therapy is justified if all other measures have failed to control the symptoms, and if there is clinical and radiological evidence of progressive disease. In particular, where the hip joint is affected and bids fair to lead to critical disability, radiotherapy should not be withheld. Finally, it may be justified in patients who cannot tolerate drug therapy, e.g. those with a peptic ulcer, or for those who perhaps live in parts of the world where access to regular supplies of drugs and medical supervision are limited.

Corticosteroid Therapy. Apart from iritis this has little place in the treatment of ankylosing spondylitis although, rarely, it may be justified for an acute exacerbation. Similarly, there may also occasionally be a place for intra-articular corticosteroid administration into an accessible joint such as the knee.

Surgical Treatment. Severe residual deformity of the spine can be corrected by spinal osteotomy. This is a major procedure of considerable risk. It is, however, occasionally impossible to prevent such deformity developing and, rarely, a case may be allowed to develop through neglect. When the patient's spine becomes so flexed that he is unable to look ahead, osteotomy may restore him to a more erect posture. Involvement of the hip joint presents a special problem. The older arthroplasties such as the Vitallium mould or cup arthroplasty unfortunately tend to ankylose again within a few years, but a total hip replacement, such as the low friction arthroplasty, may present the patient with a new, mobile and comfortable hip joint. Unfortunately, the prosthesis has a limited life and the patient who needs an arthroplasty is usually thirty or forty years of age. Thus, total hip replacement is only justified when the alternative is a wheelchair for life.

Psoriatic Arthropathy

Definition

Psoriatic arthropathy is a sero-negative, anodular, erosive arthropathy occurring in patients with the psoriatic diathesis and specifically associated with this skin condition. The latter affects the skin or the nails at some stage before, during, or after the onset of the arthritis. The pattern of joint involvement is characteristic, affecting the terminal interphalangeal joints of the fingers, the interphalangeal joint of the thumb, and the interphalangeal joints of the toes. The sacro-iliac joints and the spine are not

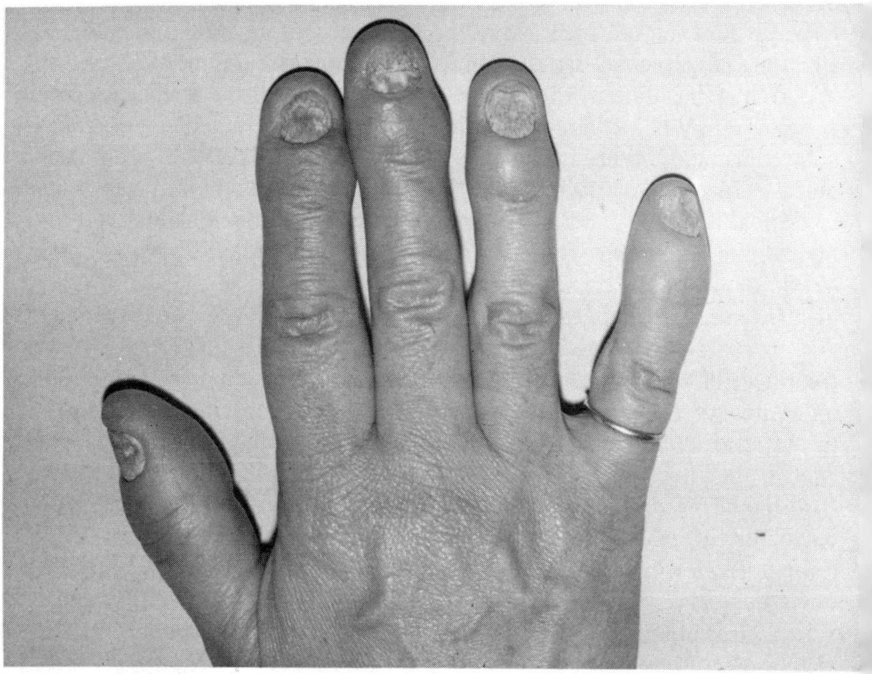

FIGURE 5.7 Psoriatic arthropathy with involvement of the nails and terminal interphalangeal joints

uncommonly affected, too. Other joints may also be affected in an indeterminate pattern. A clear distinction must be made from rheumatoid arthritis with incidental psoriasis.

DIAGNOSIS

The typical patient is one whose psoriasis has pursued the usual variable course of exacerbations and remissions. In association with a relapse of the skin condition, characteristically with involvement of the nails, the patient develops an inflammatory arthropathy of the terminal interphalangeal joint of a finger showing nail involvement (Fig. 5.7). The arthritis then spreads to other joints, especially the interphalangeal joints of the toes (Fig. 5.8), and perhaps typically, the interphalangeal joint of the big toe. The arthritis may be quite acute and 'explosive' in individual joints, with considerable swelling and synovial proliferation. Redness of the

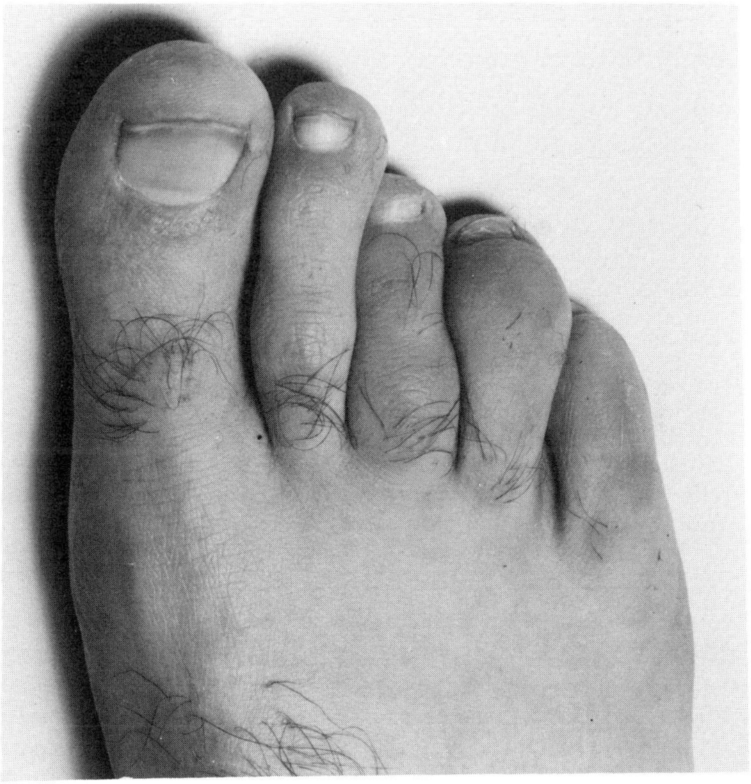

FIGURE 5.8 Arthritis of the distal interphalangeal joint of the 4th toe in psoriatic arthropathy

overlying skin often occurs. At the site of such an arthritis there may follow marked local erosive and destructive changes, with much loss of bone. Ankylosis may develop early. Later, erosive changes may occur at the sacro-iliac joints, and a characteristic spondylitis, affecting particularly the cervical spine, may develop. Occasionally, the arthritis may be of a more severe and progressive type, producing gross deformity and destruction of joints. This may be described as 'arthritis mutilans' and the hand of such a patient as *main-en-lorgnette* (Fig. 5.9). It is in this

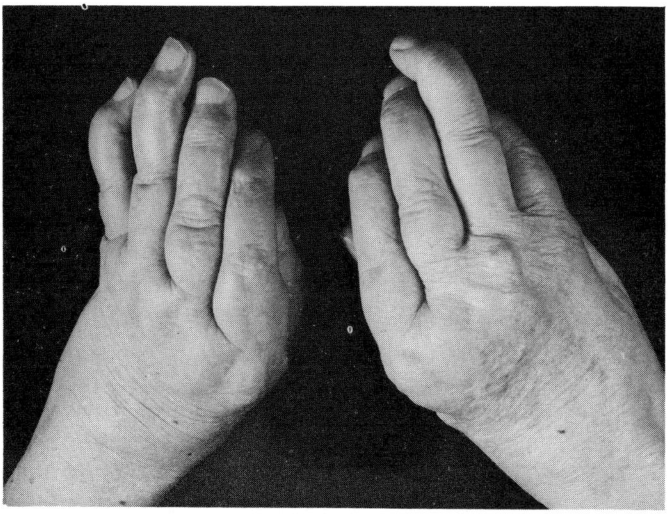

FIGURE 5.9 Arthritis mutilans in psoriatic arthropathy. Note the wrinkling of the skin which results from absorption of bone causing a surplus of soft tissue

group that spondylitis is especially common. This may be indistinguishable from ankylosing spondylitis, though the radiological appearances (*see* p. 75) may have some distinctive features. Multi-system involvement does not occur, but psoriasis may occur in association with some other forms of arthritis discussed below. In the ordinary case there is no weight loss, fever, or anaemia, and malaise is not prominent. Nodules never occur, and tests for rheumatoid serum factor are always negative. The ESR may, however, be raised, and some elevation of the plasma urate level is not uncommon (p. 159). The course of the disease is extremely variable, although it is probably true to say that this tends to be either benign or very severe, and the chronic slowly progressive disease so familiar in rheumatoid arthritis is rarely seen.

Skin and Nail Lesions
For a firm diagnosis the presence of psoriasis is mandatory. Nevertheless, the arthritis may precede the development of the skin lesions by many years. In such a case, the pattern of joint involvement may be highly suggestive, but whilst this and repeated negative tests for rheumatoid serum factor make the clinician highly suspicious, he must simply wait and watch carefully for evidence of psoriasis—the typical dry scaling rash on extensor surfaces. The rash may, however, be concealed in the scalp or misdiagnosed as 'dandruff'; flexural psoriasis affecting the natal cleft and peri-anal region, under the breasts, or in the axillae is easily missed. Similarly, psoriasis of the penis is easily overlooked. Psoriasis cannot be excluded until these areas have been carefully inspected; indeed, examination of these areas for evidence of psoriasis should always be part of the clinical examination of any patient with a sero-negative polyarthritis.

Psoriasis of the nails may be obvious, with marked subungual separation, but the characteristic pitting of the nails should be looked for—the so-called 'thimble pitting' or 'icepick' lesions may sometimes be the only manifestations of the psoriasis, and even in isolation may occasionally justify the diagnosis.

Family History
Careful epidemiological studies have shown that psoriasis occurs in about one per cent of the general population. In the relatives of patients with sero-negative polyarthritis it is some four times as frequent, so that it seems clear that there is a familial aggregation of both psoriasis and sero-negative polyarthritis. Not only does this suggest that a genetic factor is concerned in the aetiology but, in the practical problem of diagnosis, a careful family history and, if necessary, examination of close relatives may lend support to the diagnosis.

Radiology
The radiological appearances are those of an inflammatory arthropathy with erosions and periarticular osteoporosis. However, there is a greater tendency for periosteal new bone to form, and sometimes this may be very striking. The terminal interphalangeal joints are, of course, more commonly affected radiologically, as they are clinically, and here there may be considerable loss of bone ends, sometimes with remodelling and healing taking place (Fig. 5.10). The appearance in the sacro-iliac joints is entirely non-specific, but paravertebral ossification, which differs from that seen in ankylosing spondylitis, in that there is a characteristic separation of the ossification from the vertebral body, may occur (Fig. 5.11).

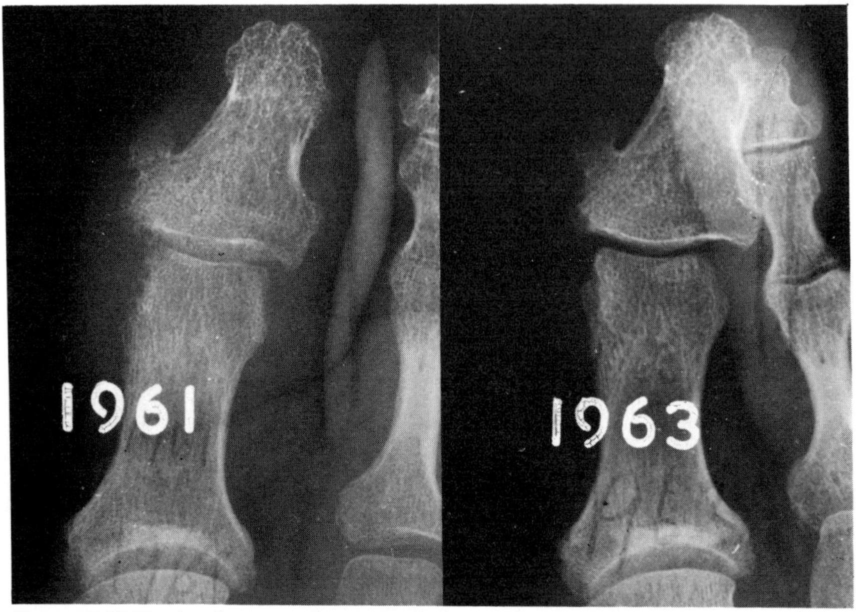

FIGURE 5.10 Erosive change can be seen in the interphalangeal joint of the big toe in 1961. This radiographic appearance is typical of psoriatic arthropathy. Within two years there has been spontaneous healing and remodelling of bone

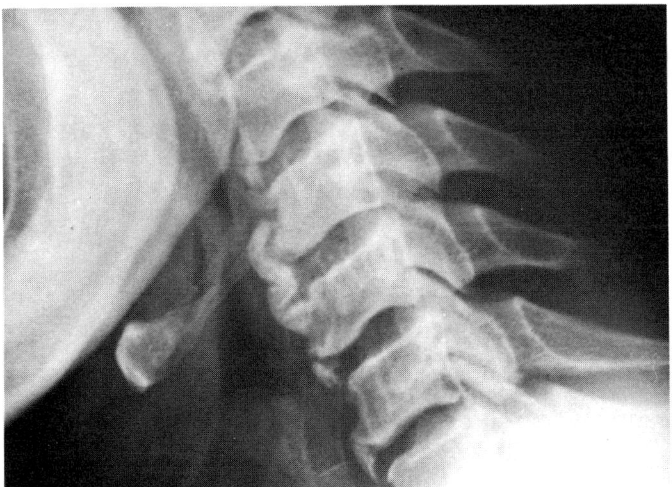

FIGURE 5.11 Lateral view of the cervical spine of a patient with psoriatic arthropathy. Compare the appearance with that of Fig. 5.5. The new bone formation is more prolific than that seen in ankylosing spondylitis and appears to be separated from the vertebral body. The facetal joints are normal

TREATMENT

The treatment of a patient with psoriatic arthropathy is very similar to that of rheumatoid arthritis or other inflammatory arthropathy. There may, however, be certain special difficulties. In rheumatoid arthritis, for example, it is often possible to form an opinion as to the likely natural history in that individual, and this may modify the degree of aggressiveness with which the patient should be treated. The natural history of psoriatic arthropathy is less easy to predict. Overall, a group of patients with psoriatic arthropathy will, on follow-up, have a better retention of function than patients with rheumatoid arthritis, and, as already pointed out, multi-system involvement does not occur. On the other hand, a small proportion of psoriatic patients will go on to develop a very destructive and crippling form of arthropathy—*arthritis mutilans*. The problem of the steadily progressive arthritis requiring continuing treatment and management, so familiar in rheumatoid arthritis, is much less frequent. In practice, therefore, therapy is likely to be required either for the mild and relatively benign case, or for the very severe problem. In the former, symptomatic treatment is usually sufficient. Gold therapy as given in rheumatoid arthritis is generally accepted as being equally effective, although this belief is not actually supported by the controlled experimental data available for rheumatoid arthritis. Antimalarial drugs—chloroquine salts—are contra-indicated since these are suspected of having the capacity to exacerbate the psoriasis. Corticosteroid therapy is valuable when applied topically to the skin, either as 0·1 per cent betamethasone-17-valerate, or as 0·025 per cent fluocinolone acetanide cream, or ointment, to small areas of psoriasis. Intra-articular corticosteroid therapy may have a temporary palliative effect in certain situations, just as in rheumatoid arthritis. Parenteral corticosteroid therapy may become necessary in the florid case, uncontrolled by conservative treatment, and the general principles for administration are similar to those in rheumatoid arthritis. However, many dermatologists believe that triamcinolone is especially useful for controlling the skin lesions in acceptable doses. Our own view is that the possible specificity of this steroid in this situation rarely justifies its use because of its marked tendency to produce myopathy as a side effect. Even when there is early improvement in the psoriasis as a result of administration of corticosteroids, subsequent exacerbations may be a prominent feature and difficult to control.

Antimetabolites and Cytotoxic Agents

Methotrexate is a folic acid antagonist which has been used in the treatment of psoriasis and psoriatic arthropathy. Its use is based on the hypothesis that the proliferation of epidermal cells known to occur in psoriasis might be inhibited by the reduction in cell mitosis consequent on the reduction of available folic acid. In addition, the arguments for using other antimetabolites (such as azathioprine) in rheumatoid arthritis, provide a theoretical basis for hoping that methotrexate may also improve the joints in psoriatic arthropathy. The drug can be administered intramuscularly, 25 mg every 7 to 14 days, or by mouth, 2·5 to 5 mg daily. In this dose it is potentially toxic and, indeed, potentially lethal. It may produce mouth ulcers, gastro-intestinal disturbance, and agranulocytosis. The results of treatment have not been entirely satisfactory, and relapses, or toxicity requiring withdrawal, are frequent. Other 'immuno-suppressive' drugs such as azathioprine or cyclophosphamide perhaps hold more promise for the future, but it remains to be seen whether any improvement in the psoriasis produced by such therapy is necessarily correlated with suppression of the arthropathy.

Surgery

There are no special orthopaedic surgical problems. Synovectomy of active joints may be justified to the same extent as it is in rheumatoid arthritis. No data are available to support the value of this form of therapy. Arthrodesis and joint replacement present exactly similar problems as in rheumatoid arthritis.

Reiter's Disease

History and Definition

Eponymous names for diseases are usually unsatisfactory, except perhaps in the early stages of characterisation of a 'syndrome'. Pathological, aetiological, or even descriptive titles are usually to be preferred. In Reiter's disease, the name remains almost universally accepted and understood although there are over twenty-five other titles for the disease – some eponymous and some descriptive. It may be briefly defined as a sero-negative arthropathy of unknown cause affecting males, predominantly in the third and fourth decades, characterised by recurrent attacks of polyarthritis with a pattern of joint involvement showing a preference for the lower limbs, the sacro-iliac joints, and the spine; it is associated with non-gonococcal inflammation of the genital tract, dysentery, or non-specific diarrhoea. Conjunctivitis, iritis, and lesions of the mucous membranes and skin are common. The name derives from the description, in 1916, by Lieutenant Hans Reiter, a German Medical Officer, of a single case occurring in a German officer serving on the Balkan front, who developed a polyarthritis following an attack of dysentery. In the same year, Feissinger and Leroy described four similar cases occurring among French troops on the Somme, during an epidemic of dysentery; hence in France, the disease is called Syndrome Feissinger-Leroy. In fact, Sir Benjamin

Brodie, Assistant Surgeon at St George's Hospital, described five cases of the disease, all associated with symptoms resembling those of gonorrhoea in 1818, and in 1824, Sir Astley Cooper,* in his surgical lectures given at St Thomas's Hospital, described a similar case which he attributed (wrongly) to gonorrhoea.

CLINICAL PRESENTATION

The patient may present in one of three ways –

1. with frank urethritis following sexual intercourse;
2. following an attack of dysentery or non-specific diarrhoea;
3. with some other manifestation of the disease, commonly articular but occasionally ocular, cutaneous, or mucosal, when the diagnosis may be made only after further manifestations of the disease have developed.

Onset

Type 1. This is the common form of presentation in the United Kingdom. The urethritis usually develops within two weeks of sexual intercourse, and is of the so-called non-specific type; that is, it is non-gonococcal. Gonorrhoea may, incidentally, be contracted at the same time and it may not be until the patient has been cured with appropriate antibiotic therapy that the diagnosis of 'non-specific urethritis' can be made. When gonococci are identified, the differential diagnosis of gonorrhoeal arthritis has to be excluded.

Type 2. The enteric type is less common in the United Kingdom but well recognised in Eastern and Northern Europe and North Africa. It is often associated with epidemics of bacillary dysentery, particularly *S. flexner* among troops, and the features of Reiter's disease develop some two to four weeks after the onset of the dysentery. It is important to appreciate that in this type, urethritis also occurs and appears to develop following the dysentery.

Type 3. In this type the patient presents with a sero-negative arthropathy, the urethritis or the dysentery being insufficient to bring the patient under medical supervision. Evidence of genital inflammation and other features of the disease are found only on careful examination.

The Arthritis

The arthritis is usually acute and polyarticular in onset with a pattern of joint involvement affecting the knees, the mid-tarsal joints, ankles, metatarso-phalangeal joints, and interphalangeal joints of the toes most commonly, although the joints of the upper limb may also be affected.

*Both these accounts bear reading as examples of masterly clinical description – abstracts from them are to be found in *Brit. med. J.*, (1960) **ii**, 1878.

These are usually acutely involved, often with erythema of the overlying skin. The affected joint tends to be more tender than is usual in rheumatoid arthritis and the tenderness may be localised to certain parts of the joint only. The pattern of joint involvement is less symmetrical than in rheumatoid arthritis. The joint fluid is characteristic of any inflammatory arthropathy and has no special macroscopic features. It is turbid with a high cell count and low viscosity. Sometimes, however, characteristic large macrophages, which appear to contain within their cytoplasm one or more intact polymorphonuclear leucocytes or other basophilic nuclear remnants with large vacuoles, are seen. These cells are some 40 μ in diameter and have been named *Pekin cells*, after the author who first described them. Tendon sheath or fascial inflammation is often a striking feature, especially Achilles tendinitis (Fig. 5.12) or plantar fasciitis producing the 'painful heel syndrome'. In severe cases, involvement of the

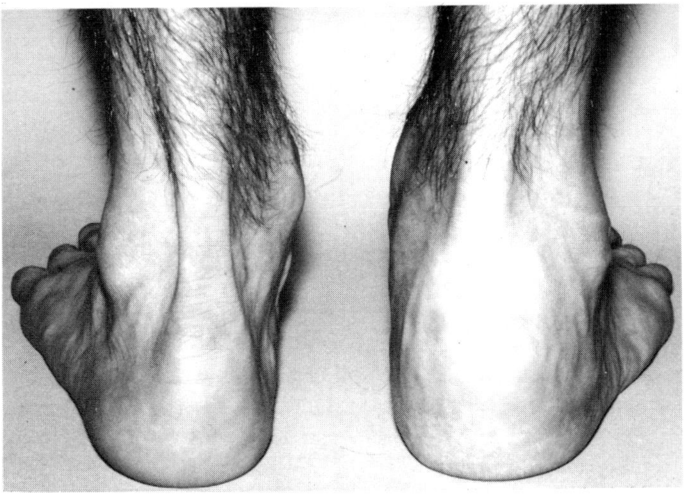

FIGURE 5.12 Achilles tendinitis causing painful swelling of the right heel in Reiter's disease

sacro-iliac joints may cause severe low backache. The initial attack tends to be self-limiting and usually subsides within three months, though relapses may occur associated with fresh attacks of conjunctivitis, urethritis, or skin eruption. The risk of relapse is probably around 15 per cent per annum and is usually associated with a fresh attack of urethritis following sexual exposure; but not necessarily so, for relapses may occur in patients who, so far as can be determined, have not been exposed to the risk of infection (whether heterosexual or homosexual). Similarly, a recurrence of dysentery or non-specific diarrhoea can trigger off a relapse of the arthritis. When the arthritis is recurrent the picture gradually becomes that of a chronic polyarthritis with sacro-iliitis becoming a more prominent feature. Subsequently, a slowly progressive spondylitis may develop, sometimes indistinguishable from classical ankylosing spondylitis.

Urethritis

Recognition of the urethritis, an essential feature of the disease in the early stages, requires careful and skilled examination. Reliance on the history alone is inadequate and will lead to the diagnosis being missed. If the urethritis is painful it may, of course, be the presenting complaint bringing the patient under observation, especially if it is associated with concurrent gonococcal infection. There may, indeed, be an associated cystitis and haematuria. But it is frequently mild and symptomless, and can be observed only by inspection of the meatus before the first morning specimen of urine has been passed, and by the two-glass test – the first few ml of the morning urine being passed into one glass and the remainder into the other. A haze of pus or clearly visible threads will be seen by naked eye in the urine in the first glass. It is important to recognise that –

1. The non-specific urethritis, which occurs in Reiter's disease following dysentery or non-specific diarrhoea, has no distinguishing features from that resulting from sexually acquired disease;
2. Co-incidental gonococcal infection occurs in about 25 per cent of cases following sexual exposure and a further significant proportion will have evidence of previous gonococcal infection, reflected in a positive gonococcal complement fixation test;
3. While there may be dysuria and, in more obvious cases, frank urethral discharge with inflammation of the urethral meatus, (in about 5 per cent of cases there may be 'abacterial haemorrhagic cystitis') the urethritis may be very mild and symptomless and diagnosed only by careful and usually specialist (venereological) examination, or identified simply as prostatitis.

Prostatitis

An almost invariable sequel to urethritis is chronic inflammation of the prostate and seminal vesicles, *prostato-vesiculitis*, often briefly referred to simply as 'prostatitis'. In those patients in whom the urethritis is so mild as to be missed, or who may present later in the disease, this may remain as the only evidence of genito-urinary involvement. The diagnosis is largely dependent on examination of the fluid expressed by digital prostatic massage. Five consecutive specimens are examined by dark-ground microscopy; prostatitis is said to be present when there are more than ten cells/$\frac{1}{12}$ field, but it is better to reserve a definite diagnosis for those cases in which there are many more cells appearing in clumps. However, it must be remembered that one-third to a quarter of healthy males in the population have a 'positive' prostatic massage by these criteria. The same frequency of prostatitis has been shown to exist in male patients with definite rheumatoid arthritis. Thus, a positive finding on prostatic massage is not a specific test for Reiter's disease, although a negative test repeated on more than one occasion by an expert is strong evidence against the diagnosis. As already mentioned, patients with ankylosing spondylitis almost invariably have a 'positive' massage. At present this observation is unexplained. The reader will already have noted that this discussion has so far been confined solely to the male sex. This is because the criteria for the diagnosis of urogenital infection in women are very much less well defined, and the significance of cervicitis, vaginitis, or even urethritis in women has not yet been adequately analysed. The diagnosis of Reiter's disease in women must depend on the other features of the disease with much less weight being attached to evidence of local inflammation. Reiter's disease is certainly rare in women although perhaps it is more common than is at present believed, for the reasons indicated.

Skin and Mucosal Lesions

The skin lesions, *keratoderma*, occur in some 10 per cent of patients with the venereal form of the disease, but are less common in the dysenteric

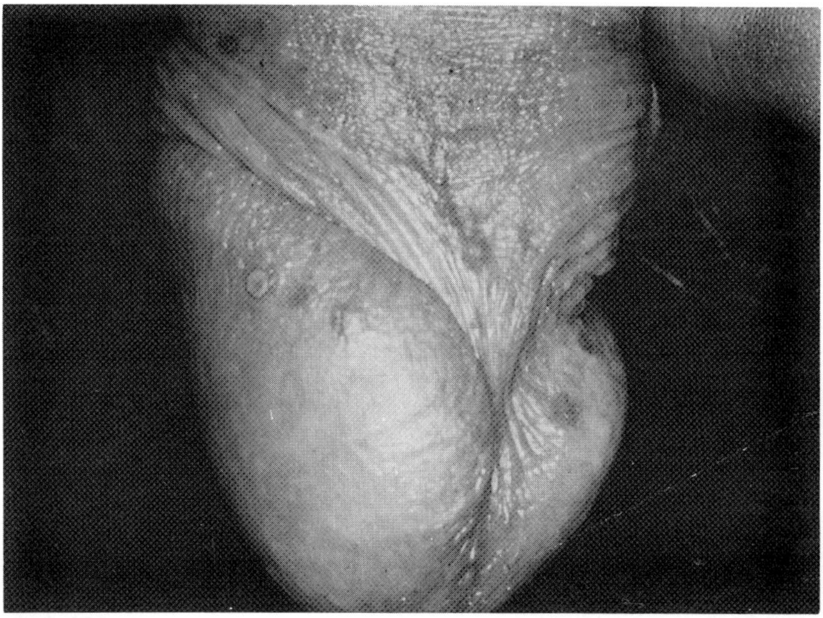

FIGURE 5.13 Circinate balanitis

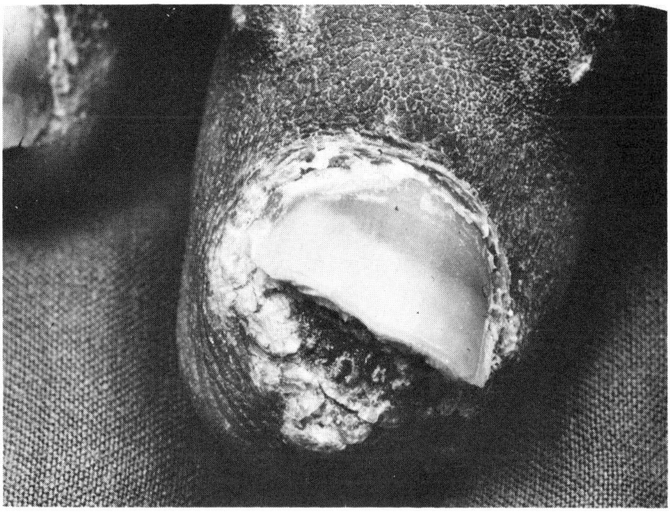

FIGURE 5.14 Keratoderma affecting the nails and causing subungual separation

variety. The soles of the feet are the most frequently involved site, and the anterior aspects of both upper and lower limbs and the scalp may also be affected. Occasionally, the lesions may be widespread, resembling an exfoliative dermatitis. Keratoderma begins as a small dull red macule, which then becomes pustular and, later, keratotic, often resembling psoriasis although it normally differs from the latter in that is usually disappears spontaneously within a few days or weeks. Sometimes, however, it becomes chronic and indistinguishable from psoriasis. Where the penis or the nails are involved there are special features. In the circumcised, involvement of the glans penis produces similar crusted lesions. In the uncircumcised, however, the local environment is different and here erosive lesions may develop, so-called *circinate balanitis* (Fig. 5.13). In the nails, the lesions take the form of a painless subungual pustule which may lead to considerable thickening of the nail and, indeed, separation of the nail may take place (Fig. 5.14). Mucosal lesions consist of transient painless superficial ulcers in the mouth affecting the buccal mucous membranes on the cheeks, the palate or the uvula; occasionally, the tongue may be affected.

Eyes

Conjunctivitis occurs in some 30 per cent of cases, usually early in the course of the disease, less commonly in association with a relapse. It is often quite mild and symptomless and only noted on careful examination.

It affects the palpebral conjunctiva of the lower lid bilaterally. When more severe it may cause discomfort in the eyes and be more obvious; occasionally, it may be sufficiently severe to cause photophobia and a purulent discharge and lead to *keratitis* and corneal ulceration. Recovery always occurs within a few weeks.

Iritis (Anterior uveitis). This is a much more serious feature of the disease. It is uncommon in the initial attack but occurs more frequently with recurrences and, in those who progress to chronic arthritis, it will develop in some 30 to 50 per cent of cases. It is a feature of severe disease and it appears to be more common in those who develop sacro-iliitis, likewise a feature of severe disease. The attacks are usually acute in onset, unilateral, and responsive to local or systemic corticosteroid therapy, but synechiae and keratitic precipitates and eventual blindness may occur.

Cardiovascular System

Lone aortic incompetence may occasionally develop in severe cases of Reiter's disease, usually as a late feature. This is an uncommon lesion, its incidence is not fully known owing to inadequate study, but it appears to be peculiarly associated with both Reiter's disease and ankylosing spondylitis. That both conditions produce this unusual lesion has been used as an argument in favour of regarding the two conditions as a single entity. The pathology has already been described (p. 64) in the section on ankylosing spondylitis. In the early stages of the disease, transient ECG changes may be observed, with prolongation of P-R interval, heart block, elevation of the S-T segment, and abnormal Q-waves. The significance of these changes is not clear, although they may presumably be associated with an underlying pathology similar to the aortic valve changes. Pericarditis has also been observed in Reiter's disease.

Central Nervous System

Neurological involvement may rarely occur, giving rise to peripheral neuritis. Optic neuritis, proximal neuro-myopathy, and meningo-encephalitis have all been recorded with recovery.

SPECIAL INVESTIGATIONS

The erythrocyte sedimentation rate, blood count, and plasma proteins all show entirely non-specific changes of inflammatory arthropathy. The serological tests for rheumatoid serum factor are negative. Examination of the joint fluid should be carried out to exclude the presence of gonococci and to look for the presence of Pekin cells. A finding of pus from the urethra, prostate, or seminal vesicles is, of course, mandatory although a positive finding does not justify the diagnosis of Reiter's disease in a sero-negative arthropathy in the absence of other characteristic features of the disease.

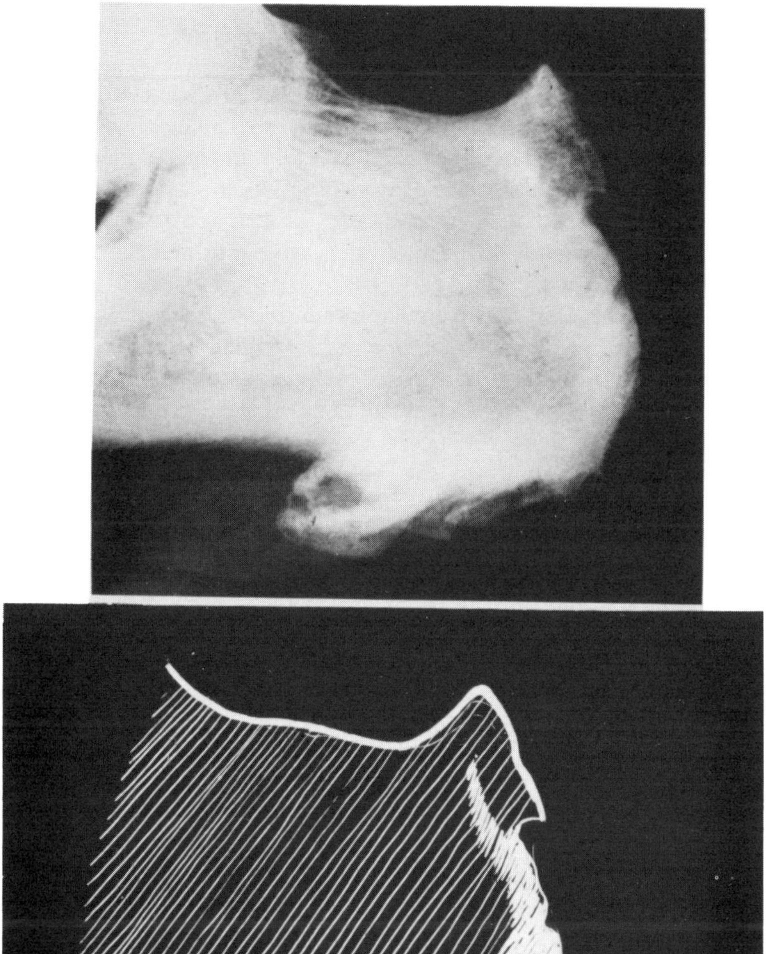

FIGURE 5.15 An example of the florid periosteal new bone formation which characteristically occurs on the os calcis in Reiter's disease and gives rise to the 'fluffy' spur. This must be distinguished from the simple spur which is common and of no pathological significance (Courtesy Dr A. C. Young)

Radiology

The radiological appearances of Reiter's disease are those of an erosive arthopathy with, however, certain distinctive features –

1. *The pattern of joint involvement* has already been described and this will, of course, be reflected in the pattern of radiological involvement. Erosive arthropathy of the interphalangeal joint of the big toe sometimes draws attention to involvement of this joint which may have been overlooked clinically.
2. *Osteoporosis* tends to be less impressive and more localised than in rheumatoid arthritis.
3. *Erosions* are often para-articular rather than subchondral.
4. *Periosteal new bone formation* is a striking feature. It is often curiously fluffy (Fig. 5.15) and may best be seen on the plantar, or less commonly on the posterior, aspect of the os calcis, producing the fluffy periosteal spur so characteristic of Reiter's disease. It is important to recognise, however, that (*a*) the fluffy spur appears only in severe longstanding disease and is not useful as an early diagnostic feature, and (*b*) it must be clearly distinguished from the simple spur with a clear outline which is seen with equal frequency in all types of arthropathy (and in otherwise normal subjects) and is of no diagnostic significance whatsoever.
5. *Sacro-iliitis* has no characteristic diagnostic features to distinguish it from ankylosing spondylitis, psoriatic arthropathy etc.
6. The *spondylitis* again has no distinctive diagnostic radiological features.

AETIOLOGY

The aetiology of Reiter's disease, especially of the 'venereal' type must ultimately be closely involved with the aetiology of non-specific urethritis, and until this is clarified it is unlikely that progress will be made. The evidence that Reiter's disease is due to an infection by some organism is based on impressive epidemiological data. Pleuro-pneumonia-like organisms (PPLO – mycoplasma hominis) have often been isolated from the urethral secretion of patients with Reiter's disease, and occasionally from joint fluids, but their pathogenicity has remained unproven for so long it seems unlikely that they are responsible. A T-strain mycoplasma (T for tiny) has also been suspect but not proven guilty. Another possibility is an organism that seems to lie halfway between the viruses and the bacteria called Chlamydia (or Bedsonia, after Professor Bedson of the London Hospital) which belongs to the psittacosis-lymphogranuloma group. These may cause trachoma and a special form of ophthalmia neonatorum. In the latter, scrapings from the conjunctiva show inclusion bodies, thus it may be termed 'inclusion conjunctivitis', and the organism as TRIC-agent (TR for trachoma and IC for inclusion conjunctivitis). Evidence that these agents are responsible for Reiter's disease is at present incomplete and certainly not proven. Just how these organisms could be responsible for the dysenteric type of the disease remains, of course, speculative although it is possible that dysentery or non-specific diarrhoea might enable these organisms to enter the body. Finally, it must be recognised that Reiter's disease remains a rare complication of non-specific urethritis or dysentery and it may be that some additional genetic predisposition to the disease is also necessary.

TREATMENT

Acute Attacks. In the absence of precise knowledge about the aetiology, treatment is at present both non-specific and of unproven efficacy. The standard treatment of urethritis is the administration of 250 mg tetracycline 6 hourly for seven to ten days. There is no evidence that other antibiotics are more effective, despite some isolated and unsubstantiated claims. Treatment of the arthritis is similar to that of any other inflammatory arthropathy and there are no special problems except that prolonged immobilisation should be avoided if possible, since muscle-wasting and joint stiffness may develop rapidly. Although phenylbutazone, oxyphenbutazone, or indomethacin may seem to be more effective than aspirin in some cases, they should, nevertheless, be regarded as purely symptomatic drugs. Corticosteroid therapy should be avoided if at all possible, since relatively larger doses may be required than are commonly needed for rheumatoid arthritis. Iritis may, however, justify corticosteroid therapy, and its use in severe cases may be essential to preserve sight. The conjunctivitis is usually mild and requires no more than half per cent chloramphenicol eye drops, to prevent secondary bacterial infection. Skin lesions commonly require no more than simple hygiene but when very severe may justify topical corticosteroid therapy.

In most cases an initial acute attack will settle within about three months, although more prolonged attacks may occur in severe cases. It remains to be seen whether the encouraging results obtained in rheumatoid arthritis following the use of cytotoxic and antimetabolic drugs extends to other forms of inflammatory arthropathy such as Reiter's disease. There is no evidence that treatment of the urethritis influences favourably or otherwise the development of the arthritis, but, traditionally, prostatic massage should be avoided in the acute phase because of the risk of an exacerbation of the disease.

Prevention. Once the diagnosis has been made, the patient must be made to realise that recurrences are likely and it seems reasonable to exhort him to avoid promiscuous sexual exposure. The consort, if identified, should be examined for evidence of genital infection, and this should be treated. The use of a condom may possibly afford some protection and, where appropriate, should be recommended. If chronic prostatitis persists, this should, again traditionally, be treated with prostatic massage and, if necessary, with further courses of antibiotics. It seems likely that if the prostatitis can be eradicated and if exposure to further infection is avoided the risk of a relapse can be reduced. But it must be accepted that recurrences and occasionally chronic arthritis may develop spontaneously despite careful attention to these precautions.

Colitic Arthropathy

The evidence for a significant association between ulcerative colitis and sero-negative arthropathy rests upon two important observations:

1. At least 10 per cent of patients with a diagnosis of ulcerative colitis develop a sero-negative inflammatory arthropathy affecting peripheral joints.
2. Over 10 per cent of patients with ankylosing spondylitis will be found to have ulcerative colitis.

As a result of several careful studies of groups of patients with ulcerative colitis it is now possible, for convenience and clarity, to regard the arthropathy as falling into two separate types—

Type 1. A recurrent mild synovitis of peripheral joints, usually oligo-articular, affecting large joints rather than small. It is often asymmetrical, affects the sexes in equal proportions, and leaves no, or minimal, residua.

Type 2. 'Ankylosing spondylitis'.

Type 1.

Usually the symptoms of ulcerative colitis precede the onset of the arthropathy, i.e. the patient commonly is already recognised as having ulcerative colitis and is under medical supervision. Often, the arthritis is associated with an exacerbation of the colitis. Sometimes, however, the arthropathy may be the presenting complaint and the colitis may be suspected only after careful history-taking. Occasionally, the colitis may be symptomless and revealed only by sigmoidoscopy or barium studies. Rectal biopsy is both a reliable and a sensitive index of the disease. In many cases in which it at first appears as if the arthritis preceded the onset of the colitis, in retrospect it seems probable that the pathological changes of colitis were present before the arthritis. The synovitis is usually self-limiting, leaving no erosive residua. The pattern of joint involvement is asymmetrical; the knee, ankle, and wrist are most commonly affected in that order, but the hip, shoulder, and elbow may also be involved, and, occasionally, the peripheral joints of the hands and feet. Erosive changes are uncommon and mild; when present they may be associated with periostitis and a tendency to healing. Involvement of the sacro-iliac joints appears to be common, although clearly this is particularly a feature of type 2 colitic arthropathy (*see* below). The significance of isolated sacro-iliitis in a patient with colitis is not certain and is of itself insufficient to substantiate a diagnosis of ankylosing spondylitis. *Erythema nodosum* is not uncommon in ulcerative colitis and may be associated with colitic arthropathy. It is not clear what relationship this arthropathy bears to that which may occur with erythema nodosum from other causes (*see* p. 277). Nodules are, of course, absent and serological tests for rheumatoid factor consistently negative. It must be remembered, however, that patients with ulcerative colitis are not prevented thereby from developing other arthropathies such as rheumatoid arthritis.

Type 2

There is no doubt that patients with ulcerative colitis run an increased risk of developing ankylosing spondylitis (the incidence being about 5 per cent), and that patients with ankylosing spondylitis have a significantly high incidence of ulcerative colitis (over 10 per cent), so that there appears to be an important association between these two diseases. Whether the spondylitis is of a different type from classical ankylosing spondylitis is speculative, but clinically and radiologically there is no distinction, either as regards the arthritis or the other systemic manifestations such as iritis. As with the peripheral arthropathy, the spondylitis may appear to antedate the development of ulcerative colitis.

Regional enteritis (Crohn's disease) may also be associated with both types of arthropathy in a manner similar to ulcerative colitis.

TREATMENT

Effective treatment of the colitis or regional enteritis appears to influence type 1 arthropathy favourably; it has no effect on type 2 (ankylosing spondylitis). In severe cases, colectomy is often followed by remission of the arthritis. In milder cases symptomatic therapy with aspirin and physiotherapy is all that is required. In the spondylitic type, phenylbutazone appears to be as effective as it is in uncomplicated types of ankylosing spondylitis, although gastro-intestinal tract intolerance may limit its use. Oxyphenbutazone or indomethacin provide possible alternatives, when intolerance to phenylbutazone occurs. As with classical ankylosing spondylitis, prolonged immobilisation of the patient should be avoided and physiotherapy should be maintained, especially if the patient is restricted to bed for more than brief periods for treatment of his colitis.

Differential Diagnosis

Ankylosing spondylitis, Reiter's disease, psoriatic and colitic arthropathy have been described as if they were entirely separate entities. It is clear, however, from the description of these diseases that many of them have very similar features although for simplicity these have not been stressed. Before discussing the problem of differential diagnosis, therefore, it may be helpful to indicate some interesting associations:

1. Patients with chronic Reiter's disease may develop a spondylitis indistinguishable from ankylosing spondylitis.
2. Keratoderma may be indistinguishable from, and is histologically indentical to, pustular psoriasis.
3. Sacro-iliitis is common in psoriatic arthropathy.
4. Iritis commonly occurs in ankylosing spondylitis, Reiter's disease, and colitic arthropathy.
5. Prostatitis is a feature of both ankylosing spondylitis and Reiter's disease.
6. Patients with ankylosing spondylitis have a high incidence of ulcerative colitis.
7. Patients with ulcerative colitis have a high incidence of 'ankylosing spondylitis'.

In addition, epidemiological studies suggest that

8. The relatives of patients with Reiter's disease have a high incidence of psoriasis, and
9. Relatives of patients with Reiter's disease have a high incidence of sacro-iliitis.

These common features suggest the possibility that these disorders represent no more than different reaction patterns (to unknown stimuli) modified by variations in the stimulus and by variations in genetic make-up which determine the host response. So long as the nature of the stimuli remains unknown, only speculation is possible. Perhaps the key lies in the identification of the agent responsible for non-specific urethritis and the mechanism whereby it initiates a synovitis in the susceptible patient. Because we believe that such speculation may produce loose thinking in the clinical field it seems justified for practical purposes to retain these various arthropathies as if they were separate entities. On this basis the differential diagnosis may be simply (or superficially) regarded along certain lines, so that when faced with a patient with a sero-negative arthropathy the following points should be considered –

Rheumatoid Arthritis is common in females and usually occurs in the older age groups; the average age of onset being 45 years. The pattern of joint involvement is symmetrical, it affects the hands as commonly as the feet, while the pattern of joint involvement of the sero-negative arthropathies all show a tendency to affect the lower limbs. Iritis and conjunctivitis, as opposed to kerato-conjunctivitis sicca, do not occur. When there are nodules and positive tests for rheumatoid serum factor the diagnosis is clarified.

Ankylosing Spondylitis. Backache due to sacro-iliitis is an early and usually a presenting feature of the disease. It may remain the only manifestation in mild examples. In Reiter's disease, sacro-iliitis is a feature of severe disease and occurs later rather than early. It is always associated with a peripheral arthropathy. Genital inflammation is commonly a presenting feature of Reiter's disease, whereas in ankylosing spondylitis it is silent and found only on special examination. Ulcerative colitis may be identified by rectal biopsy.

Psoriatic Arthropathy. Genital inflammation, buccal lesions, and iritis do not occur but the skin lesion may be identical with keratoderma.

Gonococcal Arthritis. This is very rare in the United Kingdom; it is usually monarticular or oligo-articular, but it may be preceded by generalised malaise, fever, and arthralgia. Gonococci can often be identified in the joint fluid and there is a prompt response to penicillin.

Rheumatic Fever. This may occasionally give rise to difficulty when a history of sore throat or streptococcal infection is not obtained. The skin rash of erythema marginatum is rare but characteristic. Genital inflammation and iritis do not occur, and the synovitis is non-erosive. The anti-streptolysin-O titre is raised.

Behcet's Disease. This is described on page 276. Difficulty may arise in differential diagnosis, but the mouth ulcers are characteristically painful, while those of Reiter's disease are painless. There is no urethritis, and the painful scrotal ulcers are unique. The iritis of Behcet's disease may be severe, leading to panuveitis, hypopyon, and retrobulbar neuritis.

6

Arteritis

Colin G Barnes

Inflammation involving primarily the wall of an artery is referred to as *arteritis* (or, more generally, to include all types of blood vessel—*vasculitis*). Such changes occur under a wide variety of different circumstances which, unfortunately, do not lend themsleves to any tidy system of classification. A basically similar pathological process involving blood vessels produces a variety of clinical pictures which differ because of variations in the size and type of vessels involved, the anatomical distribution of the changes, and the tempo of the inflammatory process. The clinical syndromes that have been described are not sharply defined, and the aetiology and pathogenesis of most of them is unknown. They range from fatal generalised disorders to relatively benign skin conditions, and they may occur either alone or as part of some better-defined disease.

Some examples of vasculitis are mentioned in other parts of this book; for example, anaphylactoid purpura (p. 275), rheumatoid arthritis (p. 15), systemic lupus erythematosus (p. 132), serum sickness (p. 287), and childhood dermatomyositis (p. 123). Other types of vasculitis do not have sufficient rheumatological interest to justify inclusion; for example, the arterial lesions in malignant hypertension or the various forms of isolated *cutaneous vasculitis*. Included in this chapter are, therefore, a few of the more important and better-defined examples of primary vascular disease. Their rheumatological interest is, firstly, that they may present clinically with muscle pains or stiffness, or with arthralgia; and secondly, that they overlap pathologically with conditions such as rheumatoid arthritis. Five examples of arteritis are discussed:

Polyarteritis nodosa
Giant cell arteritis (temporal or cranial arteritis)
Allergic vasculitis
Takayasu's arteritis (aortic arch syndrome, 'pulseless' disease)
Wegener's granulomatosis (midline granuloma)

The clinical syndrome of *polymyalgia rheumatica* is described in a separate chapter (p. 105), which may seem to be somewhat arbitrary since, in many instances, it is identical with *giant cell arteritis*. However, in the present state of understanding of the condition this arrangement seems to allow a clearer presentation of this somewhat confused entity.

POLYARTERITIS NODOSA

Polyarteritis nodosa (PAN), or necrotising angiitis, is an inflammatory condition of the medium-sized and small arteries, characterised by segmental vessel wall necrosis. Arteries throughout the body may be involved, leading to widespread changes in many organs.

The aetiology is unknown. Other forms of vasculitis may follow exposure to exogenous antigens or drugs, but this has not been established for classical PAN. The widespread vascular damage perhaps suggests 'immune complex' injury, of the type seen in serum sickness (p. 287), but this is at present only speculative.

PAN occurs more commonly in males than females, in a ratio of approximately 3:1. It may start at any age, but is most common in young adults.

PATHOLOGY

The lesions affect all layers of the arterial wall. Focal areas of necrosis appear with fibrinoid change and disintegration of the internal elastic lamina (Fig. 6.1). Inflammatory cell infiltration of all layers follows, and

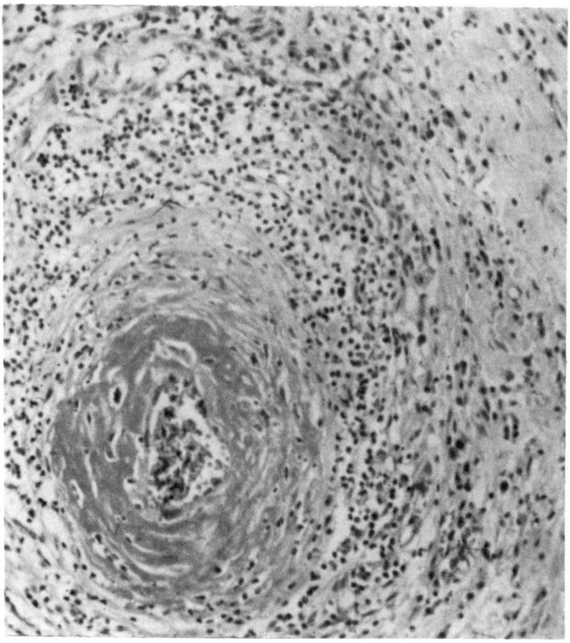

FIGURE 6.1 Necrosis of the vessel wall in polyarteritis nodosa

while this consists initially of polymorphonuclear leucocytes and sometimes eosinophils, in longer-standing lesions lymphocytes and plasma cells appear.

Healing is by fibrosis. Arterial occlusion may thus occur as a result of the inflammatory process itself, because of fibrosis, or because of intimal proliferation, each of which may be accompanied by thrombosis. Occasionally, aneurysm formation or rupture may occur at a point weakened by the inflammatory process.

Although the inflammatory lesions are widespread and may affect any small or medium-sized vessels, they are typically segmental, with lengths of entirely normal vessel between lesions. Despite the name of the disease veins may be similarly affected.

CLINICAL FEATURES

Systemic Manifestations. The disease may present as a generalised illness with fever, weight loss, malaise, lethargy, and tachycardia; and the more focal disturbances described below appear against a background of such a systemic disorder.

Skin. Subcutaneous nodules along the course of inflamed vessels give the disease its name. These nodules, which are usually tender, represent areas of inflammation or aneurysm formation in the vessel wall. They occur in a minority of cases.

Necrotic lesions result from occlusion of arteries. They vary from small ischaemic areas on the finger tips (Fig. 6.2) or ulcers on the shins, to gangrene of digits or even of entire limbs. *Skin eruptions* are common. Most characteristic is *livedo reticularis*—a purple and mottled, reticulated pattern usually occurring on the shins (not unlike the late stage of the

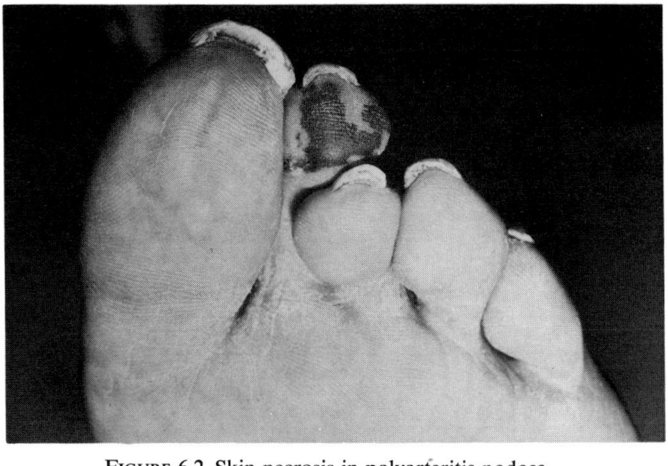

FIGURE 6.2 Skin necrosis in polyarteritis nodosa

more familiar *erythema ab igne*). Non-specific *maculopapular rashes* also occur, as may non-thrombocytopenic *purpura*.

Cardiovascular Manifestations. Arterial hypertension occurs in over half of the patients with PAN. Most, but not all, of these patients show evidence of renal disease.

Arteritis of the coronary vessels may produce all the features of ischaemic heart disease, including acute myocardial infarction, silent infarction, angina pectoris, and cardiac failure.

Abdominal Complaints. Abdominal pain is common. It results, directly or indirectly, from arteritis of intra-abdominal vessels. In the most severe cases there may be extensive infarction of the small or large bowel, while arteritis of vessels in the wall of the small intestine may produce ulceration of the intestinal mucosa. Other abdominal viscera such as the liver, pancreas, and gall bladder may also be affected, leading to hepatic infarction, or the features of pancreatitis or cholecystitis. Non-specific complaints include anorexia, vomiting, and diarrhoea.

The Kidney. Renal disease is the most important cause of death in PAN. Clinically, the first warning is usually the appearance of either proteinuria or microscopic haematuria (sometimes frank haematuria). Hypertension is common, and once there is definite renal involvement the tendency is for the condition to progress relentlessly to severe hypertension and renal failure. The tempo of this process is very variable. Occasionally, there may be acute oliguric renal failure. Renal tract infections also occur.

Pulmonary Lesions. Pulmonary involvement may be the mode of presentation of PAN. The patient will usually complain of asthma, with cough and wheezing and the expectoration of tenacious sputum. Radiologically there may be a variety of changes including occlusive lesions of the pulmonary arterial tree leading to areas of necrosis, which appear as radiological opacities, either single or multiple. Cavitation in the centre of these infarcted areas may follow (Fig. 6.3), and may present clinically as haemoptysis. Radiologically these lesions appear as multiple cavities, and the distinction has to be made from tuberculous lesions or lung abscesses. Secondary infections of these cavities with pyogenic organisms or fungi is not uncommon. Repeated radiographs of the chest show that these lesions tend to appear in crops, cavitate, and resolve; thus, lesions in all stages of evolution may be present at one time.

Central Nervous System. Ischaemic brain lesions result from arteritis of cerebral vessels. The neurological picture is therefore very variable. Sudden massive cerebral infarction leading to coma and hemiplegia or death can occur. Widespread small vessel lesions may produce epilepsy, mental disturbances, or headache. Subarachnoid and extradural haemorrhages are less common.

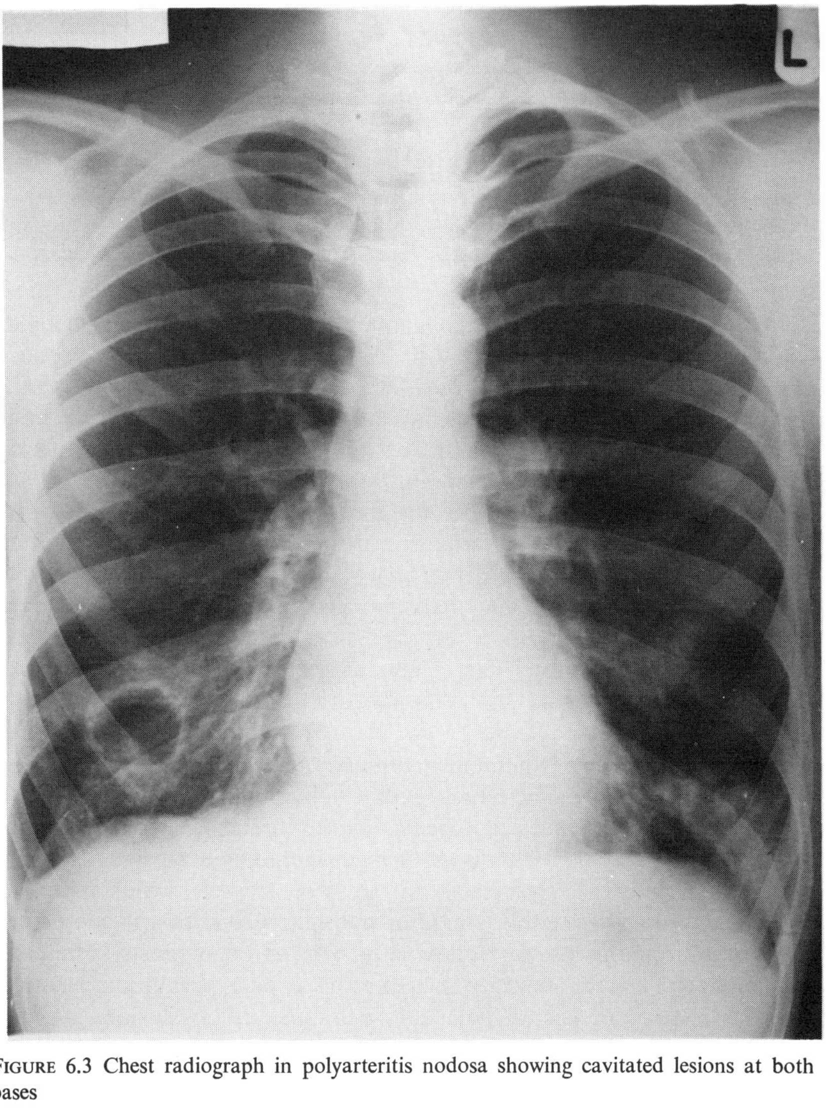

FIGURE 6.3 Chest radiograph in polyarteritis nodosa showing cavitated lesions at both bases

Peripheral Nerves. Mononeuritis multiplex due to arteritis of the vasa nervorum is the characteristic form of peripheral nerve involvement. A series of isolated nerve lesions develops in an asymmetrical pattern affecting any of the limb nerves or, less commonly, the cranial nerves. The motor and sensory neurological deficit develops in the territory of individual nerves rather than in the glove and stocking distribution characteristic of a metabolic peripheral neuropathy. However, if sufficient peripheral nerves become involved the final neurological picture may add up to one that is indistinguishable from a symmetrical peripheral neuropathy. A similar type of neuropathy may complicate rheumatoid arthritis (*see* p. 25).

Opthalmic Involvement. As in giant cell arteritis (p. 100), lesions in the distribution of the ophthalmic artery may produce blurring of vision, loss of visual acuity, formation of scotomata, or complete blindness (due to occlusion of the retinal artery).

Locomotor System. Aching girdle pains and morning stiffness with general malaise and a high sedimentation rate may produce the picture of *polymyalgia rheumatica* (p. 105). However, PAN is a less common cause of this than is giant cell arteritis. Muscle tenderness and weakness may indicate the presence of a true polymyositis.

Arthralgia commonly contributes to the general aches and pains associated with PAN. Occasionally, particularly in the early stages, a true synovitis of small joints is seen, which may be mistaken for early rheumatoid arthritis. It is non-erosive.

INVESTIGATIONS

Erythrocyte Sedimentation Rate. The ESR tends to be considerably elevated, reflecting the widespread inflammatory activity. This is extremely valuable in diagnosis. In a patient who presents, for example, with an otherwise straightforward cerebrovascular accident or myocardial infarction, or even with relatively trivial vague, unexplained, muscle and joint pain, the finding of a grossly elevated ESR may provide the clue to an underlying arteritis.

Haematology. Active phases of the disease are accompanied by a mild normochromic normocytic anaemia.

Leucocytosis is an almost invariable feature, with counts reaching 15–20,000/mm^3. This is principally due to an increase in the neutrophil polymorphonuclear count. However, in addition, an *absolute eosinophilia* accompanies over 90 per cent of those cases with pulmonary lesions, especially asthma, but is rare in their absence. The eosinophil count may reach many thousands/mm^3.

Serology and Plasma Proteins. Positive tests for serum rheumatoid factor and antinuclear factor are found in a minority of cases. Mild hyperglobulinaemia, with a rise in the gamma component, is common.

Histology. Proof of the diagnosis may require biopsy. This is most likely to be helpful if the material is obtained from a clinically involved tissue; for example a skin lesion, a kidney biopsy in a subject with renal involvement, or a sensory peripheral nerve serving an anaesthetic area. In the absence of an obvious lead, a muscle biopsy is usually undertaken. Occasionally, an unexpected histological diagnosis of PAN is made from surgical material such as an appendix or gall bladder.

DIFFERENTIAL DIAGNOSIS

When the disease involves many organs and tissues throughout the body, the diagnosis of PAN is likely to suggest itself. If, however, the picture is less complete, the diagnosis may be extremely difficult. PAN can mimic so many other diseases that no useful purpose would be served by attempting to list these. Instead, attention is drawn to a few of the more common features of PAN which, experience has shown, often provide the clue to the correct diagnosis when one or more of them (perhaps unexpectedly) forms part of the clinical picture. These are –

High ESR
Leucocytosis
Eosinophilia
Fever
Haematuria
Hypertension
Abdominal pain
Mononeuritis multiplex

Mononeuritis multiplex is also seen as a feature of severe rheumatoid arthritis. In such patients the typical picture of RA may progress to one of classical PAN with renal disease and death – *malignant rheumatoid disease*. Once this change has occurred, these cases follow the pattern of PAN and show the same histological changes. Their rheumatoid origin is shown by the erosive arthropathy, the invariably positive serological tests for rheumatoid factor, and perhaps subcutaneous rheumatoid nodules.

TREATMENT

Corticosteroid drugs are used to suppress the inflammatory activity in PAN, but their value remains somewhat controversial. The response to prednisolone is rather variable, perhaps because the healing process in the vessel wall may itself lead to occlusion. In addition, the presence of hypertension may increase the hazard of corticosteroids. On the whole, however, this drug probably provides the only useful form of treatment available at present, and should be used in full doses (prednisolone 60 mg daily initially). Concurrent anti-hypertensive therapy may be needed, but occasionally the steroids may actually lower an elevated blood pressure resulting from renal arteritis.

The use of immunosuppressive drugs is at present experimental.

GIANT CELL ARTERITIS (*Temporal* or *Cranial* Arteritis)

Giant cell arteritis (GCA) is an inflammatory, occlusive arteriopathy characterised by specific histological changes that include the presence of giant cells in the lesion. It is most commonly recognised in the superficial vessels of the scalp. However, this may merely represent an episode in the evolution of a more widespread arteritis, and while there appears to be an anatomical predilection for the branches of the carotid arteries, no vessel in the body is exempt from this change.

CLINICAL FEATURES

Age and Sex Distribution. This is a disease of the older age group, most patients being over fifty years of age at the onset. Either sex may be affected though the condition is more common in women. It is not a rare disease.

Systemic Manifestations. Systemic features are usually marked. The condition may present as fever, malaise, weight loss, or any of the manifestations of *polymyalgia rheumatica* (p. 105), of which GCA is an important cause.

Cranial Features. Generalised or temporal headache is the most common symptom. This may be severe and intractable. Pain is also frequently localised to the scalp or face and is then described as burning or shooting. It may be confused with trigeminal neuralgia. Occasionally it is localised to the tongue.

The temporal arteries may be visibly or palpably thickened (Fig. 6.4) with localised areas of tenderness and, occasionally, even redness and swelling of the overlying skin. Nodularity of these arteries and loss of pulsation are important signs. These features may be unilateral or

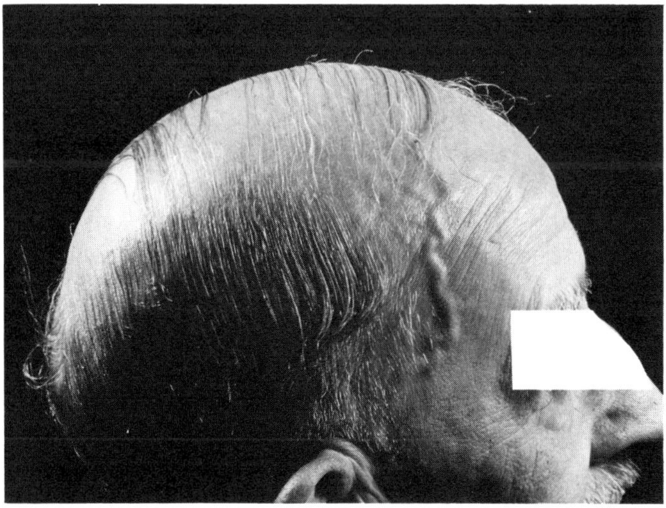

FIGURE 6.4 Thickened temporal artery in giant-cell arteritis

bilateral. They may also affect the occipital arteries. A common complaint is the discomfort produced by pressure of the pillow on an affected site in bed at night.

Involvement of the Ophthalmic Artery. Ophthalmic arteritis not only produces symptoms but is also the commonest cause of serious morbidity. It may occur at any stage of the disease. Unilateral or bilateral ocular pain, photophobia, blurring or complete loss of vision may occur, the latter often developing suddenly as a result of complete occlusion of the retinal artery (which may be confirmed by the presence of characteristic changes on retinoscopy). Weakness of external ocular muscles may also occur, producing diplopia.

Cerebrovascular Involvement. Less commonly, involvement of the intracranial arterial system leads to central nervous system disturbances. Localised lesions, depending on their site, may produce epilepsy, motor paralysis, or disturbances of sensory perception. Generalised arterial lesions may produce mental disturbances ranging from mild confusion to dementia or coma. Sudden occlusion of a main intracerebral vessel may produce a picture indistinguishable from other forms of cerebrovascular accident.

INVESTIGATIONS

Erythrocyte Sedimentation Rate. The ESR is invariably raised, reflecting the inflammatory nature of the disease. Readings in excess of 100 mm in the first-hour (Westergren) are not unusual and, in general, the ESR reliably indicates the level of activity.

Haematology. Normochromic anaemia with haemoglobin levels of the order of 10 G per cent is usual, and again reflects the inflammatory activity. It is accompanied by a moderate polymorphonuclear leucocytosis. With spontaneous or induced remissions in the disease the blood picture reverts to normal.

Plasma Proteins. Elevation of plasma globulins, particularly the gamma component, occurs, but tests for rheumatoid and anti-nuclear factors remain negative.

Biopsy. Florid inflammatory changes in a scalp vessel may establish the diagnosis beyond all doubt. Failing this, every effort should be made to establish a histological diagnosis by biopsy of a temporal or occipital artery. Local symptoms or signs may indicate which vessel to choose. If the excised artery is involved in the disease the histological changes are likely to be diagnostic. However, a negative biopsy does not exclude the diagnosis.

PATHOLOGY

The characteristic change is inflammation of small and medium-sized arteries with the formation of giant cells. This is most marked in the branches of the carotid arteries. However, identical changes may be found, usually at post-mortem, in any of the main branches of the thoracic or abdominal aorta and also, occasionally, in the pulmonary arteries. All layers of the arterial wall are involved. The intima becomes thickened and fibrotic, the internal elastic lamina is fragmented, and inflammatory cell infiltration with lymphocytes and plasma cells is present in the media. Also in the media appear areas of necrosis and giant cell granulomata (Fig. 6.5), the latter being the hallmark of this condition.

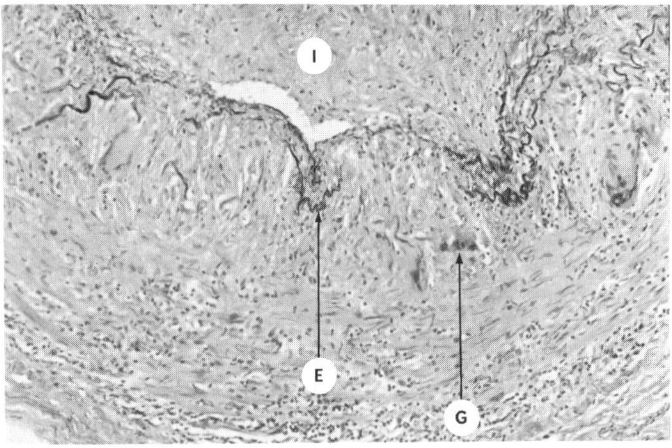

FIGURE 6.5 Histology of giant-cell arteritis showing fragmentation of the internal elastic lamina *E*, intimal occlusion *I*, and giant cells *G*

TREATMENT

A definite diagnosis of giant cell arteritis is an indication for corticosteroid therapy. The object is to prevent extension of the arterial lesions, for this disease constantly poses the threat of blindness or brain damage.

The optimal dosage is not established. It must, in any case, represent a compromise between one that is high enough to eliminate the danger of ophthalmic complications, and one that is low enough to avoid the side effects of hormonal therapy. In practice, it is usual to start with prednisolone in a dose of about 60 mg daily, unless there have been indications of ophthalmic or neurological involvement, in which case 100 mg daily is prescribed. After a few weeks the dosage is gradually reduced to that which maintains the ESR normal and the patient symptom-free. This may require about 20 mg of prednisolone daily. Complete withdrawal of prednisolone may not be possible for two or three years and, in any case, should not be attempted until the disease has been controlled for at least one year. Hormonal side effects are to be expected.

Simple analgesics may relieve the patient's symptoms, but do not protect against extension of the arteritis.

ALLERGIC VASCULITIS

Allergic vasculitis is a form of arteritis occurring during the course of allergic or hypersensitivity reactions caused by many different agents. Thus, it may develop in the course of serum sickness or reactions to drugs, including sulphonamides, gold salts, and penicillin.

It may be difficult to distinguish between allergic vasculitis and classical polyarteritis nodosa, which has led in the past to speculation that the latter is due to hypersensitivity.

CLINICAL FEATURES

The most prominent clinical features are usually skin lesions, which are often necrotic, and renal glomerular lesions, the latter presenting as albuminuria, microscopic haematuria, and the presence of granular casts in the urine.

In addition, any of the other features of polyarteritis nodosa (q.v.) may occur, although of these (after the skin and renal lesions) pulmonary involvement presenting as asthma is the most likely.

PATHOLOGY

A widespread necrotising arteritis indistinguishable from polyarteritis nodosa occurs. However, while the condition may be severe and fatal, in general the arteritis is less florid than in classical PAN.

TREATMENT AND PROGNOSIS

When the cause of the allergic reaction can be removed, e.g. the withdrawal of a drug, spontaneous resolution is common. In more severe or prolonged disease, treatment with corticosteroids is essential. Although this condition may be fatal, the majority of cases resolve completely.

TAKAYASU'S ARTERITIS

This condition, also known as *pulseless disease* or *aortic arch syndrome*, is characterised by a patchy arteritis of unknown aetiology affecting the thoracic aorta and its main branches. The vascular manifestations resulting from this form of arteritis are therefore confined to the upper part of the trunk, arms, head, and neck.

Takayasu's arteritis is much less common than either giant cell arteritis or polyarteritis nodosa. It affects, particularly, young women.

CLINICAL FEATURES

The clinical features reflect the effects of vascular insufficiency in the territory of the branches of the thoracic aorta. Claudication of the arms, necrotic ulceration of the skin of the fingers and face, and generalised wasting around the shoulder girdles and neck are usual. These may be accompanied by loss of hair.

Reduction of cerebral blood flow produces personality changes, focal neurological lesions, visual impairment and, occasionally, syncope or epilepsy.

In common with other forms of arteritis the illness produces systemic manifestations of lethargy, malaise, weight loss, fever, normochromic anaemia, an elevated sedimentation rate, and raised serum globulin levels.

Peripheral Vessels. Characteristically, pulsation in the radial, ulnar, and carotid arteries is absent. However, since this is a patchy process, in the early stages pulsation may be absent in only one or two vessels, and progressively the pulsation disappears from others with appropriate symptoms and signs related to the areas rendered ischaemic. The vessels are affected at their origins from the thoracic aorta, and the coronary arteries may be similarly affected, producing myocardial ischaemia and infarction. Partial occlusion of vessels may be indicated by *bruits*.

Joints. Small joint polyarthritis of the type occasionally seen in polyarteritis nodosa does not occur. However, cases have been reported in which there has been either radiological sacro-iliitis or even clinical ankylosing spondylitis. It is not yet clear whether this association is significant.

INVESTIGATIONS

The presence of an inflammatory process is indicated by anaemia, raised sedimentation rate, and increased serum globulin levels.

The diagnosis is established by *aortography*, which shows occlusion of branches of the thoracic aorta.

PATHOLOGY

Necrotic areas are present in the media of affected vessels, with surrounding infiltration by chronic inflammatory cells – lymphocytes and plasma cells – throughout all layers of the artery. This affects the thoracic aorta and is associated with adjacent thrombosis leading to occlusion of the branches at their point of origin from the aorta.

DIFFERENTIAL DIAGNOSIS

Takayasu's arteritis has to be distinguished from other conditions producing similar occlusive lesions. Syphilitic aortitis is characterised by positive serological tests for syphilis, while dissection of the aorta (except in Marfan's syndrome) occurs in older patients.

TREATMENT AND PROGNOSIS

The prognosis in this condition is poor, with death resulting usually from myocardial or cerebral infarction. However, it would seem reasonable to attempt to suppress the arteritis with corticosteroid drugs, and some success has been claimed for this form of treatment. Surgical reconstruction of affected large vessels is sometimes attempted.

WEGENER'S GRANULOMATOSIS

Wegener's granulomatosis or *midline granuloma* is a rare condition characterised by a combination of necrotic granulomatous lesions and arteritis. The cause is unknown. The sexes are equally affected, and the age of onset is usually between twenty and forty years.

CLINICAL FEATURES

General ill-health with fever, weight loss, anaemia, leucocytosis (often with eosinophilia), and a raised sedimentation rate is usual. Although the main features develop in the respiratory tract and kidneys, there may be generalised muscle pains and tenderness, and arthralgia. Non-specific skin rashes and peripheral neuropathy have also been reported. The condition is usually fatal.

Respiratory Tract. Necrotic granulomatous lesions develop throughout the upper and lower respiratory tract, leading to sinusitis, inflammatory lesions of the naso-pharynx, and pneumonitis. Secondary infection is common. Radiologically, widespread discrete opacities are seen throughout both lung fields. Respiratory failure is an important cause of death.

Renal Involvement. Focal glomerulonephritis leading to renal failure is an almost invariable accompaniment of this disease.

PATHOLOGY

Highly vascular, granulomatous lesions occur mainly in the upper respiratory tract. These consist of areas of necrosis with surrounding inflammatory cell infiltration. Vasculitis, affecting both arteries and veins, with necrosis and chronic inflammatory cell infiltration affects especially the vessels of the lungs and the renal glomerular loops. The latter is accompanied by cellular infiltration in the glomerular tuft and capsule, producing a true glomerulonephritis. A more generalised arteritis may produce widespread ischaemic lesions. The diagnosis is usually established by histological examination of material from the respiratory tract.

TREATMENT

Although previously regarded as invariably fatal, combined treatment with corticosteroid drugs and an immunosuppressive agent has been reported to produce a prolonged remission.

7

Polymyalgia Rheumatica

Colin G Barnes

Polymyalgia rheumatica is a syndrome consisting of aching pains in a girdle distribution, with marked morning stiffness and an accelerated erythrocyte sedimentation rate (ESR) occurring in elderly subjects for which there is no apparent pathological cause. The term polymyalgia rheumatica, therefore, must not be considered as a diagnosis in itself, since there are a number of different pathological entities that may present initially as this syndrome. This is discussed below. The confusion that has arisen in the understanding of this condition is reflected in the number of names that have been used to describe it:

Senile Rheumatic Gout (1888)
Myalgic Syndrome of the Aged with Systemic Reaction (1951)
Periarthrosis Humeroscapularis (1952)
Pseudopolyarthrite Rhizomelique (1953)
Anarthritic Rheumatoid Disease (1953)
Polymyalgia Rheumatica (1957)
Polymyalgia Arteritica (1964)

CLINICAL FEATURES

Age and Sex Distribution. Polymyalgia rheumatica occurs in the older age groups, and an onset before the age of fifty years is rare. Females are affected more commonly than males in a ratio of about 3 : 1.

Girdle Pain. The outstanding symptom is girdle pain of an aching or, occasionally, stabbing nature across the shoulders and radiating into the upper arms, and around the pelvis radiating into the legs. This is continuous, but it is characteristically worse after periods of rest or inactivity. The aching is diffuse and is not associated with true joint pain or swelling, although movements of the neck, shoulders, and hips may produce an increase in discomfort.

Morning Stiffness. Morning stiffness regularly occurs as a subjective sensation of painful immobility, and to bc significant it is usually accepted that the time taken to 'limber-up' should exceed thirty minutes. This is a similar sensation to that which occurs in association with active rheumatoid and other forms of inflammatory arthropathy.

Weakness. Subjective weakness occurs in the majority of patients and, again, is largely proximal in distribution. It does not necessarily indicate the presence of primary muscle disease (*see* below).

Systemic Manifestations. Systemic manifestations are frequently prominent. They include lethargy and general malaise, anorexia, weight loss, and fever. Headache is of great significance. While this may be diffuse and associated with the general illness, it is of particular importance if localised to the temporal or occipital regions, when it suggests a diagnosis of giant cell (cranial) arteritis (p. 98). Mental changes, usually depression or confusion, are common.

Physical Signs. Objective physical signs are inconspicuous. There may be some weakness and tenderness of girdle and proximal limb muscles, and movements of the neck, shoulder, and hip may be executed reluctantly. However, formal examination of these joints does not provide evidence of a true arthritis.

Mentally, these patients may be depressed. They may show signs of loss of weight, sometimes of anaemia.

Descriptions of this syndrome have in the past recorded the presence of features such as true arthritis, tenderness and nodularity of the temporal artery, and kerato-conjunctivitis sicca. However, as discussed below, these features are now thought not to be part of the polymyalgia rheumatica syndrome itself, but to represent features of one of the underlying diseases that may present clinically as this syndrome.

INVESTIGATIONS

Erythrocyte Sedimentation Rate. A raised ESR is the only abnormal laboratory finding characteristic of polymyalgia rheumatica. The elevation is usually impressive, sometimes over 100 mm in one hour (Westergren).

Biopsy. Temporal or occipital artery biopsy is usually considered essential. This is discussed under 'Management', below.

Haematology. A mild normochromic normocytic anaemia is common, with haemoglobin values usually about 11 G per cent. Mild elevation of the total white cell count may occur, but without any specific changes in the differential count.

Plasma Proteins. Non-specific elevations of α_1- and γ-globulin, and of fibrinogen are usually seen. These changes are in keeping with an inflammatory process. (One important reason for studying the plasma proteins is to exclude myelomatosis.)

Other Investigations. For reasons discussed under 'Aetiology' below, a wide variety of investigations are carried out in patients presenting with features of polymyalgia rheumatica. Positive results in some of these tests may lead to the patient being placed in a different diagnostic category. Thus, a diagnosis of polymyalgia rheumatica generally assumes negative results for serum rheumatoid and antinuclear factor tests, and no abnormality on X-rays of the bones or joints. Electromyography should show no evidence of polymyositis, and Bence Jones proteose should not be present in the urine.

AETIOLOGY

Polymyalgia rheumatica is a term of convenience used to describe the association, in an elderly subject, of girdle pains, morning stiffness, and high ESR, when no other pathological cause is apparent. In a sense it is a provisional categorisation, like 'pyrexia of unknown origin', which implies that further investigation and observation is likely to reveal a more precise pathological diagnosis.

Writing at a time when the condition is being intensively investigated, and when various authorities are putting forward somewhat different points of view about the exact nosological status of this syndrome, it is difficult to offer an account that allows for all the reported facts yet is sufficiently simple and clear to be practical. The following account is perhaps over-simplified, but aims at providing a practical guide in the clinical situation. It will have to be modified as we learn more about this condition.

Of the elderly patients who present initially with the syndrome of polymyalgia rheumatica, a certain number will be found, on further investigation or continued observation, to have some well-defined disease. Perhaps this means that the syndrome is a common 'reaction pattern' to a variety of different pathological processes in the elderly. Certainly, in this age group, it can be the mode of presentation of a number of diseases including rheumatoid arthritis, polymyositis, disseminated carcinomatosis, reticulosis, and myelomatosis.

However, the most important disease to present with features of polymyalgia rheumatica is giant cell arteritis (GCA). Routine temporal artery biopsies in subjects presenting with polymyalgia rheumatica have revealed that as many as 30 per cent have the typical changes of GCA, usually in the absence of any clinical evidence of this condition. This raises the question whether all patients with polymyalgia rheumatica, who do not have one of the obvious causes mentioned above, are suffering from a form of GCA.

At present there is no answer to this. A negative biopsy does not exclude GCA in other sites, for this disease is known to be patchy. Observation of 'pure' polymyalgia rheumatica shows that this condition remains active for one to six years, then remits spontaneously, although it can be dramatically suppressed at any stage by corticosteroid treatment. This holds true, of course, also for GCA. So, at present, it is not clear whether there is a 'primary' form of polymyalgia separate from GCA. This provides a therapeutic dilemma, for while a diagnosis of GCA demands corticosteroid treatment to protect the sight, polymyalgia rheumatica symptoms can usually be relieved either by simpler drugs, or by corticosteroids in small doses which may not prevent the eye complications of GCA (*see* p. 100).

MANAGEMENT

From what has been said it will be apparent that anyone presenting with the features of polymyalgia rheumatica requires urgent and thorough investigation before long-term treatment is planned. The list of diseases mentioned above that may present as polymyalgia rheumatica indicates the investigations required.

A word is necessary about temporal (or occipital) artery biopsy. Experience has shown that omitting this procedure in an effort to spare the patient discomfort is often a mistake. Carried out under local anaesthesia it is relatively atraumatic, and it can provide information of the greatest value in deciding treatment over the months and years ahead. If steroid therapy is started without first performing a biopsy doubt may always arise lest any negative result obtained later may have been influenced by the steroid. The choice of which temporal or occipital artery to biopsy is dictated by the presence of any local pain or tenderness. If none exists, then a temporal artery is selected.

If a cranial artery biopsy or other investigation establishes a definite diagnosis, then the treatment becomes that of the underlying disease. If all the investigations are negative, there remain the alternatives of supressing the symptoms which salicylates, phenylbutazone, or indomethacin (which are usually effective) and thus running the risk of retinal arteritis or, alternatively, of treating as for GCA with full doses of corticosteroids. This introduces the very real risk of serious side effects.

Opinions differ about the right course to follow, and particular circumstances may dictate the treatment in individual patients. However, other things being equal, it would seem a practical compromise to treat 'biopsy-negative' cases of polymyalgia rheumatica with a modest regimen of prednisolone and maintain them on doses similar to those used in rheumatoid arthritis. An initial daily dosage of 20 or 30 mg will usually produce a dramatic remission in symptoms and a fall in the ESR; the dosage is then gradually reduced to that which will just control symptoms and keep the ESR below, say, 30 mm. This can usually be achieved with about 10 mg prednisolone daily. Continued observation is essential. If definite signs of cranial arteritis appear, then the dosage is immediately increased to that recommended for GCA. Alternatively, if the patient remains well, attempts are made from time to time to reduce the dosage very gradually. Many patients can be weaned off prednisolone after about two years.

8

Progressive Systemic Sclerosis, Polymyositis, and Dermatomyositis

H L F Currey

These three conditions are grouped together because of certain clinical and serological similarities. Their aetiologies are unknown. Skin changes are usually the most impressive clinical feature of progressive systemic sclerosis; polymyositis affects the muscles, while in dermatomyositis both skin and muscles are involved.

Progressive Systemic Sclerosis (PSS)

This disease is often referred to as *scleroderma*, a name that emphasises the most characteristic clinical feature: a hard, waxy thickening of the skin. However, the pathological process may involve many structures, producing widely differing disturbances of function. Some of these are fatal. Hence the name 'progressive systemic sclerosis' (PSS).

CLINICAL FEATURES

The disease usually presents between the ages of thirty and fifty years, although no age is exempt. Females are affected about twice as often as males. A typical history is that of a young or middle aged woman who develops Raynaud's phenomenon, followed by a mild, small-joint, polyarthritis, and induration of the skin of the fingers. The skin changes then often spread to involve the face, and she may experience some dysphagia which results from the characteristic disturbance of oesophageal motility. The skin changes may themselves remain the main feature of the disease for a long time, but sooner or later serious visceral involvement is likely to develop in the lungs, heart, or kidneys, leading eventually to death. No effective treatment is known.

Raynaud's phenomenon is an almost invariable accompaniment of PSS, and may precede other features by months or even years. The local changes resemble those seen in the benign familial form, which starts in childhood and in which exposure to cold produces numbness and cyclical colour changes in the fingers. These changes are due to temporary spasm of digital arteries unduly sensitive to cold, and in a full cycle the fingers turn white, blue, then pink. Raynaud's phenomenon may also be the earliest symptoms of several other connective tissue disorders such as rheumatoid arthritis, polyarteritis nodosa, and polymyositis (though the incidence is lower in these conditions). It is this fact that lends such sinister significance to the appearance of Raynaud's phenomenon for the first time in adult life.

Skin Changes. Rarely, patients with PSS may die without skin changes having been recognised, the diagnosis being made post mortem from the typical histological changes in internal organs. Most patients, however, will be found to have some skin involvement. This may range in severity from mild induration of the finger tips (acrosclerosis or sclerodactyly) to extensive involvement of the arms, face and upper trunk, encasing these areas as if in a suit of armour. The basic change is a hardening and thickening of the skin, giving it a waxy, hidebound texture. This may be accompanied by loss of skin appendages, oedema, and altered pigmentation. Telangiectasia is common (*see* below). The facial appearance is characteristic, being immobile and masklike, with creases radiating from the corners of the mouth (Fig. 8.1).

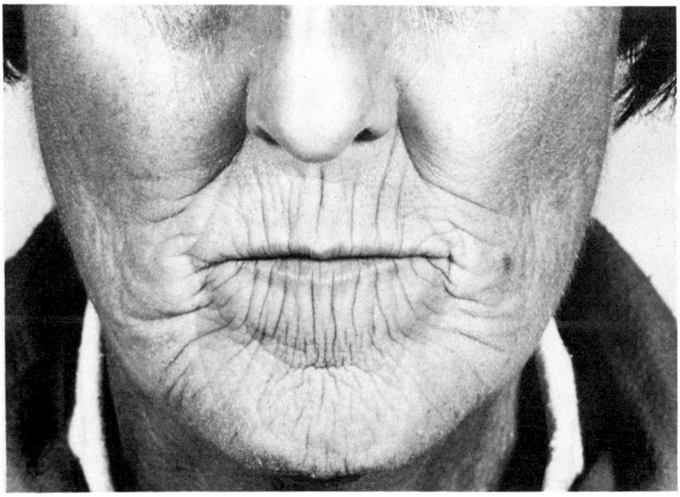

FIGURE 8.1 Progressive systemic sclerosis: fissures radiating from the mouth

In general, the areas of skin affected by PSS do not have a sharp line of demarcation from the normal skin, which serves to distinguish them from that found in two conditions, *morphoea* and *linear scleroderma*, in both of which a similar pathological change occurs, but in a localised form. The involved areas of skin in the localised forms have the same feel and appearance as that found in PSS, but there is a sharp line of demarcation from normal skin. In addition, these two conditions never involve internal organs.

Joint Changes. Particularly in the early stages, a troublesome polyarthritis may affect the small joints of the hands, occasionally other sites. There is soft tissue swelling due to a subacute synovitis which, with oedema from the skin changes, produces the typical 'sausage fingers' (Fig. 8.2). Characteristic leathery crepitus or friction rubs may arise from

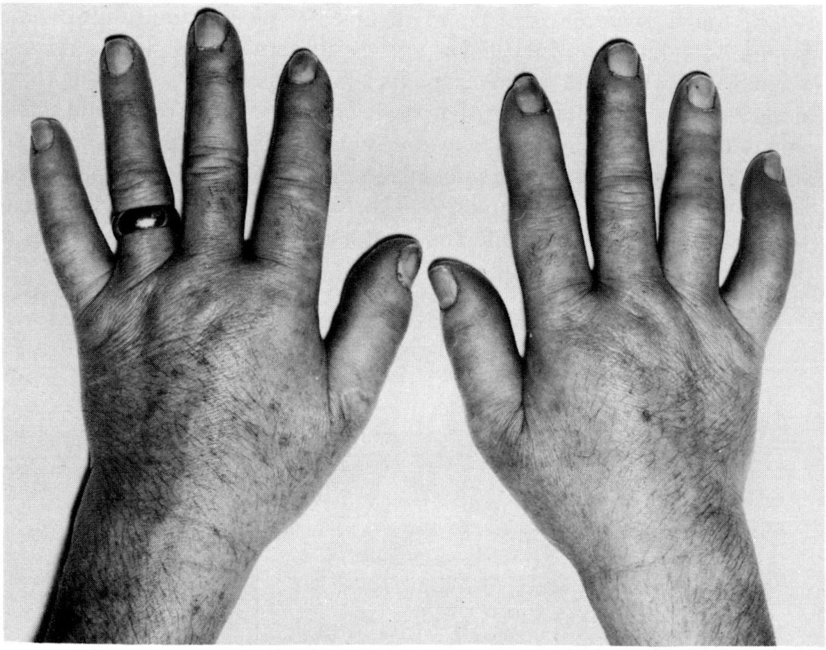

FIGURE 8.2 Progressive systemic sclerosis: skin oedema and joint swelling combining to produce 'sausage fingers'. The distal half of the right index finger illustrates the obliteration of cutaneous creases and appendages which gives the skin a smooth characterless appearance

affected joints or tendon sheaths. The joint changes may be mistaken for early rheumatoid arthritis, especially when finger joint deformities develop as a result of soft tissue fibrosis. But the steady progression with erosive changes so characteristic of rheumatoid arthritis do not occur. It is sometimes difficult to tell whether finger swelling and discomfort are due to involvement of the skin or of the joints.

Calcinosis. Subcutaneous deposits of calcific material may occur in the hands and extensor aspects of the elbows, forming palpable nodules.

These are well shown on radiographs (Fig. 8.3). The association of calcinosis with telangiectasia is recognised.

Telangiectasia. Fine telangiectasis is a common accompaniment of the skin changes of PSS. In addition, a tendency to a more widespread tel-

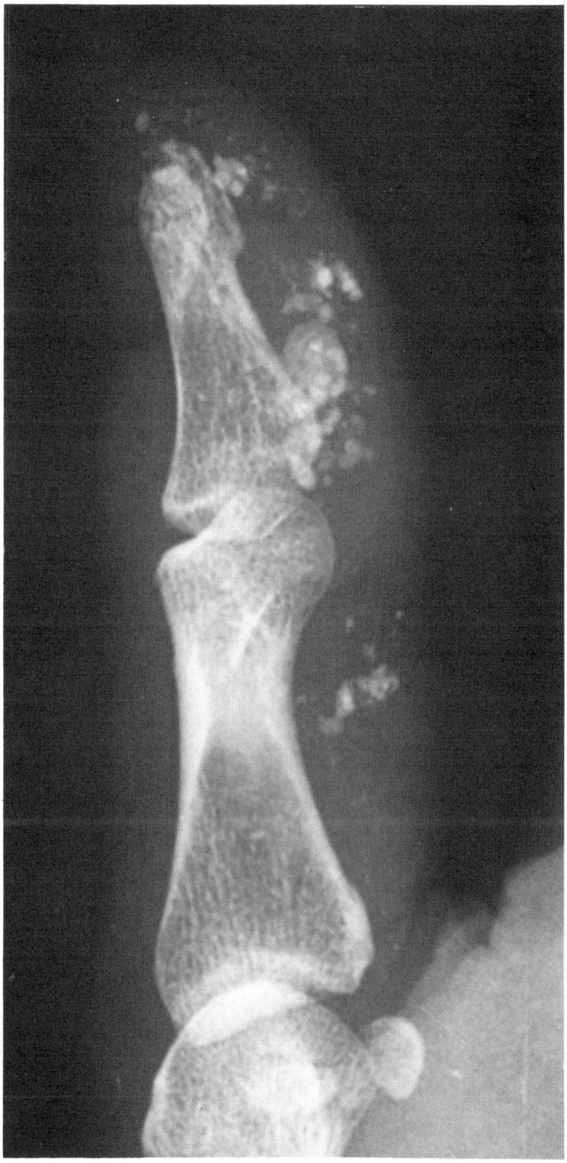

FIGURE 8.3 Progressive systemic sclerosis: subcutaneous calcinosis in the thumb

angiectasia, clinically resembling that seen in the hereditary haemorrhagic telangiectasia of Osler (but lacking a positive family history) may occur in patients with PSS and calcinosis. This association has been called the 'Thibierge-Weissenbach Syndrome'. The title *'CRST syndrome'* is useful in indicating the features (calcinosis, Raynaud's phenomenon, sclerodactyly, and telangiectasia) which together form a somewhat benign subgroup of PSS; benign in the sense that the telangiectases are less likely to produce serious haemorrhage than in Osler's disease, and in that the liability to serious visceral complications is less than in other cases of PSS.

Gastro-intestinal Tract. All levels of the gut may be involved in PSS, but only oesophageal changes are commonly recognised. Characteristically, PSS produces reduced or altered motility of the oesophagus, often with reflux at the cardia. Gross involvement produces symptoms of peptic oesophagitis, with dysphagia and acid regurgitation. Radiographic examination reveals early loss of motility when the patient attempts to swallow barium in the head-down position, showing the oesophagus to be an atonic tube, sometimes with reflux at the cardia. It is important to appreciate that this radiographic appearance is often present quite early in the disease, even in the complete absence of symptoms. It thus provides a valuable pointer to the diagnosis. However, it is not specific, for a similar appearance may be seen in other connective tissue diseases such as dermatomyositis.

Less often, PSS may involve other levels of the intestine to an extent sufficient to produce diarrhoea (sometimes constipation), or even a state of serious intestinal malabsorption and malnutrition.

Heart. Cardiac abnormalities are not infrequently seen in PSS, but are usually secondary either to systemic hypertension (from renal involvement) or to pulmonary hypertension (from lung involvement). Less often, primary sclerotic changes in the heart may lead to cardiac failure or dysrhythmias. Pericarditis may occur, and aortic valve lesions have been described. Very rarely, isolated heart involvement, without other evidence of PSS, produces fatal cardiac failure recognised only at post mortem.

Lungs. About 30 per cent of patients with PSS have evidence of pulmonary involvement; although frequently this is asymptomatic. Pulmonary function tests show the earliest changes to be a gas diffusion block. Later, there is evidence of restrictive lung disease due to peribronchial fibrosis. Physical examination occasionally reveals tachypnoea and basal crepitations, and X-rays show non-specific evidence of diffuse fibrosis. Rarely, one may get a pleural effusion, or pulmonary hypertension leading to right-sided heart failure. While signs and symptoms of pulmonary involvement tend to be inconspicuous, pulmonary function testing will often reveal unsuspected lung lesions. Exceptionally, very extensive skin involvement itself may actually restrict breathing movements. There is probably an increased incidence of both alveolar and bronchiolar cell carcinomata in patients with PSS and pulmonary fibrosis.

Kidneys. Renal involvement is the most important cause of death in PSS. At any stage of the disease it may produce hypertension associated, initially, with little if any proteinuria. Over a period, which can be as short as a few days or weeks, this may progress to severe malignant hypertension and death. It is not clear to what extent the administration of corticosteroids can contribute to this clinical picture. Certainly, rapidly fatal hypertension has occurred in patients not given this drug. In other cases, corticosteroids have clearly played at least a contributory role in producing severe hypertension, and the blood pressure has fallen on withdrawal of the drug. On the present information, there would seem to be little justification for using corticosteroids in PSS.

Muscles. Patients with PSS often have some wasting and weakness of skeletal muscles which may be due to inflammatory changes similar to those that, in more extreme form, produce the picture of polymyositis. Evidence for such myositis may be obtained by muscle biopsy, by electromyography, or by finding elevated levels of serum enzymes (creatine phosphokinase and aldolase) released from the damaged muscle fibres.

Miscellaneous. Less common manifestations of PSS include Sjögren's syndrome (*see* Chapter 10), and peripheral neuropathy.

LABORATORY FINDINGS

Active PSS may produce a modest elevation both in the erythrocyte sedimentation rate and in the level of serum globulins, but the changes are less marked than in SLE. Serological abnormalities are not at all uncommon; LE cell reactions are positive in about 5 per cent, rheumatoid factors are detectable in about 25 per cent, and about 50 per cent give positive (fluorescent) antinuclear factor tests. Occasionally, biological false positive tests for syphilis may occur.

PATHOLOGY

Common to all the structures involved in PSS is a process of fibrosis, homogenisation of collagen, sclerosis of blood vessels, and secondary atrophy. During phases of more acute inflammation there may be some infiltration with lymphocytes and plasma cells, and oedema, but this gives way later to fibrosis. The early synovitis, for example, may show lymphocyte and plasma cell infiltration and oedema; later, there is sclerosis. In the skin, the increase in collagen may be very marked, with homogenisation of the fibres, atrophy of appendages, and hyalinisation of arterioles. A fundamentally similar process of collagenous proliferation is seen when PSS involves the heart, lungs, and gut.

The kidneys of patients dying with renal PSS show focal basement membrane changes, fibrinoid necrosis of afferent arterioles and glomerular tufts, and hyperplasia of interlobular arteries. The changes tend to be focal, and are similar to those seen in 'ordinary' malignant nephrosclerosis.

Arteriolar ischaemia is clearly important in the pathogenesis of these serious renal lesions, and it is tempting to speculate that this may be essentially the same process as the digital artery spasm producing the Raynaud's phenomenon.

AETIOLOGY

The aetiology of PSS is unknown. The pattern of histological change suggests that the lesions may result from loss of control of the manner in which collagen is laid down, or from vascular occlusion. At present it is not clear what significance should be attached to the serological overlap with other connective tissue disorders, nor to the interesting observation that PSS occurs more commonly among miners exposed to dusts such as silica. The rarity of a positive family history makes it unlikely that genetic influences are important.

TREATMENT

No really effective therapy is known for this condition. Corticosteroids will suppress the early synovitis, but the hazard of producing hypertension probably makes their use unjustifiable. Theoretically interesting attempts to 'soften' the offending collagen by using the hormone relaxin and the lathyrogenic agent penicillamine have been disappointing. Nothing has been found to halt the underlying pathological process, and treatment remains symptomatic. Troublesome Raynaud's phenomenon is best treated by wearing warm gloves and avoidance of cold. Hypertension must be particularly watched for and treated vigorously along conventional lines as soon as it appears. Cardiac failure, renal failure, respiratory failure, and intestinal malabsorption may all require treatment, but do not present problems peculiar to PSS.

COURSE AND PROGNOSIS

Most patients diagnosed as having PSS will die from the effects of the disease. The duration of survival from the time the diagnosis is made varies very widely, the average being about four years. The severity of the skin changes gives no clue to the prognosis for survival, which depends on the extent of visceral involvement. Renal involvement carries a particularly bad outlook.

Polymyositis and Dermatomyositis

The term *polymyositis* is used to describe diffuse inflammatory disorders of striated muscles. The tempo of this process may range from rapid necrosis of many muscle fibres, through a subacute type with round-cell infiltration, to a chronic process in which there is no more than a very gradual fall-out of muscle fibres. When the disease process is chronic there will obviously be features in common with the (purely degenerative) heredofamilial *muscular dystrophies*. However, the two conditions are usually easily distinguished clinically, and are thought to result from different pathogenic mechanisms. The term *myopathy* embraces all diffuse disorders of striated muscles, and thus includes both polymyositis and the muscular dystrophies.

When polymyositis is associated with a particular pattern of skin eruption the condition is described as *dermatomyositis*. Together, 'pure' polymyositis and dermatomyositis form the two main diagnostic categories in the group of conditions to be described in this section. It is difficult to obtain a clear understanding of this group of disorders because of the widely differing clinical pictures that may be encountered. It is essential to appreciate that one feature is common to the group as a whole – diffuse inflammation of striated muscle. This may be acute, subacute, or chronic. Variety is introduced into the clinical picture because the pathological changes often occur in association; firstly, with features of other connective tissue disorders, secondly, with the skin changes mentioned and, thirdly, with malignant neoplasia. For this reason these disorders are customarily grouped for descriptive purposes into arbitrary categories. The following is one such classification (after Walton) –

POLYMYOSITIS

A Pure polymyositis
B Polymyositis with minor features of other connective tissue disorders or a slight rash
C Other connective tissue disorders with incidental polymyositis
D Dermatomyositis
- I Adult
  - (i) with malignancy
  - (ii) without malignancy
- II Childhood

It is important to appreciate that this classification is artificial, and that the grouping is a matter of convenience. The groups are not clear-cut, and are quite arbitrary divisions in a continuous spectrum of clinical disease. Individual cases may present intermediate pictures that make it difficult to assign them to any particular group, or may, during the course of their illness, change from one diagnostic category to another. Excluded from this classification are the myopathies of Cushing's syndrome or corticosteroid overdosage, paroxysmal myoglobinuria, and carcinomatous neuromyopathy. A more meaningful classification awaits our better understanding of these conditions. At present it is not known whether the clinical heterogeneity is due to differing aetiological factors having polymyositis as a common outcome, or whether a common pathogenic process finds different expression because of constitutional differences; i.e. whether the variation is in the seed, in the soil, or in both.

Nevertheless, the classification is valuable to the clinician in indicating the circumstances in which polymyositis may occur, and the associated conditions that need to be sought. It provides also a useful stratification for assessing prognosis and response to treatment.

CLINICAL FEATURES

These conditions are generally more common in women that men – (in the ratio of about 3 : 1). They may appear at any age but (apart from dermatomyositis of childhood, and that associated with malignancy) the mid-adult years are the most common time of appearance. For convenience, the clinical features of the different groups are described separately but, again, it must be emphasised that the groups form a clinical continuum, and the divisions are arbitrary.

'Pure' Polymyositis

The clinical features of polymyositis are a predictable reflection of the histological changes. The one constant feature is voluntary muscle weakness, usually associated with some reduction in muscle bulk. When the tempo is rapid there may be an initial period when the affected muscles are swollen, doughy, and tender, with oedema of the overlying skin. As the swelling subsides, atrophy becomes apparent. In chronic disease the patient may present simply with weakness and wasting; in these circumstances this must be differentiated from primary neurological (lower motor neurone) disorders. Points favouring a primary muscular condition are the relatively good retention of tendon reflexes, the absence of sensory loss, and the symmetrical, proximal distribution of weakness.

In a typical subacute case the patient will usually describe symptoms coming on over a few weeks or months. The girdle distribution of weakness causes difficulty to be first experienced walking up stairs, combing the hair, or getting out of the bath. As the weakness progresses the gait becomes waddling, and difficulty may now be experienced in raising the head or in turning over in bed. Involvement of pharyngeal and laryngeal muscles is indicated by weakness of phonation with a nasal quality to the voice, and with dysphagia, with choking and regurgitation of food into the nasopharynx. This difficulty with swallowing is due to weakness of the voluntary muscles of the pharynx and must be distinguished from the oesophageal atony with which it may co-exist (*see* below) and which is due to smooth muscle involvement.

In the severely affected patient the condition may progress to involve the muscles of respiration, and the combination of pharyngeal and respiratory paralysis may lead to death from inhaled secretion and respiratory failure. More commonly, the disease becomes stationary and, after a period of weeks or months there is a gradual return of power to the affected muscles. Healing is partly by fibrous replacement of muscle which may progress to calcification. Thus, the recovered patient is likely to be left with some permanent weakness in muscle groups which are somewhat wasted and indurated, and in which there may be radiological evidence of calcification. The residual functional capacity will depend both on the remaining muscle power and on the extent to which fibrous healing has produced contractures and muscle shortening. This is the natural history of the disease. Fortunately, modern methods of treatment with corticosteroid drugs (*see* below) can often cut short the course of the illness, and adequate splinting of joints can minimise residual deformities.

The tempo of the disease varies tremendously. At one end of the scale are patients in whom muscle destruction is so rapid that myoglobin may appear in the urine and in whom death may occur within weeks of the first symptom. At the opposite end of this scale are those in whom the symptoms are for many months, or even years, so slight as not to be considered abnormal by the patient. Also characteristic of polymyositis is a fluctuating course punctuated by a series of exacerbations and remissions.

By the time the patient seeks medical advice there are likely to be characteristic abnormal physical signs. Weakness is the cardinal feature, and this typically involves proximal limb and girdle muscles, the neck, and pharynx. In acute cases the affected muscles may be swollen and tender to pressure, with a doughy feel on palpation. More commonly there is only weakness and wasting, but with tendon reflexes relatively well preserved. In very mild cases the weakness may show only as inability to maintain elevation of the straightened leg or abducted arm against resistance, or as inability to rise from a supine to a sitting position with arms folded across the chest. (This useful test requires counter-pressure on the knees by the examiner.) Weakness of facial muscles may produce a characteristic facial expression.

Although polymyositis is primarily a disease of striated voluntary muscle, mention has already been made of the oesophageal smooth muscle hypomotility that may occur. In addition, electrocardiographic changes or cardiac dysrhythmias may rarely occur as a manifestation of cardiac muscle involvement.

The diagnosis of polymyositis is established by three special investigations –

1. Serum enzyme studies
2. Electromyography
3. Muscle biopsy

Since these are relevant to the other disorders mentioned in this section their description is postponed to page 123. They enable the diagnosis to be made with considerable confidence.

Polymyositis with Features of Other Connective Tissue Disorders

This is an intermediate group in which the clinical features described above under 'pure' polymyositis are accompanied by a slight rash, insufficient to justify the label dermatomyositis, or by minor features of other connective tissue disorders. The more carefully cases of 'pure' polymyositis are studied, the more often will grounds be found for including them in this second group.

An insignificant rash may be missed unless carefully sought in a good light. This may be a faint scaling eruption or transient erythema affecting the face, neck, shoulders or upper arms.

The most common accompaniments of polymyositis are features generally regarded as being more characteristic of progressive systemic sclerosis. These are *Raynaud's phenomenon, oesophageal hypomotility* and *sclerodactyly*. Raynaud's phenomenon may be the presenting symptom of polymyositis, and this is one of the conditions that has to be suspected when Raynaud's phenomenon appears for the first time in an adult. Oesophageal hypomotility is common, although usually asymptomatic. Its presence is revealed to the radiologist when the patient attempts to swallow barium in the head-down position. Skin changes in the fingers resemble those seen in progressive systemic sclerosis, and may vary from slight waxy thickening to gross sclerodactyly with poikiloderma (atrophy of the digital pulp, giving a hard, tapered finger).

Joint symptoms are not uncommon, and included in this group are patients with polymyositis in whom there are minor manifestations of rheumatoid arthritis. This is usually a mild, symmetrical, small-joint polyarthritis with some swelling, but which does not progress to erosive changes or joint deformity. Tests for rheumatoid factor may be positive. Another disorder that may be associated with polymyositis is *Sjögren's syndrome* (*see* Chapter 10). Even in the absence of a complaint of dry or gritty eyes, the Schirmer test may reveal diminished tear secretion, or instillation of a drop of Rose Bengal may show the characteristic corneal staining of kerato-conjunctivitis sicca.

Other Connective Tissue Disorders with Incidental Polymyositis

The general availability and convenience of electromyography has made it possible to screen large numbers of patients for polymyositis. Application of this test to patients with rheumatoid arthritis has shown that minor degrees of polymyositis are an occasional accompaniment of this disease, particularly in the more severe cases. In practice, the issue is somewhat confused because patients with severe rheumatoid disease tend to be treated with corticosteroid drugs. These drugs may themselves produce 'corticosteroid myopathy' (an iatrogenic form of the myopathy seen in Cushing's syndrome) with electromyographic abnormalities not always readily distinguishable from polymyositis. However, when those on corticosteroid drugs are excluded, there are still some patients with typical rheumatoid arthritis who have minor but definite degrees of polymyositis. Clinical assessment of the muscles in such patients is complicated by their joint disease, which itself may produce wasting and apparent weakness of muscles. However, it seems clear that some of these patients do have some definite weakness due to the muscle disease *per se*, while in others it is not clinically obvious. Clearly, this is extremely important therapeutically. Functionally, the rheumatoid patient is probably particularly vulnerable to a superadded myopathy, so, undue weakness in a rheumatoid patient should be regarded as an indication for electromyography, and, if polymyositis is present, relatively large doses of corticosteroids may be indicated.

Rheumatoid arthritis is only one of the connective tissue disorders that may be complicated by polymyositis. Thus, electromyographic screening of patients with progressive systemic sclerosis, polyarteritis nodosa, systemic lupus erythematosus, and Sjögren's syndrome will reveal a certain number with polymyositis. As in rheumatoid arthritis, this may or may not be associated with some degree of clinical weakness. Minor degrees of polymyositis are particularly common in progressive systemic sclerosis, and here it has been suggested that the muscle fibres are affected by the primary disturbance in the collagen of their supporting fibrous tissue. Similarly, involvement of small muscle arteries in polyarteritis nodosa may perhaps produce the electromyographic changes of polymyositis.

Dermatomyositis

In dermatomyositis the features of polymyositis occur in association with a more or less characteristic skin eruption. The typical rash is a diffuse erythema affecting the face, neck, upper arms, and upper trunk. It may be more extensive, and it may be associated with cutaneous oedema. Pruritus is variable. Characteristic features are peri-orbital oedema and a violaceous or 'heliotrope' discoloration of the upper eyelids. Over knuckles and other extensor prominences there may be atrophic scaling, producing the so-called 'collodion patch' lesions.

The muscle changes are similar to those seen in 'pure' polymyositis, but tend to be of the more acute variety, and are generally more severe. In keeping with this, local swelling of muscles, with induration, tenderness and pain are more prominent, as well as general features such as malaise, fever, and leucocytosis. Joint symptoms, in the form of a symmetrical small joint polyarthritis, may be troublesome in the early stages.

Two subgroups of dermatomyositis require special mention; they are dermatomyositis with malignant disease, and dermatomyositis in childhood.

Dermatomyositis with Malignancy. About 20 per cent of patients with dermatomyositis, who are over the age of forty years, are found to have an associated malignant neoplasm. This interesting relationship is not understood, but it is worth noting that in the condition 'carcinomatous neuropathy' there is often evidence of some muscle involvement too (hence, correctly referred to as 'carcinomatous neuromyopathy').

Dermatomyositis with malignancy has a different sex incidence from other types of polymyositis, being slightly more common in males. The most frequent sites for these tumours are the lung, ovary, prostate, breast, and gut. In some cases the malignancy may show itself at the same time as the dermatomyositis, or even earlier. More often it is not detected until the dermatomyositis has been present for anything up to three years. Dermatomyositis associated with malignancy tends to run a particularly severe course although surgical cure of the tumour has been reported to improve the myopathy. Both skin and muscle changes tend to be progressive despite treatment, and death is due usually to respiratory and pharyngeal paralysis rather than the direct effects of the tumour itself. Clearly, all patients over forty years of age, diagnosed as having dermatomyositis, require intensive and repeated investigation for treatable primary tumours.

Dermatomyositis in Childhood. Dermatomyositis is an uncommon disease in childhood, but it is important because of the severe deformities that may result. The clinical features resemble those seen in the adult, but there is no increased incidence of malignancy. The first symptoms may occur at any age, the average being about eight years. As in the adult, the proximal muscles are affected more than the distal, and the tempo may vary from rapid progression over a few weeks, producing paralysis of chewing, swallowing, phonation, and respiration, to the gradual development of a mild weakness over a number of years. Some have a fluctuating course in which there are repeated unpredictable exacerbations and remissions. In many there is a marked tendency for muscles to atrophy and shorten, with the development of crippling contractures. Good physiotherapy, with correct splinting, can do much to minimise this.

The cutaneous lesions also resemble those seen in the adult, but 'collodion patch' lesions over the extensor surfaces of joints are particularly characteristic. Mild joint pains are also common. Unique to childhood polymyositis is the occurrence of abdominal pain, sometimes associated with gastro-intestinal bleeding, and even perforation, due to vasculitis in the gastro-intestinal tract. In children (but not in adults) a similar vasculitis may, not infrequently, be found in voluntary muscles. Almost all these children, if followed long enough, will be observed to develop subcutaneous calcification. This may produce obvious subcutaneous nodules of plaques, or be detected only radiologically.

LABORATORY INVESTIGATIONS

When the disease is chronic, polymyositis may produce little, if any, change in the sedimentation rate and blood picture. When it is more acute there is usually a moderate elevation in the sedimentation rate, a mild anaemia and, occasionally, a leucocytosis. Serum proteins may show a slight reduction in albumin and a mild increase in most globulin fractions.

Patients with polymyositis have an increased incidence of positive serological tests for rheumatoid factor, antinuclear factors, and LE cell factor (even excluding those with obvious rheumatoid arthritis, systemic lupus erythematosus, or Sjögren's syndrome). Anti-muscle antibodies have also been detected in the serum of some of these patients, but they are equally common in patients with neurogenic and other causes of muscle wasting; they probably represent a result, rather than the cause, of polymyositis.

Serum Enzymes. The destruction of muscle fibres brought about by polymyositis releases a variety of enzymes from the muscle fibre; these may then be detected in the serum in increased concentrations. This method of detecting cell damage by serum enzyme determinations (of value also in diseases of the liver, heart, and pancreas) depends on the tissue specificity of the enzyme measured. The following enzymes tend to be elevated in polymyositis –

Creatine phosphokinase
Aldolase
Lactic dehydrogenase
Transaminases

The first two are perhaps the more nearly specific for muscle damage, while the last is more convenient for serial studies. It is advisable to use more than one test if possible. In practice, such enzyme studies are of the greatest value in the diagnosis of polymyositis, and in following the progress of the disease. They provide a yardstick against which to titrate the dose of corticosteroids, and they may give early warning of a relapse. The older biochemical measures of muscle damage – increased creatine and decreased creatinine in the urine – are of much less value than the enzyme determinations.

Electromyography. In the great majority of patients with polymyositis electrodiagnostic studies of a clinically affected muscle will establish the diagnosis with certainty. The characteristic features include –

Spontaneous fibrillation
Short-duration polyphasic potentials of low amplitude
Salvos of repetitive potentials

When the findings are characteristic it is possible to differentiate muscle weakness due to polymyositis from that due to lower motor neurone lesions or muscular dystrophy. Occasionally, the EMG may reveal a myasthenic element in polymyositis.

PATHOLOGY AND AETIOLOGY

Biopsy of a clinically affected muscle (but avoiding the track of EMG needles) provides a valuable method of establishing the diagnosis of polymyositis. The changes, some of which are illustrated in Fig. 8.4.,

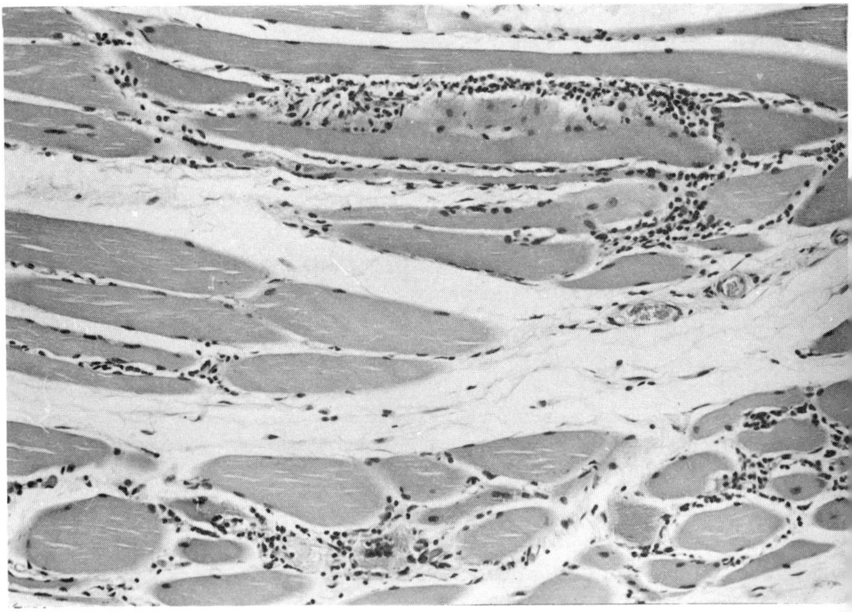

FIGURE 8.4 Polymyositis. Biopsy of deltoid muscle; degeneration of muscle fibres and cellular infiltration

include muscle fibre degeneration, with or without evidence of phagocytosis and regeneration. Infiltration with round cells is often the most striking feature. In longstanding disease there may be fibrosis and also calcification. Biopsy of involved areas of skin shows only non-specific evidence of inflammation.

In children with dermatomyositis coming to post mortem there is often evidence of widespread vasculitis ('systemic angiopathy'), with perivascular collections of inflammatory cells, intimal hyperplasia, and thrombosis.

The aetiology and pathogenesis of polymyositis is unknown. Some of the histological features and serological changes suggest that there is at least some immunological overactivity, and polymyositis certainly occurs in association with conditions such as systemic lupus erythematosus and Sjögren's syndrome, in which there is a strong suspicion that immune processes play a pathogenic role. In polymyositis there is no direct evidence of this. If altered immunity is important, it is not clear whether it operates by initiating the disorder or by maintaining a process started by some other agent. The interesting association with malignant disease can be made to fit an 'autoimmune' hypothesis by arguing that the neoplasm releases cross-reacting antigens which (perhaps like streptococci in rheumatic fever) break down the tolerance for normal body tissues.

TREATMENT

The prognosis in polymyositis has been appreciably improved by the use of corticosteroid drugs. Prednisolone is the preferred drug, and given in a daily dose (for adults) of about 60 mg, it will predictably improve 60 to 70 per cent of cases. In some, the response is dramatic and may be life-saving. Inexplicably, a minority of patients show no response. All severe cases justify a trial of the drug. If a response is obtained, the dose is then titrated down to that which will maintain reasonable suppression (as judged clinically and by serial enzyme studies). Prednisolone may have to be continued for months or even years, and the patient is quite likely to be more troubled by the side effects of the drug than by the underlying disease. This problem is discussed at length in Chapter 3.

Physiotherapy has an important role to play in avoiding deformities. During active phases the joints are probably best put gently through a full range of movement passively each day, and splinted where necessary to prevent muscle-shortening deformities such as foot-drop. Later, active exercises will be needed, and rehabilitation may involve functional re-education of depleted musculature.

Paralysis of swallowing and of respiration will involve, to a greater or lesser extent, the routine of intensive total patient care needed for completely paralysed patients. The maintenance of artificial respiration, bronchial toilet, and nutrition do not present problems peculiar to polymyositis, and will not be discussed here.

Attempts have recently been made to treat polymyositis with immunosuppressive drugs such as azathioprine. There are, as yet, no adequately controlled data to allow evaluation of this form of therapy.

PROGNOSIS

Of all patients diagnosed as having polymyositis, about 30 per cent are likely to die from the results of the disease. Of the survivors, a majority will eventually achieve a reasonably normal functional capacity, but an appreciable minority will be left with some degree of disability.

The presence of a malignancy is the most ominous prognostic sign. Older patients, and those with a rapid and severe onset, also do less well. Childhood polymyositis is rarely fatal, but may produce significant permanent disability.

9

Systemic Lupus Erythematosus

Graham R V Hughes

Systemic lupus erythematosus (SLE), possibly more than any other disease discussed in this book, presents a challenge to the physician, not only in diagnosis and management, but also in his study of the pathogenesis of the rheumatic disorders in general.

It is a disease of unknown aetiology, commonly affecting many systems of the body. It oftens presents with an erythematous skin rash and may produce prolonged fever, arthralgia and arthritis, lymphadenopathy, polyserositis (especially pleurisy and pericarditis) and renal, neurological, and cardiac damage. Untreated, its course is punctuated by exacerbations and natural remissions, but eventually it usually kills the patient. It affects women more commonly than men (between 80 and 90 per cent of patients affected are female) and negroes more commonly than white people.

Kaposi, in 1875, gave the characteristic facial 'butterfly' rash its name, and noted that 'various grave and even dangerous constitutional symptoms may be intimately associated with the process in question'.

In 1895, Osler described: 'a disease of unknown aetiology with polymorphic skin lesions – hyperaemia, oedema, and haemorrhage – arthritis occasionally, and a variable number of visceral manifestations of which the most important are gastro-intestinal crises, endocarditis, pericarditis, acute nephritis and haemorrhage from the mucous surfaces. Recurrence is a special feature of the disease, and attacks may come on month after month or even throughout a long period of years'.

Despite these detailed clinical descriptions, the disease remained poorly understood and infrequently recognised. It was not until 1948, when Hargraves and his colleagues discovered the LE-cell phenomenon, that it became possible to define the disease more precisely.

This discovery was important for two reasons. First, it gave the clinician a valuable laboratory aid to the diagnosis of SLE; its help in the recognition of atypical presentations of lupus has largely been responsible for the increasing frequency with which the disease has been diagnosed during the past two decades. Secondly, it provided an important clue to the aetiology of the disease.

AETIOLOGY

IMMUNITY

SLE is thought to occupy a central position among the so-called autoimmune diseases. In these disorders the body appears to mount an immune response against some part of itself, there being no recognisable outside antigen. The result is usually a widespread and damaging inflammatory reaction.

These diseases have several features in common—the so-called 'markers' of autoimmune disease—and SLE is no exception. They are—

High titres of circulating antibodies.
Raised serum levels of gamma globulin.
Lymphoid and plasma cell hyperplasia.
A tendency to occur together with other diseases in the group.
Responsiveness to steroids.

In SLE there is abundant evidence that a number of antibodies are concerned in the tissue damage. The LE-cell phenomenon results from damage to the cell nucleus by a circulating humoral antibody—a 7-S gamma globulin, or IgG. The frequently occurring haemolytic anaemia is also secondary to attachment of immune globulin, this time on the surface of the red cell. In addition to humoral antibody, cellular reactions (lymphocytes) are probably also important, and antigen/antibody complexes have been shown to take part in the tissue damage (*see* p. 6).

The finding of antibodies to white cells and to platelets, the 'false positive' Wasserman reaction, and the demonstration of antibodies to muscle and to thyroid all underline the disturbances in immune mechanisms present in this disease.

SENSITIVITY

Despite the absence of a known extrinsic cause for SLE there are several factors that in some cases undoubtedly precipitate an exacerbation. In particular, patients with SLE are commonly light or drug sensitive.

Light. Many patients give a history of lifelong skin sensitivity to sunlight. In the established disease, exposure to sunlight may produce not only exacerbations of the skin eruption but a generalised systemic flare-up of the condition. This tendency is more common in white than in coloured races.

Hydrallazine. This drug, introduced in 1951 for the treatment of hypertension, was found to produce an illness characterised by fever, malaise, arthralgia, lupus-like rashes and, sometimes, LE-cells in the blood. The symptoms subsided when the drug was stopped. This raised the possibility that lupus might be a form of hypersensitivity to drugs, the apparent increase in the incidence over the past two decades resulting from the ever-increasing variety of new drugs to which the body is exposed.

Other Drugs. Sulphonamides, the anti-epileptic drugs, antituberculous drugs, procainamide, and penicillin have all been implicated in the pathogenesis of SLE. It is, however, extremely difficult to prove that these are not merely producers of sensitivity reactions in a patient already suffering from, or developing, SLE. In the large majority of patients with SLE there is no obvious causative factor.

ENDOCRINE

Sex Incidence. Between eight and nine out of every ten patients suffering from SLE are female. Although this might suggest an endocrine basis for the disease, no consistent endocrine abnormality has been discovered, neither has any X-chromosome defect been found with consistency. Treatment with testosterone has proved ineffective.

Pregnancy. Not only is the incidence of SLE highest in women in the child-bearing years, but the disease is sometimes exacerbated by pregnancy. Again, the reason for this is not known.

GENETIC FACTORS

There are many reports of more than one member of a family suffering from lupus, which has led to the suggestion that the disease might be genetically determined, possibly on the basis of an inborn error of protein metabolism, or a hereditary abnormality in gamma globulin (especially hypergammaglobulinaemia). While these have been found in some cases, the vast majority of patients have no such family history.

GEOGRAPHICAL FACTORS

The apparent geographical and racial prevalence of any disease is to some extent a reflection of its clinical recognition. This, in SLE, depends to a certain extent on laboratory and hospital facilities. It is certainly a clinical impression that lupus is seen more commonly in the USA than in Britain, and the largest series of cases have all been reported from North America. Most workers agree that the disease is commoner in negroes than in white populations. Again, the reasons for these differences, are not known.

RELATIONSHIP TO OTHER CONNECTIVE TISSUE DISEASES

In many ways lupus resembles the other so-called 'connective tissue' diseases. The basic pathology is similar, and the clinical pictures overlap. The antibodies found in SLE may be found in other members of the group – particularly rheumatoid arthritis, Sjögren's syndrome, and progressive systemic sclerosis. There is a higher than expected incidence of 'connective tissue' diseases in the families of SLE patients, and, rarely, a patient with, for example, progressive systemic sclerosis may progress to SLE, or vice versa.

The relationship is probably greater than mere resemblance. As always, the more that is known about each of these diseases, particularly in their atypical forms, the more the overlap between each, and the less clear the spectrum.

Clinically, however, the differences in the vast majority of cases are clear cut, and there is no excuse for the term 'connective tissue disorder' as a definitive diagnosis.

RELATIONSHIP TO DISCOID LUPUS ERYTHEMATOSUS

Chronic discoid lupus erythematosus (CDLE) is a skin disease characterised by a persistent erythematous rash, often circular or oval in pattern, with scaling, telangiectasia, follicular plugging and scarring (Fig. 9.1). Its course may be protracted or it may heal, leaving scarring or pigmentation. These changes are identical with those of the chronic skin lesions of SLE, and a great deal of confusion has surrounded the relationship between the two diseases. During the past few years it has become increasingly recognised that CDLE is not purely a skin disease. Approximately half the cases have positive tests for anti-nuclear factor (ANF)

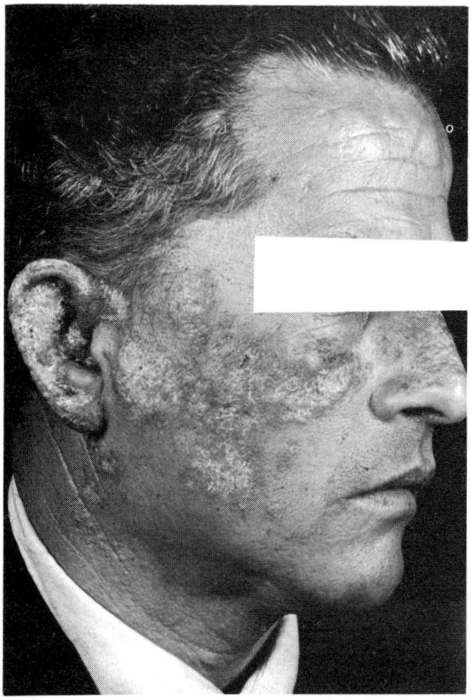

FIGURE 9.1 Chronic discoid lupus erythematosus (CDLE) showing follicular plugging and scarring. This patient suffered no systemic features (Courtesy Dr B. Russell)

though the titres are seldom high. Between 5 and 10 per cent have positive LE-cell tests. More significantly, over half appear to suffer, on closer investigation, from a mild form of systemic lupus, with arthralgia, pleurisy, fever, and Raynaud's phenomenon.

It seems likely, therefore, that CDLE is fundamentally a form of SLE, occupying the benign end of the disease spectrum, but worth separating for clinical purposes because of its excellent prognosis.

PATHOLOGY

Systemic lupus erythematosus may affect most organs and tissues of the body. Understanding of the pathology is simplified if it is realised that three or four basic microscopic changes occur, and that most damaged organs show one or more of these. The following are the most important –

Fibrinoid change.
Sclerosis of collagen.
Haematoxylin bodies.
Vascular lesions.

FIBRINOID

This is an acellular, deeply eosinophilic material occurring in threads and bands, superficially resembling fibrin. It is thought to result from damage to the ground substance of connective tissue, possibly to fibrin itself, by the deposition of plasma proteins. Around the areas of fibrinoid, a mild inflammatory reaction occurs, with lymphocytes and plasma cells predominating. This inflammatory reaction appears to be more intense on the serosal surfaces, such as the pleura, following fibrin deposition.

SCLEROSIS OF COLLAGEN

As a result of the chronic inflammatory reaction around fibrin the nearby collagen fibres become swollen and altered. Fibroblasts grow in, with resultant increase in connective tissue formation. A peculiarly marked example is seen in the spleen, where concentric fibrosis encircles the splenic arterioles, giving the so-called *onion-skin* appearance (Fig. 9.2), one of the two findings almost pathognomonic of SLE.

HAEMATOXYLIN BODIES

Foci of basophilic staining material are the other characteristic feature. These so-called 'haematoxylin bodies' probably consist of desoxyribonucleic acid (DNA) released from nuclei damaged by the antibody. The material is possibly identical with that in the LE-cell.

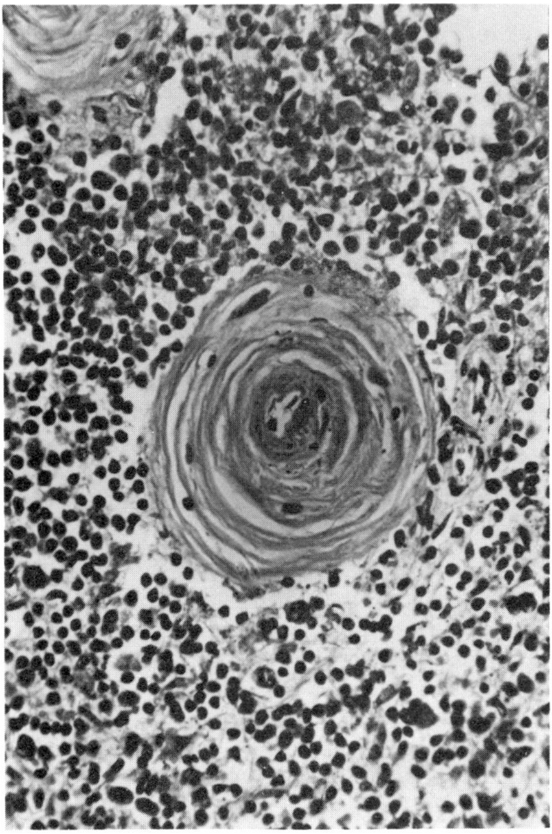

FIGURE 9.2 'Onion skin' lesion of splenic arteriole. Prior to splenectomy, the diagnosis had been 'idiopathic thrombocytopaenic purpura' (Courtesy Dept. of Morbid Anatomy, The London Hospital Medical College)

VASCULAR CHANGES

Widespread lesions in the arterioles and capillaries are, possibly more than any other changes, responsible for the clinical picture of SLE. Fibrinoid change appears in the intima, with narrowing of the lumen of the vessel. The formation of new collagen adds to this tendency. Further, the endothelial cells of small arterioles and blood vessels are almost always swollen and thickened. Despite these changes, thrombosis is surprisingly uncommon.

ORGAN CHANGES

Heart. All elements of the heart may be affected in SLE. Fibrinoid deposition occurs in the pericardium, the surrounding reaction leading to chronic pericarditis. In the myocardium, fibrinoid deposition leads to a focal myocarditis with fibrosis and atrophy of myocardial fibres, sometimes leading to cardiac failure. On the endocardium vegetations are occasionally found, usually on the valves, especially the mitral. These superficially resemble those of bacterial endocarditis. This so-called *Libman-Sacks* endocarditis rarely leads to flow disturbances, but may itself become infected.

Kidneys. The mildest lesion is confined mainly to the renal endothelial cells, the capillary basement membrane being thickened. There may also be mild proliferation of cells within the glomerular tuft. These changes may affect only a few glomeruli, or only a part of each glomerulus. At this stage the lesion may pass unnoticed clinically, and be picked up only on renal biopsy. It is reversible.

If epithelial cells are heavily involved, the renal lesion becomes irreversible. Depending on the stage at which the kidney is examined, all grades of damage may be found. Glomeruli, tubules, and interstitium are involved. The changes are numerous and include local necrosis with obliteration of capillaries, fibrinoid change, increase in cellularity, and haematoxylin bodies. A characteristic finding is the *wire-loop* change, so-called because the fibrinoid change affecting capillary walls in the glomerulus causes the thickened loops to stand out prominently. The final picture is often indistinguishable from chronic glomerulonephritis with widespread glomerular and secondary tubular damage.

There is good evidence that the damage to the glomerular basement membrane results from the deposition in it of immune (antigen/antibody) complexes and complement.

Skin. There is an increase in keratin, with plugging of hair follicles, vacuolar degeneration in the basement layer, vascular changes, and infiltration of the dermis with lymphocytes.

Other organs. Similar changes may occur in most organs of the body. In *joints* fibrinoid appears in the synovium and is associated with a mild plasma cell and lymphocyte inflammatory response in the loose connective tissue of synovial villi. The only finding specific for SLE is the presence of haematoxylin bodies.

The *lungs* are affected both by pulmonary vascular changes and pneumonitis, with thickening of the alveolar septa. The *lymph nodes* are enlarged but usually preserve their normal architecture. The *liver* frequently escapes being affected, or shows only a mild perihepatitis. Fibrinoid has been found in the *meningeal* and *cerebral vessels*, as well as in the vessels supplying *peripheral nerves*. In addition to this, non-specific changes, including demyelination and gliosis, are frequently seen in the *central nervous system*.

CLINICAL FEATURES

The widespread tissue involvement in SLE permits an enormous number of possible clinical permutations. The diagnosis depends largely on the recognition that a multi-system disease is present, and on a knowledge of the more common patterns with which the disease presents (Fig. 9.3).

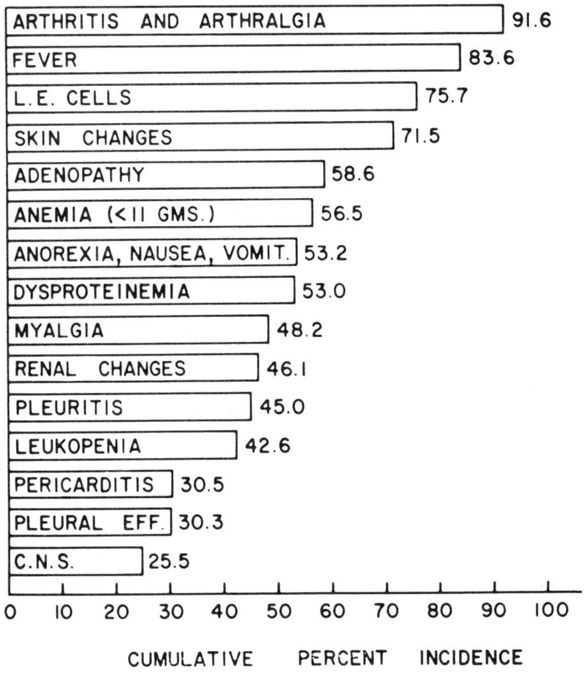

FIGURE 9.3 Commonest clinical manifestations. 520 cases of systemic lupus erythematosus (*From* Dubois, E. L. *Lupus Erythematosus.* McGraw-Hill, New York, 1966)

Faced with only a few features of the disease, the physician can often be helped by one or two clues. *Fever* is particularly common and may antedate the presenting complaint by many months. In addition, there may be a long history of *drug sensitivity* or of *joint pains*, or a few *low white cell counts* may be found in the patient's medical record.

JOINTS

Far and away the most common complaint in SLE is joint pain, and the rheumatologist is often the first to be presented with the diagnostic problem of this disease.

Commonest is a mild flitting arthralgia, often mistaken for early rheumatoid arthritis or rheumatic fever. As with light and drug sensitivity, the patient may give a history of such pains going back over many years, perhaps dismissed as 'fibrositis' or 'rheumatism'. Many, however, progress to a more serious polyarthritis. True synovitis is common. It tends to be periodic, and rarely causes underlying cartilage destruction. Any joints may be involved, especially the hands, wrists, knees, and ankles.

Permanent deformity occurs in up to one-third of patients; while this resembles rheumatoid arthritis in some respects, it differs in that true X-ray erosions are extremely rare.

In large joints, especially the hip or the knee, aseptic necrosis of bone may occur. This is possibly secondary to arteritis; it may certainly be hastened by steroid therapy.

SKIN

The skin manifestations of SLE are frequent and variable (*see* Table 9.1). The classical erythematous rash across the bridge of the nose and the cheeks ('butterfly rash') is the commonest change (Fig. 9.4). Worth pointing out, however, is the frequency of hair changes – sometimes leading to total baldness. In milder form, the hair resembles that in myxoedema, being coarse and dry, but later there is a tendency for hair to fracture, with loss particularly in the frontal region.

Subcutaneous nodules do occur but are rare.

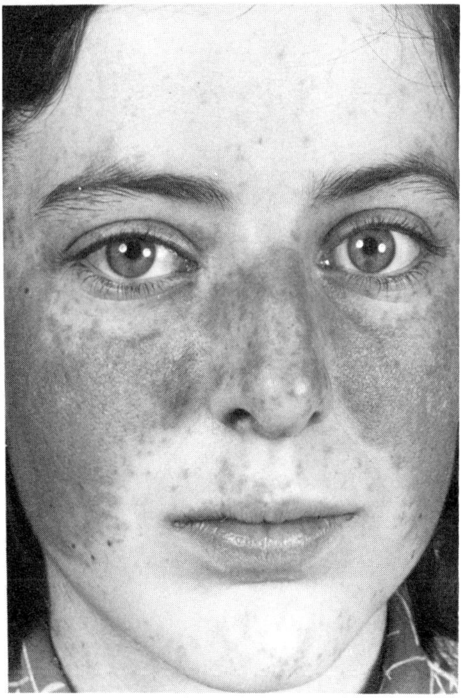

FIGURE 9.4 Facies in SLE

TABLE 9.1

*Systemic Lupus Erythematosus—Cutaneous Manifestations**
(520 patients)

	Per cent
Butterfly blush	36·7
Photosensitivity	32·7
Chronic discoid lesions	28·6
Alopecia, nonscarring	21·3
Butterfly eruption	20·9
Petechiae, purpura, and ecchymoses	19·8
Maculopapular lesions, non-specific	19·0
Raynaud's phenomenon	18·4
Conjunctivitis	10·0
Maculopapular lesions, sun-exposed areas	9·1
Mucous-membrane lesions	9·1
Diffuse hyperpigmentation	8·4
Urticaria	6·9
Erythema, articular	6·5
Fractured frontal hair	5·6
Leg ulcer	5·6
Subcutaneous nodules	5·0
Periorbital oedema	4·8
Thrombophlebitis	4·6
Facial oedema	4·6
Jaundice	3·8
Alopecia, scarring	3·6
Pruritus, marked	2·8
Gangrene, digital	1·3
Palatal erythema	1·3
Periungual erythema	1·1
Bullae	0·4

* (*From* Dubois, E. L. (1966) *Lupus Erythematosus*. New York: McGraw-Hill)

HEART

The most common cardiac manifestation of SLE is pericarditis; this may be so mild as to be missed, but probably occurs in up to one-third of all patients. In fact, ECG changes consistent with pericarditis are found in the majority of patients at some time during the course of their disease. The clinical picture is usually that of a 'dry' painful pericarditis, producing a pericardial friction rub, though large effusions may also occur.

It has become increasingly recognised that myocardial disease is frequent in SLE. This commonly produces little more than cardiac enlargement recognised by radiography, but may sometimes lead to arhythmias and even signs of cardiac failure, although the latter may be due largely to hypertension, anaemia, or pericardial tamponade.

Libman-Sacks endocarditis is usually haemodynamically insignificant, and is not easily diagnosed in life. Murmurs are frequently heard in SLE, often in the absence of any anatomical proof of endocarditis, and are an unreliable guide to its diagnosis.

PERIPHERAL VASCULAR SYSTEM

While many of the visceral changes in SLE are themselves due to vasculitis, more obvious evidence of blood vessel disease may be present. Raynaud's phenomenon is common, though not as prominent as in scleroderma. Occasionally, peripheral vascular disease can be extremely serious, resulting in gangrene and loss of digits, or even limbs. Less serious vascular disturbances include livedo reticularis, chronic leg ulcers, and recurrent thrombophlebitis.

RESPIRATORY SYSTEM

Pleura. Clinically detectable pleurisy develops in approximately half of all cases of SLE, and most of these develop effusions. A point worth remembering is that such an effusion may be the first manifestation of the disease. The fluid is clear yellow, and the effusions are rarely very large.

Lungs. Despite the frequency of pathological pneumonitis in this disease, X-ray changes are comparatively uncommon. Plate-like areas of atelectasis are sometimes seen and 'antibiotic resistant pneumonia' occasionally suggests the diagnosis. Dyspnoea, when it occurs, is more commonly due to pleural or pericardial effusions. Respiratory function tests may be abnormal, even early in the disease, and provide a useful ancillary investigation. The picture is one of diffusion block, associated with a reduced vital capacity, the latter especially being found if there is X-ray evidence of lung involvement.

KIDNEYS

While changes are found in the kidneys of almost all patients dying of this disease, correlation of the clinical findings with the degree of renal damage is often difficult. Generally, definite evidence of renal disease affects the prognosis profoundly.

The commonest urinary abnormality is proteinuria, occurring in about 50 per cent of patients with the disease. This may become gross, with the patient losing as much as 10 G protein a day, and presenting the full nephrotic syndrome, sometimes with extreme oedema which may be very resistant to treatment. In addition, red cells and granular and hyaline casts are found in the urine with increasing frequency as the disease progresses. The patient may develop acute renal failure, requiring dialysis, or may progress more insidiously to chronic renal failure and uraemia.

Hypertension is a common and serious complication of SLE. It is almost invariably secondary to renal damage. Its presence always raises the question of whether or not steroids should be withheld. Acute rises in blood pressure are certainly sometimes seen when steroids are introduced in SLE, although these are rarely as dramatic as in progressive systemic sclerosis (Chapter 8). In general, provided that effective hypotensive therapy is given, hypertension is not necessarily a contra-indication to the use of steroids.

MUSCLES

Muscle pains and tenderness are common, and sometimes there may be true *polymyositis* with wasting and weakness of proximal muscles. This diagnosis can be established by serum enzyme determinations, electromyography, or muscle biopsy (*see* Chapter 8). Some fall-out in muscle bulk and weakness may also occur due to *myopathy* secondary to corticosteroid (or, rarely, chloroquine) therapy.

A rare but very interesting association is the occurrence of both SLE and *myasthenia* in a patient with a tumour of the thymus gland (thymoma).

NERVOUS SYSTEM

It is no exaggeration to say that almost any neurological picture may result from SLE, and that none is particularly diagnostic. Especially important is the recognition of psychosis. In some studies as many as 20 per cent of patients suffered from episodes of psychosis, varying from mild behavioural abnormalities to gross psychotic episodes, indistinguishable from florid schizophrenia.

These attacks are probably due to organic brain damage, the most frequent pathological change being cerebral arteritis. Psychotic episodes in SLE were recognised before the introduction of corticosteroids, and have conclusively been proved to be distinct from so-called steroid psychosis. This point is important as a *psychotic episode in a patient on steroids for active SLE is a clear indication for raising the dosage of steroids rather than for their withdrawal.*

Other CNS manifestations include peripheral neuropathy, myelopathy, epilepsy, hemiplegia, vertigo, and choreiform movements. In the CSF there may be a small rise in cells (usually lymphocytes) and in protein.

RETICULOENDOTHELIAL SYSTEM

The spleen is sometimes palpable, though rarely is it grossly enlarged. More common is lymphadenopathy, and while lymph node biopsy appearances are non-specific, this investigation is sometimes useful in the differentiation from a reticulosis.

EYES

A number of ophthalmological complications are recognised. The most important are the association with Sjögren's syndrome (*see* Chapter 10) and the occurrence of *cytoid bodies* (Fig. 9.5). These are fluffy white exudates that occur in the nerve fibre layer of the retina and are indistinguishable from the exudates of hypertension or diabetes.

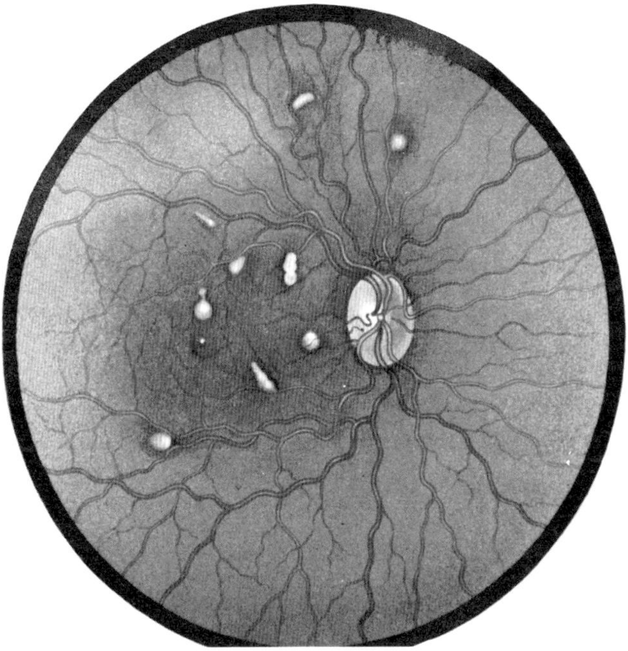

FIGURE 9.5 Cytoid bodies (Courtesy Professor J. Ledingham)

ALIMENTARY SYSTEM

Gastro-intestinal symptoms are particularly common and variable, and include anorexia, nausea, diarrhoea, gastro-intestinal bleeding, and abdominal pain.

Abdominal pain and tenderness, sometimes amounting to an 'acute abdomen', are not uncommon in SLE and may be due to a wide variety of lesions, including arteritis, peritonitis, perisplenitis and perihepatitis, gastro-intestinal infections, pancreatitis (secondary to arteritis), and cholecystitis (secondary to gall stones resulting from haemolytic anaemia). In addition, patients on corticosteroid drugs are liable to the gastric complications of this form of therapy.

LIVER

Although the liver is often slightly enlarged, liver damage is surprisingly rare in SLE. The organ may be involved by arteritis or perihepatitis, but jaundice, if it occurs, is usually due to haemolytic anaemia.

RELATIONSHIP TO 'LUPOID HEPATITIS' (active chronic hepatitis)

This rather uncommon liver disease occurs predominantly in young women (80 per cent) and is characterised by recurring jaundice and a marked increase in serum gamma globulin. The liver is initially enlarged. Clinically, the picture is one of recurrent hepatitis (anorexia, jaundice, abdominal pain) and of endocrine disturbances. A well-marked feature is the large number of spider naevi found. The serum transaminase level is generally high (SGOT: 300–500 units) and the gamma globulin level is usually between 2 and 8 G/100 ml. Pathologically there is marked liver cell necrosis, plasma cell infiltration, and fibrosis. Some of these patients are found to have a positive LE-cell test (hence the term 'lupoid hepatitis'). In addition, many clinical similarities to SLE have been noted, particulary arthralgia (in half the cases), enlarged spleen, rashes, pleurisy, and haemolytic anaemia. Clinical renal complications, however, are rare.

These features, together with the predominantly young female distribution, and the finding of positive antinuclear factor and LE-cell tests, has led to protracted debate as to the relationship of the two conditions. At present it seems wise to regard them as two quite separate diseases; although there is no obvious explanation why hepatitis occurring in young females should produce lupus-like and 'autoimmune' features.

SJÖGREN'S SYNDROME

This is described in Chapter 10. SLE is one of the conditions with which Sjögren's syndrome may occur, and even when the syndrome occurs without other evidence of SLE, there is a high incidence of positive ANF and LE-cell tests.

INVESTIGATIONS

ANTINUCLEAR FACTORS AND THE LE-CELL PHENOMENON

These two laboratory tests together form the cornerstone of diagnosis. The antinuclear factor (ANF) is the most useful screening test for SLE, for it is almost invariably positive in active stages of the disease. A negative ANF test makes the diagnosis very unlikely. The only drawback is that it is sometimes positive in other diseases, particularly progressive systemic sclerosis, Sjögren's syndrome, rheumatoid arthritis, and Still's disease. To complete the list, positive ANF tests have been described in –

Polyarteritis nodosa.
Polymyositis.
Dermatomyositis.
Chronic 'lupoid hepatitis'.
Occasional cases of chronic liver disease.
Hyperglobulinaemic purpura of Waldenstrom.
Myasthenia gravis.
Thymoma.
Hashimoto's thyroiditis and other thyroid disorders.
Pernicious anaemia.
Ulcerative colitis.
Chronic membranous glomerulonephritis.
Lepromatous leprosy.
Tuberculosis (and patients on anti-tuberculous treatment – *see* above).
Diffuse interstitial pulmonary fibrosis.
Lymphoma and lymphosarcoma.
Some normal (especially elderly) persons.

In most of these conditions, however, ANF when found is present only in low titre.

LE-cell Phenomenon. A positive ANF test should automatically lead to a search for LE-cells. Careful searching (if necessary, up to a half a dozen blood smears should be performed) generally reveals a positive test in up to 80 per cent of cases with systemic involvement. LE-cells are also found in chronic active ('lupoid') hepatitis, in 10 per cent of patients with rheumatoid arthritis (*see* below), and in some cases of ulcerative colitis and of leprosy.

Steroid therapy tends to lessen the number of LE-cells found, and high doses almost invariably cause their total disappearance from the blood. Although this is often taken as a guide to the adequacy of steroid dosage, it is somewhat unreliable, since the number of LE-cells does not necessarily reflect the severity of the disease.

ERYTHROCYTE SEDIMENTATION RATE

The ESR is frequently raised, sometimes well above 100 mm/hr (Westergren). Although it is usually lowered by effective treatment, it is not always a useful guide in this respect.

HAEMATOLOGICAL FINDINGS

As with the clinical findings, these are very variable. Haematological abnormalities are common, and may actually be the presenting feature of the disease.

Anaemia is common. Usually, this is a mild non-specific, normochromic anaemia, unless there is an added factor of iron deficiency due to gastro-intestinal blood loss. Less common, but more important, is the *autoimmune type of haemolytic anaemia* which develops because of the appearance within the patient's circulation of antibodies directed against her own red cells. This antibody becomes attached to the surface of the red cell, which it damages, resulting in the removal of the cell from the circulation by the spleen. The antibody is of the IgG class of immunoglobulin, and its presence free in the circulation and attached to the red cells can be shown by the *indirect* and *direct Coombs' tests* respectively.

Autoimmune haemolytic anaemia may be severe and life-threatening. While corticosteroid therapy and even splenectomy can be helpful, some cases are very resistant to treatment. As with thrombocytopaenic purpura, it may occur without any other manifestations of SLE, or be the first evidence of multiple system lupus. It also occurs in association with other disorders of the reticuloendothelial system.

Leucopenia is also common. It often affects especially the lymphocytic series, and it may be persistent or variable. A review of the case notes of any patient with SLE will generally reveal at least one white cell count between 2,000–4,000 mm^3. However, steroid therapy, as well as the frequent infections to which these patients are prone, are able to induce a leucocytosis.

Thrombocytopenia occurs less commonly but may be very severe, and again thrombocytopenic purpura may be the presenting sign of the disease. For this reason a diagnosis of 'idiopathic thrombocytopenic purpura' carries the reservation that the disease may later turn out to be SLE. Both the leucopenia and the thrombocytopenia of SLE may well be mediated by the type of autoantibody responsible for the haemolytic anaemia, but directed in these instances against the leucocytes and the platelets respectively.

Coagulation defects due to circulating anticoagulants are among the rarer manifestations of SLE.

PLASMA PROTEINS AND ELECTROPHORESIS

The gamma globulin level is almost always raised, while the albumin level is generally lowered. Serum electrophoresis, however, gives no specific pattern in SLE.

SERUM COMPLEMENT

Many of the antigen-antibody reactions (for instance the LE-cell phenomenon) take up complement from the serum. Though not yet performed routinely, estimation of serum complement activity may prove to be a useful investigation. There is a tendency to lowered serum complement activity in SLE (as opposed to RA where it is normal or high). When there is renal involvement in SLE very low levels may be found.

OTHER SEROLOGICAL CHANGES

A wide range of antibodies (mainly 'autoantibodies') may be found in the serum of patients suffering from SLE. These include the factor responsible for the Wassermann reaction, and antibodies against globulin (rheumatoid factors), thyroid and muscle, as well as the more specific antibodies already mentioned.

BIOPSY

Renal Biopsy. Renal biopsy is relatively simple to perform, but carries a definite slight risk. It is carried out only when the result is likely to contribute information relevant to planning therapy. For establishing a specific diagnosis of lupus nephritis it is often not particularly helpful, the histological changes not infrequently being indistinguishable from other types of glomerulonephritis. Renal biopsy finds its main usefulness in establishing whether, in a known case of SLE, there is histological nephritis and, if there is, its degree of severity. This is fundamental to prognosis.

Skin Biopsy. Skin biopsy may be diagnostic, and is of value if the disease presents with an atypical skin rash.

Muscle Biopsy. Muscle biopsy will reveal whether there is any evidence of polymyositis. A proximal muscle is chosen (and the track of electrodiagnostic needles must be avoided!).

DIFFERENTIAL DIAGNOSIS

Just as the list of organs and systems involved by lupus is seemingly endless, so also is the list of diseases with which it may be confused. Possibly even more than syphilis, SLE is a mimic and a test of diagnostic skill.

The florid case is unmistakable. The young, toxic, febrile woman with the characteristic facial rash, leucopenia, joint pains, and palpable spleen should invariably lead to the finding of LE-cells in the peripheral blood.

Similarly, the patient with a long history of drug or photosensitivity and nephrotic syndrome, or the woman with haemolytic anaemia, pleurisy, Raynaud's phenomenon, and skin and hair changes should be equally quickly diagnosed.

Diagnosis is often more difficult in the insidious case, or in the older patient, and may depend on a prolonged search for LE-cells.

Some diagnostic situations are difficult. A patient with lymphadenopathy, fever, and splenomegaly may be misdiagnosed as having a reticulosis, septicaemia, or miliary tuberculosis. One with pleural effusions and mental changes may be diagnosed as carcinoma of the lung. The person with neurological changes and a positive Wassermann reaction may be diagnosed as syphilitic, and given penicillin.

In childhood, the disease may be mistaken for viral pneumonitis, rheumatoid arthritis, or rheumatic fever, depending on the organs involved. Sarcoidosis may be diagnosed, especially if there are chest X-ray changes, lymphadenopathy, splenomegaly, and atypical skin changes.

Perhaps the most difficult differential diagnosis is from other members of the group of so-called connective tissue disorders, especially as the ANF and LE-cell tests may be positive in the other members of the group. Conditions such as progressive systemic sclerosis and polymyositis may so overlap with SLE that a sharp differentiation is not always possible. The most important diagnostic problem within this group is the differentiation of SLE and rheumatoid arthritis.

SLE AND RHEUMATOID ARTHRITIS (RA)

Occasionally, the differentiation between these two diseases may be difficult. The complications of RA include not only arteritis, neuropathy, and leucopenia, but pulmonary, pleural, pericardial, and even cardiac involvement, which may all add up to a picture closely resembling SLE. The development of the LE-cell test has not resolved this difficulty, for some one in ten patients with RA will be found to have a positive test. Indeed, it is just this group that is particularly liable to the visceral manifestations just mentioned, and it is in these patients, where one disease appears to shade into the other, that the differential diagnosis may be difficult, or impossible.

Is it important to differentiate? It might be argued that both diseases are part of a spectrum and that some examples of RA develop into a picture indistinguishable from SLE. For the clinician, however, working rules are essential. SLE, in general, is a serious, commonly fatal disease, often ending in renal failure. Rheumatoid arthritis, in itself, is rarely fatal. Table 9.2 lists some of the differences between the two diseases.

In our experience the most useful guide has been the presence or absence of radiographic erosions. Though there are exceptions to the rule, if erosions are present the diagnosis is almost certainly RA.

TREATMENT

GENERAL MANAGEMENT

Lupus may be a protracted and serious disease, the patient's existence sometimes appearing to consist of a series of medical crises. The age incidence of the disease is such that it often strikes tragically at the young mother or breadwinner.

TABLE 9.2

SLE and Rheumatoid Arthritis

	SLE	RA
Age of onset (years)	20–40	All ages
Sex incidence (F:M)	9:1	3:1
Morning stiffness	Moderate	Prominent
Arthritis	Mild	Severe
Erosions	Rare	Common
Fever	Common	Rare
Skin rashes	Common	Rare
Subcutaneous nodules	Rare	Common
Renal involvement	Common	Primary renal involvement rare
Cytoid bodies	Sometimes present	Absent
Autoimmune haemolytic anaemia	Common	Rare
ANF positive	99%	Up to 50%
LE-cells	80–100%	10–20%
Pregnancy remission	No	Yes
Histology	Usually differentiates	

The emotional problems are great. It has been estimated that 50 per cent of married women with SLE obtain divorces. The high incidence of psychotic episodes, alopecia, skin changes, and steroid side effects must in themselves lower the patient's tolerance to the physical pain of the disease.

The many facets of SLE will each need separate consideration. Thus, the hypertension or renal failure will need treatment in their own right; the Raynaud's phenomenon may lead to peripheral gangrene that may require surgery; rarely, a constricting pericardial effusion will require tapping. The frequency with which superinfection occurs means a careful watch for this, and its immediate treatment.

One question about which the patient may seek advice is that of the advisability of embarking on a pregnancy. The effect of pregnancy on the mother is variable, and the presence of SLE is itself not a contra-indication to pregnancy unless there is definite renal disease, or serious cardiac involvement. Foetal mortality is higher than normal, but some 60 per cent of pregnancies will produce a live infant. Congenital malformations do not appear to be associated with corticosteroid therapy, which should be continued during pregnancy when necessary.

DRUG THERAPY

Corticosteroids. Corticosteroid preparations form the basis of the drug treatment of SLE. Their effects are often dramatic, and they may be life-saving. Most of the symptoms and signs will disappear within two weeks if dosage is adequate. This, in turn, depends on the clinical state of the patient. The absolute indications for steroids include the patient critically ill in a general sense, the pericardial effusion threatening tamponade critical thrombocytopenic purpura or haemolytic anaemia, and the psychotic episode signalling the threat of a possibly fatal cerebral arteritis For these emergencies, up to 100 mg of prednisone a day may have to be used.

Less reliable indications are the myocardial and renal lesions. Myocarditis often fails to respond to steroid therapy alone, and the value of steroids in renal lupus is still disputed. The patient with early uraemia often responds to a course of 20 to 40 mg prednisolone daily for two to three months, though there is little to suggest that steroids halt the progress of the kidney pathology.

The frequent necessity for prolonged high dosage steroids means that the physician is in the invidious position of trying to balance the high morbidity and mortality from these drugs against the serious but far less predictable effects of the disease itself.

There seems to be little doubt that the long-term prognosis is improved by steroids, though to what extent this is so it is impossible to say. While it is clear that high-dosage prednisolone can damp-down life-threatening complications and so keep the patient alive until the disease goes into remission again, what is not clear is whether lower doses given at other times, and titrated against evidence of disease activity, favourably influence the prognosis.

Salicylates. In the mild case, or during remission, symptoms may be controlled by aspirin alone. The arthralgia and fever generally respond to 3 to 4 G a day, but the more serious systemic changes are unaffected.

Indomethacin and Phenylbutazone. The same applies to these drugs, which may be substituted for the patient intolerant of salicylates.

Chloroquine Compounds. Since 1951, chloroquine has been used widely and successfully in the management of SLE. It may be effective in controlling the skin changes and is sometimes dramatic in relieving the joint syptoms. It has little use in the management of the systemic disease Unfortunately, the relapse rate is high following cessation of the drug, and retinal damage is common following its prolonged use (*see* p. 47).

Immunosuppressive Therapy. Drugs such as cyclophosphamide and azathioprine are being increasingly tried in all disorders thought to have an immunological basis. In SLE the results are mixed, but on the whole fairly encouraging. Certainly, in a few patients the steroid requirements fall when this form of therapy is added, and occasionally a patient with nephrotic syndrome resistant to all other therapy responds to these drugs. Great care is necessary in the administration of these agents, and their use should still be regarded as experimental.

COURSE AND PROGNOSIS

Until the use of the LE-cell test became standard, the prognosis was thought to be uniformly poor. The average life span from time of diagnosis was three years, and many instances occurred of patients with catastrophic spread of disease dying within a month of diagnosis.

It is now recognised, however, that this group of patients represents the severe end of a spectrum, at the other end of which are patients with one or two features of the disease only, who can expect a normal life span.

For all patients the advent of corticosteroid drugs has improved the prognosis. It is difficult to compare pre-steroid and post-steroid figures, but now, patients who might previously have died during exacerbations of the disease can be kept alive until remission occurs.

In those with clinically obvious renal involvement the prognosis is poorer and depends directly on the degree of such involvement. It is also worse in those diagnosed within two years of the onset of symptoms, such patients presumably suffering a more stormy course.

For the remainder, the earlier diagnosis, the carefully regulated steroid therapy, and advances in the control of individual complications have meant that the physician can now give a hopeful prognosis in what was, until recently, a dread disease.

10

Sjögren's Syndrome

Colin G Barnes

Sjögren's syndrome (SS) is define as a combination of *keratoconjunctivitis sicca* (dry eyes), *xerostomia* (dry mouth), and a *connective tissue disorder*, of which rheumatoid arthritis is the most common. It is accepted that the syndrome may be diagnosed when only two of these features are present. Thus, the eye and mouth manifestations may be present in the absence of any generalised connective tissue disorder. This is then known as the *sicca syndrome*.

CLINICAL FEATURES

The clinical features of the 'sicca' components of the syndrome result from a failure of mucous gland secretions affecting particularly the salivary and lachrymal glands. Usually, the affected glands remain normal in size but they may become enlarged and firm, although not tender. Females are affected more commonly than males in a ratio of about 9:1.

Eyes. The main symptoms are grittiness and soreness of the eyes due to reduction of lachrymal secretions. Rather surprisingly, however, the patient will often not have appreciated her reduced capacity to produce tears. This dryness of the eye may lead to conjunctivitis, corneal erosions or fibrillary keratitis, with blurring of vision. Rarely, the outcome may be severe impairment of vision or even blindness.

Gastro-intestinal Tract. While dryness of mouth is the most important gastro-intestinal feature, diminution of gastric and pancreatic secretions have also been described. Discomfort and dryness of the mouth may be sufficiently severe to cause difficulty in swallowing. On close questioning it is apparent that this is due to difficulty in forming a food bolus because, owing to the lack of lubrication, the food sticks to the palate, tongue, and teeth. The lips-and tongue become smooth, dry and painful, and fissured cracks that are slow to heal may appear. The gastric and pancreatic 'dryness' rarely produce clinically recognisable abnormalities.

Respiratory Tract. In common with other mucous glands, those of the nose, pharynx, larynx, and bronchial mucosa are also affected. Thus, nasal and pharyngeal irritation may occur, together with episodes of sinusitis, laryngitis, and tracheitis. There is an increased predisposition to chest infections.

The Kidneys. A variety of renal tubular defects have been described in patients with SS. Most commonly this amounts only to a reduced capacity to acidify the urine following an oral acid load. Occasionally, however, the full clinical picture of renal tubular acidosis and/or nephrogenic diabetes insipidus may occur. Amino-aciduria is not a feature.

The mechanism of this tubular defect is unknown. Somewhat similar changes may occur in patients with systemic lupus erythematosus or myelomatosis, and it has been suggested that the pathogenesis is related to the hyperglobulinaemia common to these conditions.

Genital Tract. Vaginal dryness may lead to atrophic vaginitis and dyspareunia.

Other less common clinical features are lymphadenopathy, sometimes of considerable degree (*see* below), splenomegaly, and peripheral neuropathy. An increased tendency to allergic reactions to drugs has been recorded, particularly to gold salts and penicillin. Skin dryness is common, and an unexplained, non-thrombocytopenic purpura may also occur.

PATHOLOGY

The specific pathological changes of SS are confined to the mucus secreting glands. In the early stages of the disease the glands may be enlarged. This is due to an inflammatory reaction with extensive infiltration by lymphocytes and plasma cells, mainly concentrated around the ducts, together with oedema of the parenchyma.

Subsequently, the glands shrink as the acini atrophy and the normal architecture is lost. Fibrosis follows, narrowing the lumen of the ducts. It is uncertain whether the loss of acinar pattern is due to the inflammatory process itself, or whether it is secondary to back-pressure behind blocked ducts.

Proliferation of the duct cells occurs, and the infiltrating lymphocytes become aggregated into follicles with germinal centres. Thus, the final picture is a small disorganised, fibrotic gland with lymphoid follicles and islands of proliferated duct epithelium surrounded by lymphocytes ('epi-myoepithelial islands').

Generalised lymphoid hyperplasia is not uncommon, and there is an increased incidence of conditions such as reticulum cell sarcoma. Cases have been reported which, on histological grounds, appeared to be examples of widespread malignant lymphomata, but which went into complete remission on corticosteroid therapy. Into what pathological category these 'pseudo-lymphomata' should be placed is not yet clear.

The pathology of associated connective tissue disorders (e.g. rheumatoid arthritis) does not differ from the changes seen in these conditions occurring without the features of SS.

ASSOCIATION WITH OTHER CONDITIONS

Approximately one-third of patients with SS are found to have the sicca components alone, without evidence of other connective tissue disorders. Rheumatoid arthritis is the most commonly associated condition, being found in half the patients with kerato-conjunctivitis sicca and/or xerostomia. Conversely, in patients with rheumatoid arthritis the incidence of SS is between 10 and 15 per cent. The association with rheumatoid arthritis is limited to patients with positive tests for rheumatoid factor and with longstanding joint involvement. However, there does not seem to be any particular correlation with the activity of the synovitis, since many cases of SS develop in patients in whom the articular manifestations of the disease appear to have burnt out.

The remaining 20 per cent of cases of SS are associated with a variety of other disorders, including progressive systemic sclerosis, polymyositis, Hashimoto's thyroiditis, and systemic lupus erythematosus.

SPECIAL INVESTIGATIONS

Serological Tests. Rheumatoid factor tests are positive in over three-quarters of the patients, some estimates being as high as 97 per cent. When the sicca syndrome occurs alone, or in association with rheumatoid arthritis, the test is invariably positive.

Antinuclear antibodies are found in the serum of two-thirds of patients with SS. Only a minority of these patients show evidence of having systemic lupus erythematosus.

LE-cell tests are positive in some 15 per cent of patients with SS.

Other antibodies found are those reacting with salivary duct cells (in approximately 50 per cent of these patients) and against thyroglobulin (in approximately 35 per cent).

The Eye. Schirmer's test is designed to measure the rate of secretion of tears. Two strips of filter paper 5 mm wide are folded 3 to 4 mm from one end; one is hooked into each of the lower conjunctival sacs, then left in position with the eyes lightly closed for five minutes. The length of the paper along which tears have soaked is measured from the fold and should normally exceed 15 mm. In practice, there is rarely any difficulty in interpreting the results since either the 15 mm length is achieved well within the time limit, or at the end of five minutes only a few millimetres of wetness are seen.

Rose Bengal dye or *fluorescein* instilled into the conjunctival sac will reveal the superficial corneal erosions typical of kerato-conjunctivitis sicca.

Slit lamp examination may enable strands of mucus and corneal epithelium to be seen adhering to the cornea and bulbar conjunctiva. This is the *filamentary keratitis* characteristic of SS. When much of this mucus material is present it may be seen macroscopically or with the aid of a hand lens, using light directed tangentially to the cornea.

Plasma Proteins. In most cases globulin levels are raised, particularly the gamma components. This may be associated with hypoalbuminaemia.

Haematology. Haematological changes are usually unimpressive. There may be a mild normochromic, normocytic anaemia, a leucopenia affecting both neutrophil and lymphocyte series, or an absolute eosinophilia.

Sialography. Sialography is rarely indicated. When performed it shows dilatation of the smaller-sized ducts (sialectasis) with the formation of sizeable cavities. *Salivary flow rates* can also be measured, and show considerably reduced values compared with controls.

AETIOLOGY

SS occupies a position in the spectrum of immunologically determined diseases midway between those characterised by organ specific antibodies (e.g. Hashimoto's thyroiditis) and those with non-organ specific antibodies (e.g. systemic lupus erythematosus). It can be classified as one of the former group on the grounds that the pathological changes are confined to mucus secreting glands and that salivary autoantibodies are present. On the other hand, it frequently occurs in association with conditions such as rheumatoid arthritis and systemic lupus erythematosus.

DIFFERENTIAL DIAGNOSIS

In practice, most cases of SS are mild, and the condition has to be differentiated from other causes of irritable eyes in rheumatoid subjects. Reliance cannot be placed on the patients' subjective impression of tear production; this should be measured by the Schirmer test. Reduced tear secretion and characteristic appearances with the Rose Bengal or slit-lamp examinations establish the diagnosis.

Occasionally, SS produces a localised swelling in one salivary gland. This has to be differentiated from a neoplasm (mixed parotid tumour or carcinoma). Ophthalmological examination, serological testing, and the presence or absence of a generalised connective tissue disorder, will usually clarify the diagnosis. However, biopsy may be necessary.

Diffuse enlargement of salivary and lachrymal glands with reduced secretions may be produced by leukaemic or lymphomatous infiltration – the so-called *Mickulicz's syndrome*. (The terminology is confused because SS was at one time referred to as Mickulicz's *disease*.) *Sarcoidosis* may produce a similar picture. Differentiation between these conditions and SS is usually clear from other features of the diseases but, again, biopsy may be necessary.

PROGNOSIS

SS usually remains a benign condition, producing no more than discomfort in the form of a dry, gritty sensation in the eyes, and a dry mouth occuring during the course of rheumatoid arthritis.

However, in a minority of cases the syndrome progresses to severe ocular damage – corneal ulceration and opacity – recurrent upper and lower respiratory tract infections, and severe dryness and cracking of the buccal mucosa, with the difficulty in swallowing already described. The development of a malignant reticulosis, 'pseudolymphoma' or peripheral neuropathy is rare. Amyloid disease has also been recorded during the course of SS both in those with and those without an associated rheumatic disorder.

TREATMENT

Treatment is largely symptomatic. Ocular symptoms may be relieved by the regular and frequent use of 1 per cent methyl-cellulose eye drops – 'artificial tears'. Unfortunately, the effect of these is very shortlived. Spectacle frames fitted with reservoirs of methyl-cellulose and capillary tubes for constantly wetting the conjunctival sac via the inner canthus are being developed at present. Dryness of the mouth may be temporarily relieved by the use of glycerine mouth washes. Respiratory tract infections require treatment along conventional lines.

There is no evidence that corticosteroid drugs have any beneficial effect in SS, except for the very rare 'pseudolymphoma'.

The treatment of any associated rheumatic disease need not be modified because of the presence of SS.

11

Crystal Deposition Diseases – Gout and Pyrophosphate Arthropathy (Pseudogout)

H L F Currey

In both the conditions described in this chapter, a metabolic product is laid down in crystalline form in or around the joints. This may cause an arthropathy in one of two ways: either the crystals enter the joint space to provoke an acute *crystal synovitis*, or the presence of this crystalline material within articular cartilage leads to chronic degenerative changes.

In gout, the responsible crystals are known to be urate, while in pseudogout they consist of calcium pyrophosphate dihydrate. These two conditions are, therefore, grouped together as the *crystal deposition diseases*, subdivided into *type urate* and *type pyrophosphate*.

Less formally, while 'gout' remains a convenient clinical description for the one, neither 'pseudogout' nor 'chondrocalcinosis' is really satisfactory for the other. We would suggest *pyrophosphate arthropathy* as the most generally useful term for this condition.

Gout

The term *gout* defines an arthropathy resulting from the deposition of urate crystals in and around joints. It is but one hazard of a sustained abnormally high level of uric acid in the plasma (hyperuricaemia). Plasma uric acid (PUA) levels depend on the interaction of many different variables, and whether or not hyperuricaemia leads to the joint involvement that we call gout probably depends both on the degree and on the duration of PUA elevation.

PURINE METABOLISM AND HYPERURICAEMIA

Uric acid is a divalent weak organic acid with pK_a values of 5·75 and 10·30. It has the following formula:

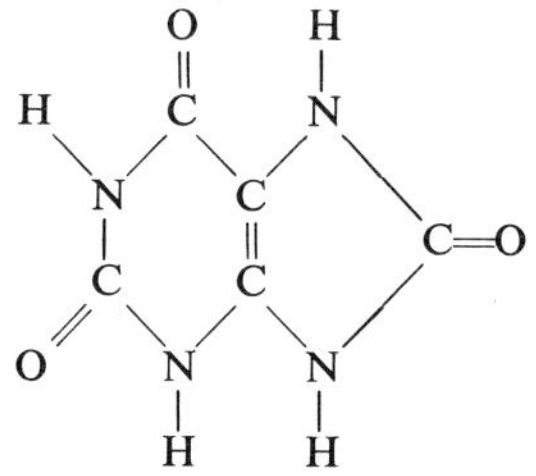

In the body it exists either as uric acid itself or as a monourate salt, depending on the local pH. Uric acid is produced by the degradation of the purine bases adenine and guanine (constituents of nucleic acids and nucleotides) according to the following scheme –

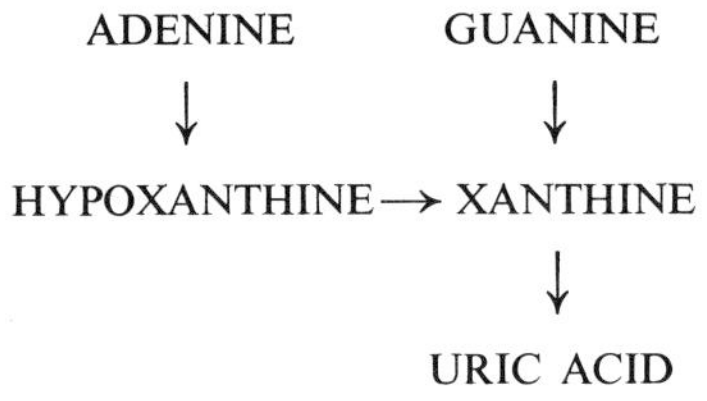

In lower mammals this sequence is carried a stage further by the enzyme *uricase*, converting uric acid to *allantoin*, which is then rapidly eliminated through the kidneys. Man, however, has suffered an apparently disadvantageous evolutionary mutation resulting in the loss of uricase, and leaving uric acid as the end-product to be eliminated. To understand the implications of this it is necessary to consider how urate is excreted.

Renal Handling of Urate. In the mammalian kidney, urate, a relatively small molecule mostly not bound to protein, is freely filtered through the glomerulus. It is then completely (or almost completely) reabsorbed in the proximal tubules by a process of active tubular transport. In those species possessing uricase this process is advantageous in that it prevents a relatively insoluble compound entering the distal nephron where increasing urinary concentration might produce precipitation and stone formation; instead, the uric acid is re-circulated, to be acted on by uricase and eliminated as soluble allantoin. In man, however, the loss of uricase has not been accompanied by any compensatory adjustment in renal function, and the reabsorption of urate now means that blood urate must rise to a level at which another process – proximal tubular secretion – operates sufficiently to eliminate the necessary amount of uric acid. (A minor pathway of elimination is excretion into the gut, followed by bacterial uricolysis.) Thus, man achieves a steady state at the expense of relatively high levels of both plasma and urinary urate. Both levels are uncomfortably close to those at which urate precipitates out of these two fluids.

Deposition of Urate. Sustained hyperuricaemia (the critical level is about 7 or 8 mg/100 ml) leads to deposition of urate in the tissues. In severe, longstanding cases the miscible pool of urate may increase from about 1 G to as much as 30 G, and the total urate mass to a much greater quantity. Deposition occurs particularly in relation to avascular tissues: articular cartilage, the pinna of the ear, the olecranon bursa, and tendons generally. The renal parenchyma is another favoured site.

The result of this urate deposition is seen most dramatically in the joints, where crystals may enter the synovial cavity to provoke an *acute synovitis*, or the articular cartilage deposits may lead to *osteoarthrosis*. Larger deposits may be clinically obvious as *tophi*, and renal deposits may be associated with *nephropathy*. Those subjects in whom the urinary urate load also is increased (*hyperuricosuria*) are exposed, in addition, to the risk of *urate urolithiasis*.

The Aetiology of Hyperuricaemia. The total load of urate carried by the plasma (and hence the PUA level), in the simplest terms, depends on the factors illustrated in this scheme –

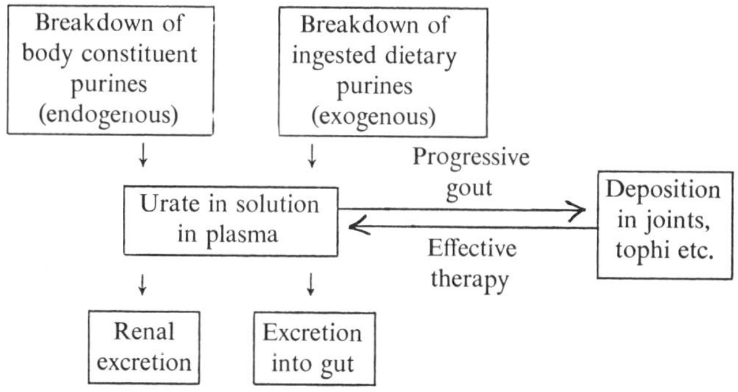

The three important variables determining the PUA level are the rate of endogenous purine breakdown (a reflection of purine turnover), the amount of purines in the diet, and the rate of renal clearance of urate. (The modest gut elimination probably does not vary much.) There is no direct physiological control of PUA levels apart from the influence that this itself has on the rate of tubular secretion, a mechanism which (in this sense) provides only a crude 'spill over', and which is itself influenced by many variables. Hence, the PUA level in an individual at any one time is the result of the interaction of many variable factors. The distribution curve of PUA levels in population samples reflects the interaction of these random influences, and the 'upper limits of normal' (in men about 6, and in women about 5 mg/100 ml) represent only arbitrary points on this curve, indicating levels above which some subjects may develop gout.

It has been customary to divide gout into primary and secondary forms. *Secondary gout* refers to cases in which the underlying hyperuricaemia is due mainly to a single well-defined cause. This may be a condition producing an increased turnover of purines, such as one of the myeloproliferative disorders or other neoplastic disease. Or it may be due to a condition reducing renal urate elimination, such as the chronic administration of thiazide diuretics, or to intrinsic renal disease (although the mode of urate handling by the kidneys is such that gross hyperuricaemia usually occurs only late in renal disease). In *primary gout*, by contrast, the hyperuricaemia is the result of multiple interacting variables. Clearly, such a distinction between primary and secondary forms is somewhat artificial, and hyperuricaemia is always, in a sense, *multifactorial*. Another over-simplification in classifying patients with gout is to divide them into *over-producers* or *under-excretors* of urate. In the former hyperuricaemia is associated with an increased urinary urate output (on a low purine diet the upper limit of normal is about 600 mg/24 hr), while in the latter it is associated with a normal or low output. In practice, a combination of factors often operates, increased urate production being associated with a reduced renal urate clearance.

Control of the Rate of Purine Synthesis. Recent studies into the intermediate metabolism of purines have clarified one mechanism by which patients with 'primary' gout may 'overproduce' uric acid (Fig. 11.1). The first step in *de novo* purine biosynthesis, which is unique to this pathway, is catalysed by the enzyme *phosphoribosyl-pyrophosphate amidotransferase* (PRPP-ATase). Predictably, this is the site of action of a feed-back control mechanism by which the end-products of this biosynthesis (adenine and guanine nucleotides) regulate the rate of their own production. It is now clear that at least some overproducers of uric acid have a deficiency of another enzyme, *hypoxanthine-guanine phosphori-*

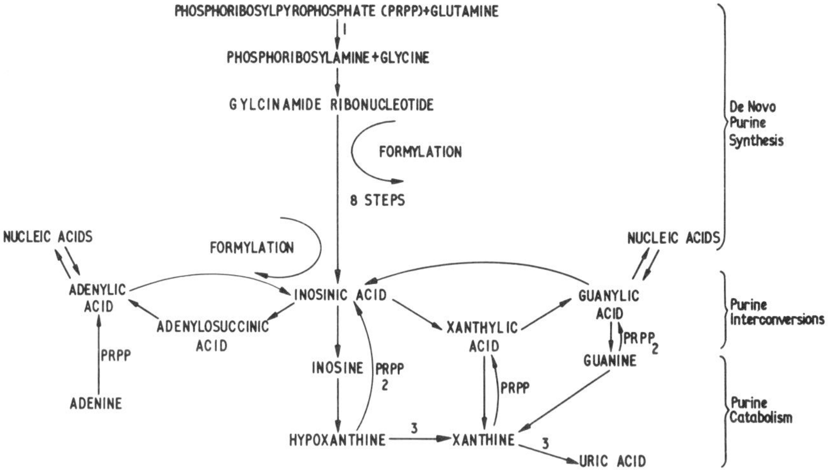

FIGURE 11.1 Some pathways of purine metabolism in man. The sites of action of three enzymes are indicated: (1) Phosphoribosylpyrophosphate amidotransferase (PRPP-ATase), (2) Hypoxanthine-guanine phosphoribosyltransferase (HG-PRTase) and (3) Xanthine oxidase. (*After* Kelley, W. N., Rosenbloom, F. M. and Seegmiller, J. E., *J. Clin. Invest.*, **46**, 1518, 1967)

bosyl-transferase (HG-PRTase). This catalyses the reactions converting hypoxanthine and guanine to their respective nucleotides (Fig. 11.1); reactions which, in a sense, salvage these purines for reutilisation as nucleotides or in nucleic acids, instead of allowing them to be irreversibly degraded to uric acid. A deficiency of HG-PRTase therefore results in wastage of purines along this latter pathway (a so-called *shunt pathway*) which normally operates only for the disposal of purines that are in excess of the body's needs. The consequential reduction in nucleotide production operates via the feed-back mechanism to speed up *de novo* purine synthesis. The end result of HG-PRTase deficiency is, therefore, a greatly increased purine turnover and excessive urate production.

HG-PRTase occurs in many body cells, and can conveniently be assayed in erythrocytes. Complete absence of the enzyme is the cause of the gross hyperuricaemia in children suffering from the rare *Lesch-Nyhan syndrome* (*see* p. 166). Reduced, but not absent, enzyme activity has been found in gouty subjects in whom the disease starts at an earlier age than usual and in whom there may be minor neurological defects (suggesting that this may represent a partial expression of the Lesch-Nyhan syndrome). A simple *screening test* for HG-PRTase deficiency is the determination of the urinary uric acid/creatinine ratio. A figure of 0·76 or over suggests a partial deficiency.

HG-PRTase deficiency also accounts for some variation in the influence of certain drugs on purine metabolism. Both azathioprine (Imuran) and allopurinol (*see* p. 175) reduce the rate of *de novo* purine synthesis in some, but not all, subjects. It is now clear that HG-PRTase is necessary to convert both drugs to their respective nucleotides, in which form they can then inhibit PRPP-ATase, thus operating the feed-back control mechanism. Reduced HG-PRTase activity may therefore account for the failure of these drugs to inhibit purine synthesis.

It is necessary to point out that, at the time of writing, these observations on the intermediate purine metabolism of subjects over-producing uric acid are very recent, and work is currently continuing in this field. Much remains to be explained, and the simplified account given above is likely to require modification in the light of research now in progress.

Other Factors Influencing the Plasma Uric Acid Level. Population surveys show that the distribution of PUA levels vary significantly with sex, age, race, and social grade. In addition, hyperuricaemia tends to run particularly in certain families. The incidence of gout follows a similar pattern. As mentioned above, the PUA level in an individual is the result of the interaction of many variables, although all must operate finally by modifying one of three factors: dietary purine intake, *de novo* purine synthesis, or renal urate clearance. Some of the more important variables have already been mentioned. A number of others are known.

Dietary purine intake exerts a modest influence on PUA levels. Changing from a normal to a 'low purine' diet produces a fall in PUA of about 1·3 mg/100 ml, and vice versa. In general, high income groups tend to have a higher purine intake than low income groups. This factor was probably of much greater significance 200 years ago when gout was 'the rich man's disease'. Today, this is not so, although it remains a commoner disease in affluent than 'developing' countries, with certain exceptions due to racial differences, e.g. it is very common among the Maoris of New Zealand.

Renal urate clearance is highly variable. The mode of handling urate by the kidneys has already been mentioned. It seems likely that, other factors being equal, the basic clearance rate for urate is a genetically determined attribute. However, it can be modified by a great many factors. A number of drugs influence urate clearance. The most obvious examples are the *uricosuric drugs* (such as probenecid – *see* p.174) which paralyse both tubular absorption and tubular secretion of urate, so that most of the filtered load is excreted. *Salicylates* in very large doses have a similar uricosuric effect, but in normal analgesic doses produce selective suppression of tubular secretion. This results in marked urate retention, and is an obvious pitfall in interpreting random PUA determinations. Both *thiazide diuretics* and the anti-tuberculous drug *pyrazinamide* cause urate retention, and continued therapy with either may produce clinical gout. Conditions of *ketosis* produce urate retention, and this is known to be due to β-hydroxybutyrate. Lactic acid has a similar effect. The elevated PUA levels found during starvation and in patients with *glycogen storage disease* are thought to be due to the associated ketosis. Similar effects are probably at least partly the explanation of hyperuricaemia following *alcoholic excess*. Other diseases may influence renal clearance of urate. In primary renal disease the rise in PUA is usually late, and clinical gout is uncommon. *Lead nephropathy* may lead to 'Saturnine gout', and both *hyperparathyroidism* and *hypothyroidism* may reduce renal urate clearance and result in clinical gout. By contrast, certain types of *renal tubular defect* may produce a urate leak and hypouricaemia. *Wilson's disease* is one example.

Purine turnover rate is the third variable. This may be increased by complete or partial lack of the enzyme HG-PRTase, as described above. There may well be other genetically determined variations in intermediate purine metabolism yet to be identified. *Neoplastic diseases* may also increase purine turnover, particularly the *myeloproliferative disorders*, and this effect is exaggerated by any form of therapy that produces cell necrosis. Extensive *psoriasis* may produce hyperuricaemia, presumably by the increased proliferation of epidermal cells, and this may lead to confusion in diagnosis if the patient has *psoriatic arthropathy* (q.v.).

PATHOGENESIS OF ACUTE URATE ARTHROPATHY

Acute gouty arthritis is an inflammatory response to the presence of microcrystalline urate within the synovial fluid. Whether these crystals are precipitated in the fluid *de novo* or arise from ruptured microtophi is uncertain. During an acute attack, many of the crystals lie within leucocytes, and this has led to the widely held view that the urate crystals are phagocytosed by neutrophils which then die and rupture, releasing the enzymes contained within their lysosomes to act as the chemical mediators of the inflammation. Small crystals may possibly be digested by *myeloperoxidase* contained within the leucocytes, but the larger crystals probably kill successive leucocytes as they are ingested in turn by each, leaving a trail of ruptured cells whose lysosomal enzymes add to the inflammatory reaction and call forth more neutrophils. This inflammation is thought to be a non-specific reaction to the physical presence of microcrystals of a critical size, rather than to any chemical irritant properties.

Hence the description *crystal synovitis*. A similar mechanism operates in pyrophosphate arthropathy (*see* below) and also, probably, in the acute reaction that occasionally follows intrasynovial corticosteroid injections. This scheme fails to explain two facts known about gout: firstly, that joints may contain tophaceous deposits of urate actually bathed by synovial fluid, yet never be the site of acute attacks; secondly, that measures such as uricosuric therapy, which rapidly lowers plasma urate levels, frequently precipitate acute attacks of gout.

An entirely different hypothesis about the mechanism of acute crystal synovitis postulates that the urate crystals activate *Hageman factor*, present in the synovial fluid, to activate, in turn, *bradykinin*, which then acts as the mediator of inflammation. However, there is good experimental evidence that this is at most no more than a contributory mechanism.

CLINICAL FEATURES

The age and sex incidence of primary gout was noted by Hippocrates, and recorded in his now famous three aphorisms –

Eunuchs do not take the gout or become bald.
A woman does not take gout unless her menses be stopped.
A young man does not take gout until he indulges in coition.

These observations remain broadly true today. Primary gout is a disease mainly of post-pubertal males and, less often, post-menopausal females. Predictably, this is reflected in a slightly higher mean PUA level in these two groups, and it is clearly an expression of hormonal status, although how this operates is uncertain. Thus, in a narrow sense, the main features of the epidemiology of primary gout (age and sex incidence, and familial grouping) can, like frontal baldness, be explained on the basis of a genetically determined variation, the clinical expression of which is 'permitted' by a particular hormonal status. In practice, over 50 per cent of patients with primary gout have a positive family history.

Gout usually presents as an attack of acute monarticular crystal synovitis, which settles in a week or two to leave a perfectly normal joint. This is followed by further similar attacks at intervals of weeks, months, or even years. After a time, in the more severe cases, tophaceous deposits appear on the pinna of the ears and in relationship to tendons and joints. Affected joints become distorted, and function is impaired. The final picture may be one of severe deforming polyarthritis. As the disease evolves, the acute attacks may become less severe and are replaced by local subacute exacerbations of a generalised chronic arthropathy. A minority of gouty patients pass urinary urate calculi, but most long-standing cases show evidence of renal impairment.

The Acute Attack. First attacks of gout usually affect the metatarsophalangeal joint of the big toe—*podagra*. This site may be favoured because of the trauma to which it is subjected. Subsequent attacks may return to the same joint, the opposite joint, or elsewhere. But the hips and shoulders tend to be spared and are never affected in the first attack.

The attack is often dramatically acute. Pain, tenderness, and swelling appear, and over a few hours increase until the joint is tensely swollen, and exquisitely painful and tender. The tense skin overlying the joint is warm, red, and dry (contrasting with the moist skin over the acute rheumatic fever or septic joint). There is often a systemic reaction, with malaise, fever, tachycardia, raised sedimentation rate, and leucocytosis. Untreated, the severe pain persists for a few days, then gradually subsides over a week or two, to leave a perfectly normal joint.

Attacks may be precipitated by trauma, surgical operations, alcoholic excess, or the administration of diuretics. The most potent provoking factor is probably the initiation of therapy to reduce PUA levels (allopurinol or uricosuric agents).

Chronic Gouty Arthropathy. Pathologically, the first sign of chronic urate arthropathy is a 'sugar icing' of the joint cartilage with urate crystals. Next, deposits of urate appear within the joint cartilage, and these grow to form larger deposits, replacing areas of cartilage and bone around the joint. These growing tophaceous deposits interfere with joint function both by the destruction of the joint-bearing surfaces, and by mechanically obstructing joint mobility. On the whole, small rather than large joints bear the brunt of this tophaceous, deforming process (Fig. 11.2); and the

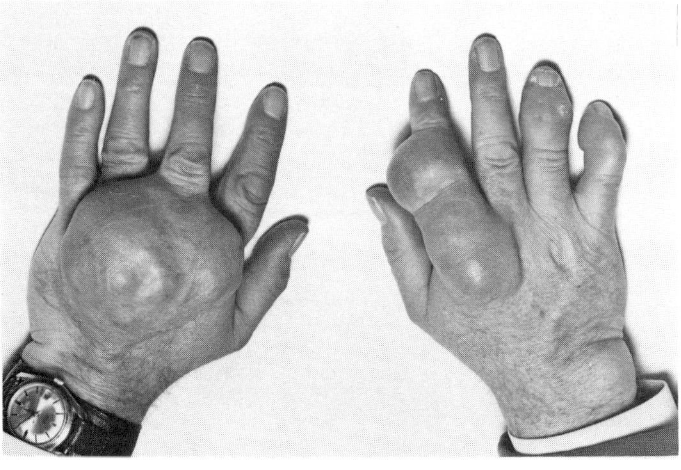

FIGURE 11.2 Gouty tophi related to small joints of the hands

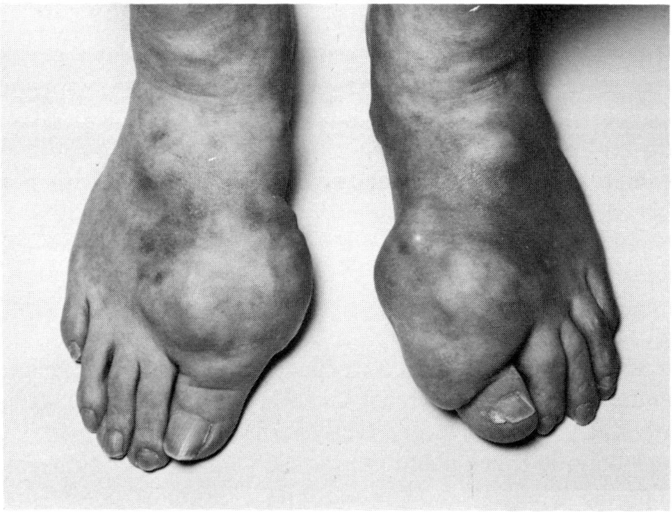

FIGURE 11.3 Gouty tophi in the first metatarsophalangeal joint and in the tarsus

tarsus is often the worst affected site (Fig. 11.3). Very rarely, bony ankylosis may occur.

Clinically, chronic gouty joints present the features of osteoarthrosis in association with tophaceous swellings in and around the articulation. In severe cases the gross deformity, with chronic sinus formation, may render a limb useless, and even necessitate amputation (Fig. 11.4).

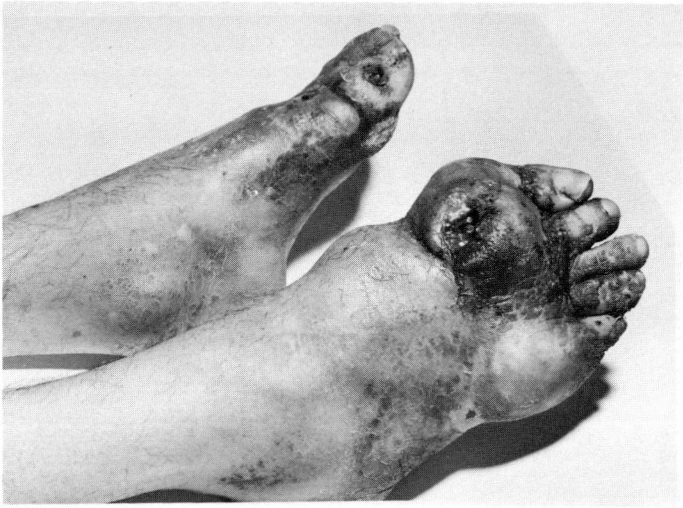

FIGURE 11.4 Rarely, gross deformity of the feet and sinus formation may necessitate amputation

Tophi. The presence of tophi is a measure of the severity of gout. The young man who develops tophi within a few years of his first attack of arthritis is likely, if untreated, to progress eventually to joint deformities. Hence, gout is classified clinically as 'tophaceous' or 'non-tophaceous'.

Tophi are often first discovered in a characteristic position on the helix of the ear (Fig. 11.5), a site where they should always be sought.

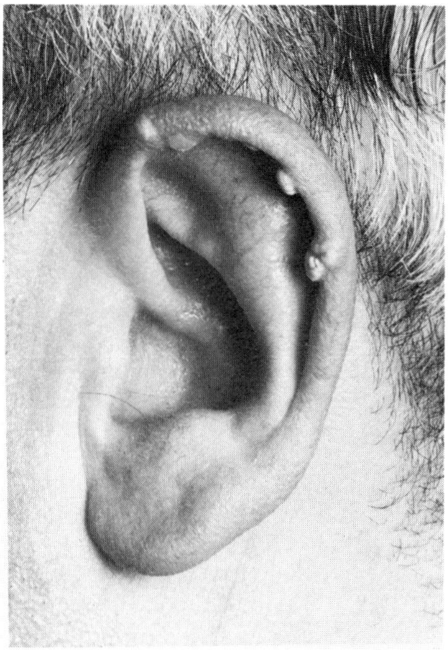

FIGURE 11.5 Gouty tophi on the helix of the ear

However, they may occur in relationship to cartilage anywhere (Fig. 11.6), particularly joint cartilage. Bursae and tendon sheaths are other favoured sites (Fig. 11.7).

Tophaceous deposits contain crystalline and amorphous urate salts which, in small deposits, are solid; but larger deposits often develop areas of softening. They are usually painless, but may themselves become the site of an acute gouty attack. With increasing growth of a tophus there may be necrosis of overlying skin to reveal the chalky contents. Semi-solid urate masses may then be extruded. For diagnostic purposes, material obtained from a tophus may be identified as urate by polarised light microscopy (*see* below) or by the chemical *murexide test* (*see* Appendix B). In severe cases, secondary infection and discharging sinuses may complicate the picture (*see* Fig. 11.4).

Renal disease and Urolithiasis. Urate urolithiasis occurs in about 20 per cent of gouty subjects. It is also seen in subjects with neither gout nor hyperuricaemia. The formation of urate stones is favoured by a

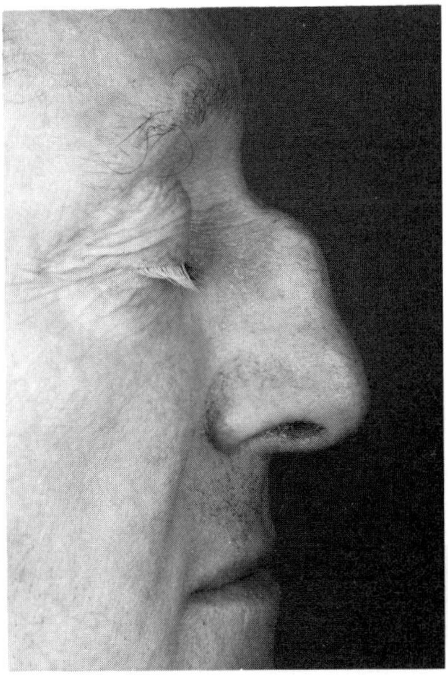

FIGURE 11.6 Gouty tophus of nasal cartilage

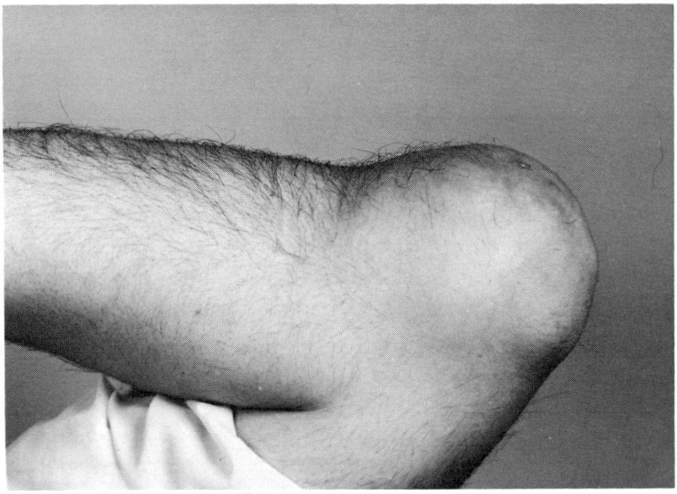

FIGURE 11.7 Gouty tophus associated with an olecranon bursa

high urinary urate output, a concentrated urine and, particularly, by a highly acid urine (for urate solubility increases greatly with increasing pH). Precipitation of urate within the urinary tract may result in stone formation, or in the passage of finer 'gravel'. The clinical features and complications of urate urolithiasis are similar to those of other urinary calculi. In contrast to calcium containing stones, pure urate calculi are, of course, radiolucent on X-ray.

Treatment of conditions such as leukaemia with cytotoxic drugs or irradiation may result in the death of large numbers of cells over a short period of time. Breakdown of the released nucleic acids can then lead to a vastly increased urinary urate load. The result is sometimes an acute obstructive anuria due to blocking of the whole urinary collecting system by urate crystals. The introduction of allopurinol (*see* below) has provided a method of avoiding this hazard.

The most common renal complication of gout is the one whose pathogenesis is least well understood, and indeed it is not even certain whether the *'gouty kidney'* represents a single entity or not. What is clear is that subjects with tophaceous gout of some years duration usually show evidence of renal disease even in the absence of the obstructive complications mentioned above. Proteinuria is the first evidence of this nephropathy. Later, there is impaired concentration, decreased clearance values and, finally, nitrogen retention and hypertension. Directly, or indirectly, renal disease is the most important cause of death in gouty subjects. The rate of the progression of gouty nephropathy is often surprisingly slow, and even established renal impairment may apparently remain unaltered over a few years. For this reason the prognosis in gouty nephropathy is usually better than it would be if the same degree of renal impairment were due to some other cause.

Pathologically these kidneys show urate deposits within the interstitial tissues, and a variety of histological changes which are patchy and not clearly related to the urate deposits. Most obviously, there are shrunken, fibrosed areas in the cortex suggestive of old infarcts, and the collecting system may show atrophy and changes characteristic of pyelonephritis. Actual bacterial infection may be present. Glomerular lesions are variable; there may be patchy sclerotic changes. The interstitial tissues show variable round cell infiltration and fibrosis, and arteriosclerotic changes are common.

These changes are too variable and non-specific to provide a clear interpretation of the pathogenesis of gouty renal disease. Nor do they establish whether it is a single condition or a number of different pathological processes. The appearances are not those of a simple reaction to the presence of urate crystals within the interstitial tissue, and while there can be little doubt that abnormal uric acid metabolism does produce parenchymal renal damage, it is still not clear whether *hyperuricaemia* or *hyperuricosuria* is responsible. This distinction is important when treatment is considered.

'Secondary Gout'. The distinction between 'primary' and 'secondary' gout has been discussed above in connection with the aetiology of

hyperuricaemia. Clinically, these two groups are similar, except that the age and sex incidence of secondary gout is that of the underlying disease. Secondary gout can be classified as follows –

A. *Increased purine turnover*
   Myeloproliferative disorders
   (polycythaemia vera, myeloid leukaemia, myelosclerosis).
   Other types of leukaemia.
   Other neoplasms.

B. *Decreased renal urate excretion*
   Primary renal disease.
   Drugs producing urate retention, e.g. thiazide diuretics, pyrazinamide.
   Diseases producing urate retention, e.g. hyperparathyroidism, hypothyroidism, glycogen storage disease.

This is the 'check-list' of conditions to be excluded each time that a diagnosis of gout is made.

LESCH-NYHAN SYNDROME

This very rare inborn error of metabolism provides 'an experiment of nature' that has greatly advanced the understanding of purine metabolism. It is encountered in male children in certain families, being inherited as an X-linked recessive trait.

These children present in infancy with a neurological syndrome of choreo-athetosis, spasticity, and mental retardation. The most striking feature is an extraordinary compulsive self-mutilation, in which they will chew their own fingers, despite the obvious pain this produces. Biochemically they have excessively high levels of PUA and a high urinary urate output. Acute and chronic gouty arthritis, tophi, and urate urolithiasis may all occur.

The disease is due to a lack of the enzyme hypoxanthine-guanine phosphoribosyltransferase (HG-PRTase); the resulting alteration in purine metabolism is discussed on page 157. The neurological damage is probably not due to the very high PUA levels, but may result from the (predictably) increased concentrations of hypoxanthine and guanine in those tissues that normally contain HG-PRTase. These include the brain (particularly the basal ganglia), and a considerable increase in oxypurine concentration has been demonstrated in the CSF and the basal ganglia. If this hypothesis is correct it follows, incidentally, that it would be unwise to treat these children with the xanthine oxidase inhibitor allopurinol, a drug that inhibits oxypurine degradation (*see* below).

Partial expressions of this same enzyme defect may account for some cases of adult gout, which may have an unusually early onset of arthritis and mild neurological abnormalities. A simple screening test (p. 158) is now available to detect this condition, which is confirmed by erythrocyte enzyme determinations. This is another metabolic abnormality for which all mentally retarded and spastic children should now be screened.

DISEASES ASSOCIATED WITH GOUT

Among gouty subjects there is an increased incidence of *hypertension*, *diabetes*, and *ischaemic heart disease*. The significance of this relationship is at present not clear. Obviously, there is occasionally a simple explanation; for example, the occurrence of hyperuricaemia secondary to anti-hypertensive drug therapy or chronic diabetic ketosis; or hypertension due to gouty nephropathy. On the other hand, families have been described in which gout, hypertension, ischaemic heart disease, and diabetes occur in successive generations with such regularity and severity as to leave no doubt that this grouping is genetically determined. Usually, however, the familial clustering of these conditions is less clear-cut and may well depend on a number of variables, some inherited, others environmental. Studies on subjects in whom these various conditions co-exist have suggested that raised *serum triglyceride* levels may be the common biochemical feature they share.

Interestingly, there is one condition, *rheumatoid arthritis*, which is associated with gout so infrequently as to suggest that the two diseases may be mutually exclusive. If this is so the mechanism is unknown.

INVESTIGATIONS

The most important laboratory investigations in gout are plasma and urinary urate determinations and examination of joint fluids for crystals. Special tests are also needed to exclude the various causes of 'secondary gout' and to assess renal function.

Urate Levels in Plasma and Urine. Modern techniques for *plasma* urate determinations are accurate and reproducible. However, it is necessary to be certain that the results are not influenced by irrelevant factors such as drugs (salicylates, thiazide diuretics, pyrazinamide etc.) or starvation ketosis. An arbitrary upper limit of normal is usually accepted as 6 mg/100 ml for men, and 5 mg/100 ml for pre-menopausal women. A strict low purine diet will reduce this level by about 1 to 1·5 mg/100 ml.

Determinations of *urinary urate* are usually carried out on an aliquot of the 24 hour collection. A simultaneous creatinine estimation allows the urate/creatinine ratio to be calculated (*see* p. 158). The upper limit of normal for the total 24 hours urinary urate on a low purine diet is about

600 mg. Figures above this indicate 'overproduction', while a normal value in association with an elevated PUA indicates 'underexcretion'. Isotope studies indicate that, very generally, PUA levels are a reflection of total body urate, while urinary urate levels reflect purine turnover.

Examination of Synovial Fluid for Crystals. The most positive method of diagnosing gout is to identify urate crystals within synovial fluid from an affected joint.

Examination of joint fluids for crystals involves the use of the *polarising light microscope* (Fig. 11.8). This differs from a standard instrument in

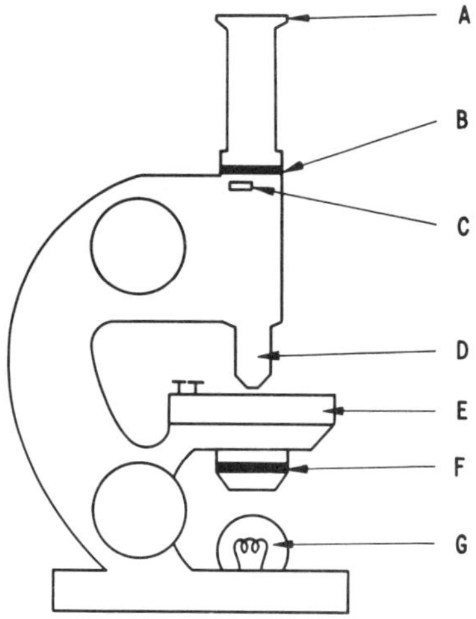

FIGURE 11.8 Polarising light microscope: *A* Eyepiece with cross-hairs. *B* Analyser. *C* Slot for insertion of either quartz wedge or first-order red plate. *D* Eyepiece of strain-free glass. *E* Objective centred, rotating stage. *F* Polariser. *G* Light source providing randomly orientated white light

having two polarising filters, or polars, placed one above (analyser) and one below (polariser) a rotating mechanical stage. Each polar allows through only that light that is polarised in one particular plane. The relationship of the planes of polarisation of the two polars to each other can be varied. In practice, the most useful position is that in which they are at right angles to each other—*crossed polars*. Under these circumstances the randomly orientated light reaching the polariser is selectively filtered so that only light polarised in a particular plane is transmitted. Travelling upwards, this polarised light then encounters the analyser, which is orientated in the opposite plane; so no light gets through, and to the observer the field appears dark.

Urates belong to a class of crystals that, because of asymmetrical internal molecular structure, will transmit light at one of three different speeds, depending on the plane of polarisation of the light waves. These crystals thus have three different refractive indices. Optically, this endows them with the property of *birefringence*, and when viewed between crossed polars they stand out brightly against the dark background.

Rotation of the mechanical stage shows that this brightness varies with position (Fig. 11.9). In each 360° rotation there are four positions in which the crystal appears bright, and four intermediate positions in which it is dark. The exact relationship of the dark position to the planes of the polars (indicated by hair-lines) is the *angle of extinction* of a particular crystal (Fig. 11.9).

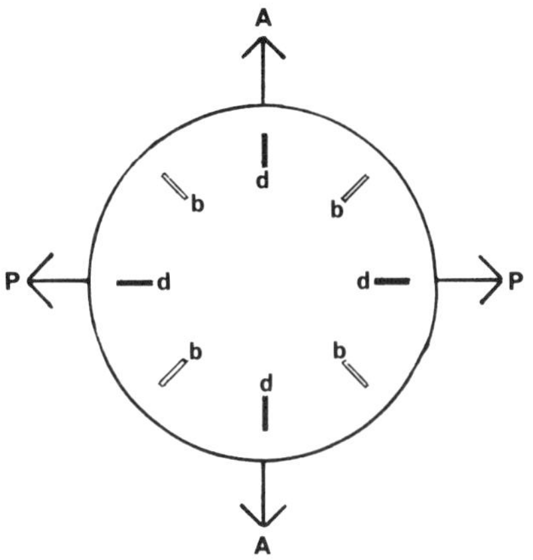

FIGURE 11.9 Appearance of a birefringent crystal during rotation between crossed polars. *P-P* Plane of polariser. *A-A* Plane of analyser. (*b*) Positions in which crystal appears bright. (*d*) Positions in which crystal appears dark. The crystal illustrated has an angle of extinction which is parallel (with *P-P* and *A-A*), as in the case of urate. (*From* Currey, H. L. F., *Proc. Roy. Soc. Med.*, **61**, 969, 1968)

For the further identification of birefringent crystals, use is made of the fact that such material alters the colour of light passing through it. Thus, a wedge-shaped piece of birefringent material, such as quartz, inserted obliquely between crossed polars will change the dark background into a series of colour bands, actually a sequence of repeated 'orders' of colour, similar to Newton's rings. Urate microcrystals are themselves too small to produce an obvious colour change, being, as it were, off the scale at the thin end. However, when viewed between crossed polars, with a quartz wedge in position, they take on a colour different from that of the background. This 'colour-shift' is more easily appreciated by replacing the wedge with a flat quartz plate ground to such a thickness that the most sensitive tint—*first order red*—appears throughout the field. Under these circumstances the crystal can be regarded as increasing or decreasing the birefringent colour effect of the quartz. By convention, those crystals that turn yellow when their long axis is parallel with the 'slow component' of the first order red plate (the orientation of which is indicated on the mounting), and blue when lying at right angles to it, are said to be negatively birefringent (Fig. 11.10). Urate crystals produce a marked shift of this type (*strong negative birefringence*), while crystals

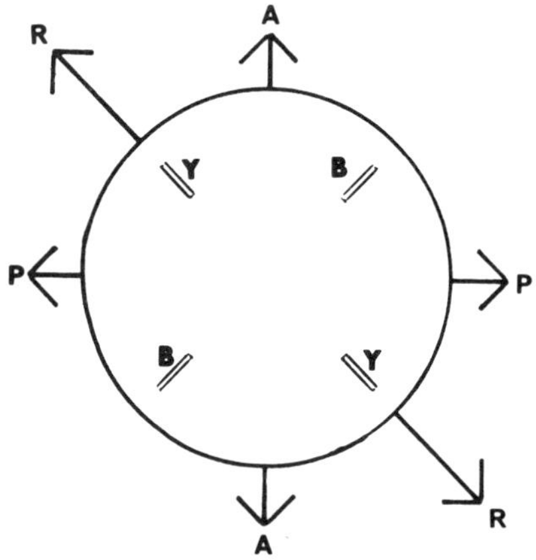

FIGURE 11.10 Appearance of a birefringent crystal during rotation between crossed polars with the first-order red compensator in position. *P-P* Plane of polariser. *A-A* Plane of analyser. *R-R* Orientation of slow component of first-order red compensator. *B* Positions in which crystal appears blue. *Y* Positions in which crystal appears yellow. The crystal illustrated is negatively birefringent as in the case of urate. (Adapted from Currey, H. L. F., *Proc. Roy. Soc. Med.*, **61,** 969, 1968)

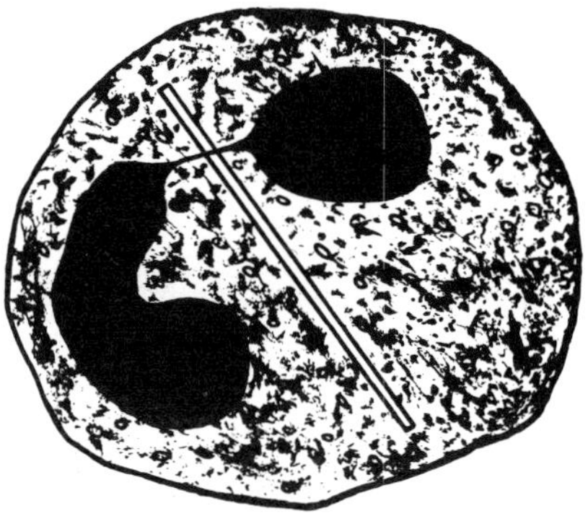

FIGURE 11.11 Sketch of a polymorphonuclear leucocyte containing a urate crystal. The typical appearance seen in synovial fluid from an acute gouty joint

of *calcium pyrophosphate dihydrate*, exhibit opposite and less-marked colour changes – *weak positive birefringence* (*see* p. 181 and Fig. 11.12). The optical principles underlying the application of polarised light microscopy to crystal identification are fully described in standard textbooks.*

Synovial fluid for crystal examination is collected without added anticoagulant. When immediate examination is not possible the specimen should be collected and stored under sterile conditions – ideally at 4°C.

*Bunn, C. W. (1961) *Chemical Crystallography.* 2nd ed. London: Oxford University Press. Chamot, E. M. & Mason, C. W. (1958) *Handbook of Chemical Microscopy.* Vol. 1. 2nd ed. New York: Wiley.

	CALCIUM PYROPHOSPHATE DIHYDRATE. (CPPD)	SODIUM URATE.
Class of Crystal	Biaxial Monoclinic & Triclinic	Biaxial Monoclinic & Triclinic
Birefringence	Weak positive	Strong negative
Extinction	Oblique	Parallel
Twinning?	Yes	Yes
Morphology	Rods Tablets Parallelepipeds 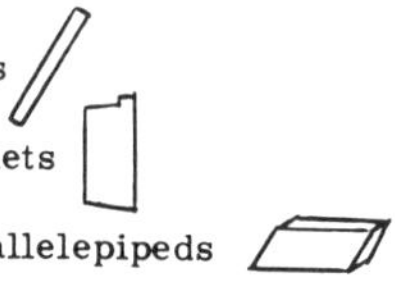	Needles 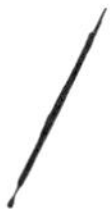

FIGURE 11.12 Table comparing the optical properties of the two types of crystal found in synovial fluids

If a clot forms it will enmesh both crystals and cells, so part of any such clot must be included in the drop of fluid placed on a glass slide under a coverslip. A search is then made for crystals using crossed polars; this allows rapid scanning of the slide. Slight rotation of either polar admits more light for identification of cells, etc. Once crystals are observed, the stage is rotated to find the angle of extinction. The first order red plate is then inserted, and the sign of birefringence determined as described above.

Morphologically, urate crystals are rods or needles with an average length approximately equal to the diameter of a leucocyte. During acute attacks of gout numerous urate crystals are found in the fluid, many situated within leucocytes (Fig. 11.11). Fluid from subacute joints may still contain enough crystals to be diagnostic, but these are likely to be mainly extracellular. The finding of scanty crystals is of doubtful significance and should probably be disregarded. There are only two natural diseases known to produce crystal synovitis, hence the identification of synovial fluid crystals involves only the differentiation between urate and calcium pyrophosphate dihydrate crystals. The points of difference are listed in Fig. 11.12. The same principles of crystal identification can also be applied to material obtained from a suspected tophus, or to biopsy material. Such material should be fixed in alcohol, *not in formalin solution* (which may dissolve the crystals).

X-rays in Gout. Uric acid and urate salts are translucent to X-rays. Tophaceous deposits therefore appear as clear areas, unless secondary

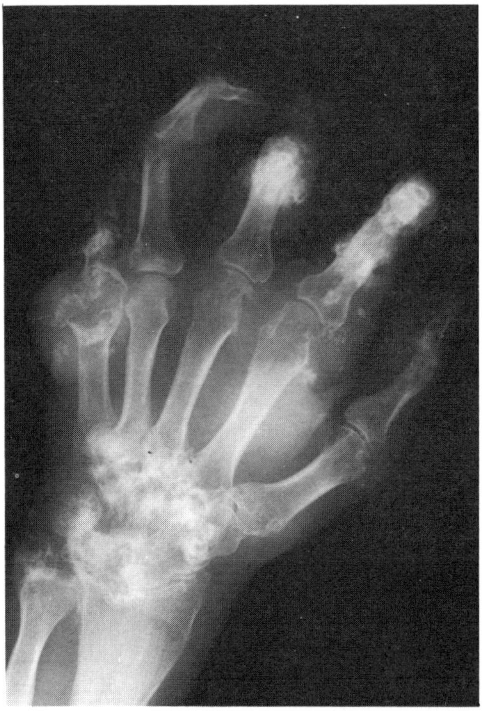

FIGURE 11.13 The hand in advanced tophaceous gout; radiograph showing tophi with secondary calcification

calcification has occurred. This may be present in advanced cases (Fig. 11.13). Small tophaceous deposits in bone may produce punched-out areas occasionally resembling rheumatoid erosions, but tending to be larger. In practice, confusion seldom arises, for these radiological changes do not appear until there is already clinical evidence of tophi. Hence, the truth of the observation that *the diagnosis of gout is never established initially by radiology*.

DIAGNOSIS

The most positive method of diagnosing gout is by the identification of urate crystals in synovial fluid, in biopsy material from a joint, or in material from a tophus. In doubtful cases every effort should be made to confirm the diagnosis by crystal identification. Failing this, the occurrence of podagra or typically acute arthritis in other sites, in a patient with a raised PUA, provides presumptive evidence of gout. Other helpful points are a positive family history, and the unequivocal response of an acute attack to colchicine (*see* below). Although raised PUA levels are often encountered in non-gouty subjects, the converse does not hold, and a diagnosis of (untreated) gout is untenable in a persistently normouricaemic subject.

PROGNOSIS

Primary gout ranges in severity from a disease that shows itself during the whole life of the patient only as a few attacks of acute crystal synovitis, to one that starts at puberty and cripples the patient by the time he is forty, finally killing him from renal disease.

Certain features may indicate the course the disease will take. The presence of tophi indicates a more severe form of the disease; a very high mean plasma urate level has the same significance. Other bad prognostic signs are the appearance of the first attack at an early age, and a short interval between the first attack and the appearance of tophi. Evidence of renal disease is obviously a bad prognostic sign but, as mentioned above, the expectation of life is usually rather better than the degree of renal failure might otherwise suggest. These observations apply to untreated gout. The development of effective drug therapy has certainly improved the overall prognosis to an extent that it is not yet possible to assess.

TREATMENT

Therapy in gout aims at preventing attacks of crystal synovitis, or terminating them once they have started. In the more severe cases treatment should, in addition, lower the PUA level to normal, and reverse the process of urate deposition so that tophi are reabsorbed.

The Acute Attack. For many years the accepted treatment of acute urate crystal synovitis was colchicine, given at frequent intervals (0·5 mg every 2 hours by mouth) until either the attack cleared, or toxic effects in the form of vomiting and diarrhoea supervened. Colchicine is without effect on purine metabolism, and its therapeutic effect may depend on some action by which it inhibits the phagocytic activity of leucocytes, thus breaking the pathological cycle in crystal synovitis. Its effect in gout is sufficiently specific for a clear-cut response to be regarded as confirmatory evidence of this diagnosis. Colchicine has now, however, given way to other forms of therapy for the acute attack. As far as drugs are concerned, both *phenylbutazone* and *indomethacin* given in large initial doses (phenylbutazone 600 mg and indomethacin 150 mg daily) then reduced over the next few days, seem more effective than colchicine, and gastro-intestinal disturbances are avoided. Gouty subjects should have one or other of these drugs always on hand to start at the earliest sign of an attack.

If the affected joint is accessible to drainage by aspiration, then this, combined with a *local corticosteroid injection*, is the most certain and rapid method of terminating the acute attack. Exceptionally, if other measures fail or are impractical, corticotrophin by injection, or corticosteroid drugs by mouth, may provide relief.

Prophylaxis Between Attacks. Colchicine, displaced from its traditional role in the treatment of acute attacks, has now found a new usefulness in the prevention of such attacks. Taken regularly in doses of 0·5 to 1·5 mg daily it definitely reduces the frequency of acute attacks and, in this dosage, does not produce gastro-intestinal side effects. It is compatible with all other drugs used in the treatment of gout; so, if other measures do not competely prevent attacks, a 'background' of colchicine should be added. It is of particular value during the period when treatment with uricosuric drugs or allopurinol is being started, when there is a greatly increased liability to acute attacks.

Reduction of Plasma Urate Levels. The above measures alone may be all that are needed in the mildest cases of gout. When, however, there is evidence that the disease is more severe, it becomes essential to provide treatment aimed at compensating for the underlying metabolic abnormality. This involves lowering the plasma urate levels to a point where the process of urate deposition is reversed. The indications for such treatment are the persistence of acute attacks, the development of tophi, or a PUA level consistently over 8 mg/100 ml. Two types of drug therapy are capable of reducing the PUA level. One is the group of uricosuric drugs, the other is allopurinol.

Uricosuric drugs act by paralysing renal tubular transport of urate, which effectively prevents urate being either reabsorbed or secreted in the proximal tubule, and the full filtered load is theoretically available to pass on for elimination in the urine. Even the lesser degree achieved in practice can represent a marked urate diuresis. The following are the three most useful uricosuric drugs and their usual daily doses:

Ethebenecid	(Urelim)	1–2 G
Probenecid	(Benemid)	1–2 G
Sulphinpyrazone	(Anturan)	200–400 mg

Any of these drugs, given in the doses shown, may be expected to produce a urate diuresis and to lower the PUA level. Unfortunately, the initiation of this therapy may provoke attacks of acute gout (even in patients on prophylactic colchicine), and the increased urinary urate load represents an added risk of stone formation. The latter hazard is minimised by reducing the acidity of the urine and increasing fluid intake. Patients on this form of therapy require periodic PUA determinations. The aim is to increase the dose until the level of PUA falls below 6 mg/100 ml. Salicylates (which themselves modify the renal handling of urate—*see* p. 159) effectively block the action of the uricosuric drugs, so must be avoided by patients on this form of therapy. Uricosuric drugs become progressively less effective in the presence of renal damage.

Another development in the treatment of gout is the introduction of the drug *allopurinol*, an inhibitor of the enzyme *xanthine oxidase*. Figure 11.1 indicates the reactions catalysed by xanthine oxidase, and shows how inhibition of this enzyme blocks the final stages in the degradation of oxypurines to uric acid. The effect of giving allopurinol is therefore to reduce the production of urate, so that both the PUA level and the urinary urate load fall. Instead, levels of oxypurines rise, although not to the predicted extent, for allopurinol also exerts a variable inhibition on *de novo* purine synthesis (explained on p. 158). This drug, therefore, achieves a more complete adjustment of the metabolic defect than the uricosuric agents. In addition to lowering the PUA level it actually reduces the hazard of urolithiasis by spreading the reduced total purine load between three compounds, urate, xanthine, and hypoxanthine, each of which has its own independent solubility limit. It also has the advantage of being effective in the presence of renal failure. These effects are achieved with doses of about 200 to 500 mg daily. Initiation of therapy often provokes acute attacks of gout, and some patients develop rashes; otherwise allopurinol appears relatively free from serious toxic effects.

Up till now, there has been some hesitation about using allopurinol as the drug of first choice in all cases for lowering the PUA level because of doubts about long-term toxicity which attend the introduction of any new, potent drug. So far these fears have proved unfounded, and the uricosuric drugs are soon likely to give way almost completely to allopurinol. The present policy is to use one of the uricosuric drugs initially in the uncomplicated case, reserving allopurinol for the following circumstances—

Failure of adequate control by uricosuric drugs.

An added liability to urolithiasis (a history of passing stones, renal colic, haematuria, or a very high urinary urate output).

The presence of renal failure.

In the severe case, difficult to control, uricosuric drugs and allopurinol therapy can usefully be combined. It is in this situation that the prescription of a *low purine diet* is necessary.

Allopurinol finds a special use in the treatment of childhood leukaemias and other highly cellular neoplasms. Irradiation or cytotoxic drug therapy in such patients may produce so much nucleic acid breakdown that the PUA level may rise to exceptional heights, and the great outpouring of urate through the kidneys can lead to massive precipitation and an acute obstructive anuria. Allopurinol minimises this risk, and it follows that the drug should be used as prophylactic cover in these patients. It needs to be remembered that antipurine drugs such as 6-mercaptopurine are themselves degraded by xanthine oxidase, and their action is thus significantly potentiated by simultaneous allopurinol administration.

Prevention of Urate Urolithiasis. For patients liable to stone formation, preventative therapy aims at producing a dilute urine which never becomes strongly acid. Avoidance of dehydration, and an ample fluid intake, combined with an alkali such as sodium bicarbonate 2 to 6 G daily, will usually achieve this. Ideally, the pH of the urine should occasionally be monitored (using an indicator method on each specimen passed in the 24 hours) to ensure that the pH remains above 6·5. Restriction of dietary purines alone is unlikely to make a decisive difference. Allopurinol therapy is the most certain way of reducing urinary urates, and is indicated when urate urolithiasis is not prevented by simple measures.

Surgery in Gout. Prior to the introduction of modern drug therapy, the surgical removal of tophaceous deposits gave disappointing results, the operation being commonly followed by re-accumulation of the deposit and, occasionally, leaving discharging sinuses. The ability of drug therapy to achieve effective metabolic control has changed the situation. In the majority of gouty subjects it is now possible to reduce the PUA to a level at which urate leaves the tissue deposits to enter the plasma, and such treatment can be shown actually to reduce the size of tophi. But the process is slow, and in these circumstances surgery becomes a much more attractive proposition. Once metabolic control is achieved, and urate begins to leave the tophi, there would seem to be good reason to resect any large and unsightly deposits or those interfering mechanically with function, for even the most vigorous and successful drug therapy would take many years to dissolve away the extensive deposits seen in advanced tophaceous gout.

Pyrophosphate Arthropathy

Unlike true gout, descriptions of which appear in the most ancient medical writings, pseudogout has been identified as a separate disease entity only during the past decade. It was the application of polarised light microscopy to the examination of joint fluids for urate crystals that provided the essential clue. Using this technique, it was found that some synovial fluids contained crystals that were clearly not urate. These specimens came from patients experiencing attacks of acute gout-like arthritis (*pseudogout*), but whose plasma uric acid levels were regularly normal, and in whom there was radiological calcification of joint cartilage or *chondrocalcinosis*. The calcific material in the cartilage, like the synovial fluid crystals, has been shown to consist of a calcium salt of pyrophosphate, and it is becoming clear that *pyrophosphate arthropathy* is a quite important cause of joint pathology.

CLINICAL FEATURES

Pyrophosphate arthropathy is usually first diagnosed in the middle-aged or elderly. It lacks the male predominance seen in true gout, and a positive family history is relatively uncommon. A notable exception has been reported in certain Czechoslovakian families in whom a very high incidence of the disease is associated with the onset of symptoms in early adult life.

The clinical course is very variable. Some patients experience only episodic acute attacks, others develop progressive degenerative joint disease without acute attacks, while perhaps the most common picture is one in which the gradual development of osteoarthrosis is punctuated by acute episodes. Occasionally, in patients with a longstanding subacute polyarthritis, the disease may mimic rheumatoid arthritis.

The Acute Attack. Acute pyrophosphate synovitis may be as severe as that described above for true gout, or it may be less dramatic. One or a few joints are affected at a time. Podagra has been described but, unlike urate gout, large joints are affected more commonly than small joints, and the hips and shoulders are not spared. Much the commonest site is the knee joint. Acute attacks may be precipitated by surgical operations or by the taking of diuretics. The untreated acute attack usually subsides after about ten days, but may then grumble on subacutely for a month or two. During the acute phase there is often a systemic reaction, with malaise, fever, elevated sedimentation rate and, sometimes, a leucocytosis. These features, in association with an acutely inflamed joint, may lead to an erroneous diagnosis of septic arthritis. The correct diagnosis will, however, be suggested by the presence of radiological chondrocalcinosis (best sought in the knee joints), and will be confirmed by observing the responsible crystals within the synovial effusion.

Chronic Arthritis. Radiological chondrocalcinosis has been observed in patients with severe progressive osteoarthrosis of one or a few joints, and also in subjects with otherwise typical nodal multiple osteoarthrosis who never experience acute attacks. When progressive osteoarthrosis occurs in joints that are also the site of acute attacks of pyrophosphate synovitis, then there seems little reason to doubt that the pyrophosphate is responsible for the degenerative changes. When, however, chondrocalcinosis is observed in patients with generalised osteoarthrosis without acute attacks it becomes more difficult to decide whether the pyrophosphate deposition has contributed to the cartilage degeneration. Minor degrees of calcification (particularly in knee menisci) are a not uncommon asymptomatic finding in elderly subjects. Experience suggests that radiological calcification that is heavy and extensive is usually associated with, and responsible for, definite joint pathology. Whether or not lesser degrees of (perhaps radiologically inapparent) pyrophosphate deposition may contribute to what is regarded as 'primary' osteoarthrosis is unknown.

Associated Conditions. In most patients with pyrophosphate deposition disease there is no evidence of any underlying biochemical abnormality. However, in a definite minority it occurs in association with hyperparathyroidism, haemochromatosis, or true urate gout. Thus, like true gout, pyrophosphate arthropathy may, in a sense, exist in a primary or secondary form.

RADIOLOGY

Chondrocalcinosis affects both hyaline and fibro-cartilage. In the latter

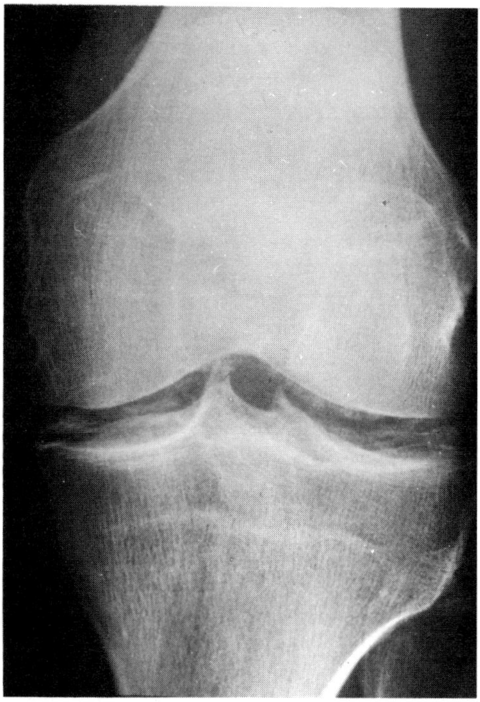

FIGURE 11.14 Chondrocalcinosis of the knee joint. Radiograph showing calcification both in the menisci and in the hyaline cartilage covering the femoral condyles

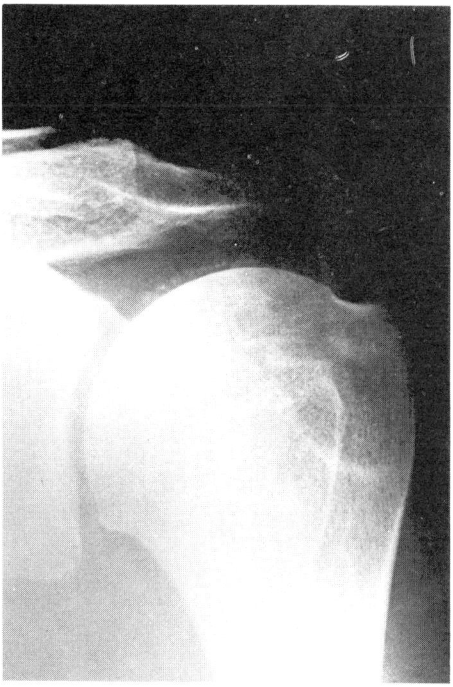

FIGURE 11.15 Chondrocalcinosis of the shoulder joint. Radiograph showing calcification in the hyaline cartilage covering the humeral head. (*From* Currey, H. L. F. and Mason, R. M. in *Recent Advances in Orthopaedic Surgery*, 1969, Ed. A. G. Apley. London: Churchill)

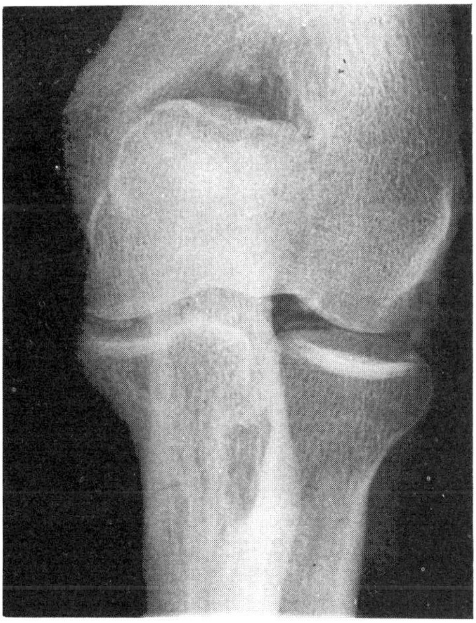

FIGURE 11.16 Chondrocalcinosis of the elbow joint (*From* Currey, H. L. F. and Mason, R. M. in *Recent Advances in Orthopaedic Surgery*, 1969, Ed. A. G. Apley. London: Churchill)

it appears as diffuse or mottled patches in the knee menisci (much the commonest site), in the labrum of the acetabulum and glenoid cavity, in the triangular ligament of the distal end of the ulna, and in the symphasis pubis. In hyaline cartilage it appears as a fine, stippled line parallel to, and narrowly separated from, the underlying bony cortex. Again, the most common site is the knee, but the hip, shoulder, elbow, wrist, and even the finger joints may be affected. Figures 11.14 to 11.16 show some typical examples. Clearly, radiological evidence of osteoarthrosis is to be expected in some of these joints. Occasionally, the intervertebral discs are involved, but the familiar costal cartilage calcification appears to be independent of pyrophosphate deposition.

Because of the frequency with which the knee joint is the site of calcification, X-rays of this joint alone constitute a useful routine screening test for chondrocalcinosis.

Is radiological chondrocalcinosis always significant in indicating pyrophosphate deposition disease? The fact that minor degrees of chondrocalcinosis, particularly affecting knee menisci only, are relatively common among the elderly, raises the question whether this may not occur secondary to normal senescent changes in cartilage. This question is not yet answered. It does appear, however, that when calcification affects multiple joints, or when hyaline cartilage is clearly involved, this should be regarded as indicating pyrophosphate deposition disease. Isolated meniscal calcification may or may not be significant.

THE IDENTITY OF THE CRYSTALS

Precise identification of the crystalline material involved requires the use of X-ray diffraction techniques. Using this method it has been shown that crystals from both synovial fluid and cartilage consist of *calcium pyrophosphate dihydrate* (CPPD). Considering that almost all other abnormal calcifications in the body consist of hydroxyapatite, the consistency with which chondrocalcinosis is due to deposition of CPPD is impressive. (Rarely, asymptomatic isolated meniscal calcification may be due to an orthophosphate or to hydroxyapatite in an atherosclerotic vessel wall.)

INVESTIGATIONS

The most important investigations in establishing a diagnosis of pyrophosphate arthropathy are radiological screening for articular chondrocalcinosis (described above), examination of synovial fluid for crystals and, occasionally, the examination of biopsy material by polarised light microscopy. Once the diagnosis is established it is necessary to exclude the various conditions that may be associated with chondrocalcinosis.

Polarised light microscopy has been described in the section on gout. The same technique is employed for joint fluids from patients suspected of suffering from pyrophosphate synovitis. Like urate, CPPD crystals are birefringent, and so are easily detected using 'crossed polars'. Morphologically they exist as rods or more bulky parallelepipeds, and the main point of differentiation from urate crystals is that they exhibit *weak positive birefringence*. The main characteristics of the two types of crystals are set out in Fig. 11.12.

As in the case of gout, synovial fluid from a joint that is the site of acute pyrophosphate synovitis usually contains numerous CPPD crystals, mainly in rod form, with many of the crystals within leucocytes (Fig. 11.17). Fluids from subacute joints may still be diagnostic. In this case,

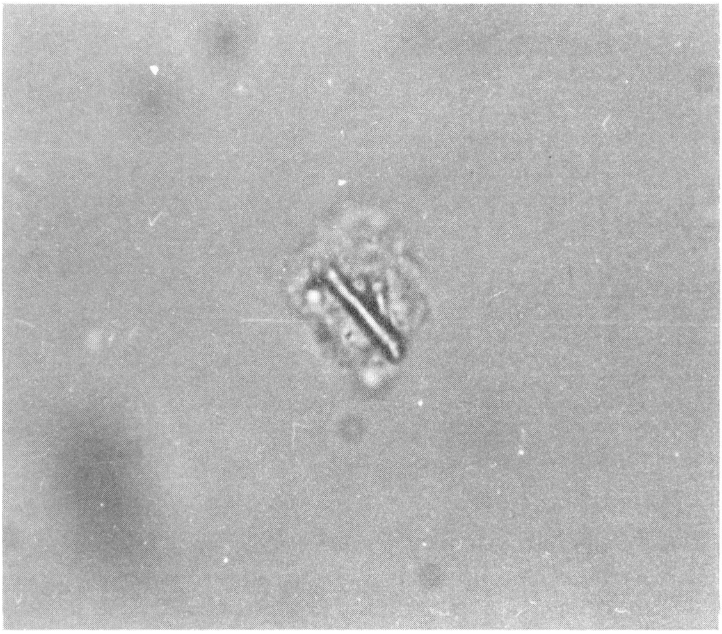

FIGURE 11.17 Polymorphonuclear leucocyte containing a crystal of calcium pyrophosphate dihydrate. This is the typical appearance seen in synovial fluid from a joint affected by acute pyrophosphate arthropathy. (Polarised light microscopy with polars partially crossed.) (*From* Currey, H. L. F. and Mason, R. M. in *Recent Advances in Orthopaedic Surgery*, 1969, Ed. A. G. Apley. London: Churchill)

the crystals tend to be less numerous and are mainly extracellular, parallelepiped forms. Experience has shown that the occurrence of only occasional crystals of either type in a synovial fluid is not necessarily significant, and should be disregarded. The main value of polarised light microscopy is in the examination of fluid from acutely inflamed joints.

Here it provides positive evidence of crystal synovitis, and it should now be regarded as a routine technique for the investigation of synovial fluids.

Crystal deposition arthropathy can also be diagnosed from biopsy material. To avoid dissolving the crystals, the tissue is placed in absolute alcohol, then sectioned in the normal way. Provided that all embedding wax is removed in processing, crystals can be readily identified in both unstained and stained sections (Fig. 11.18).

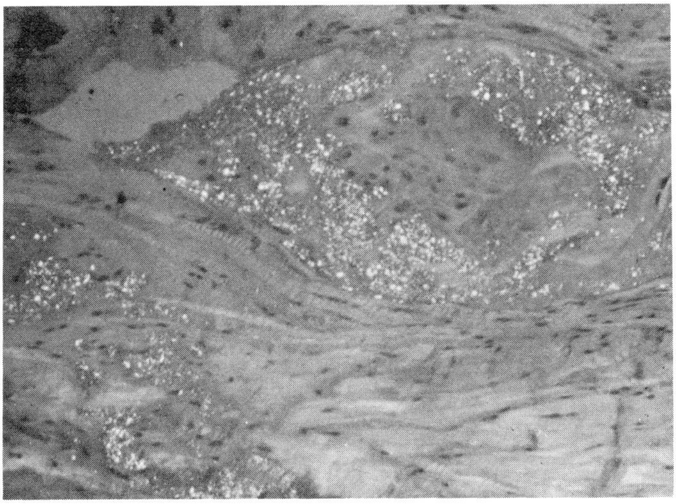

FIGURE 11.18 Crystals of calcium pyrophosphate dihydrate lying within the fibrocartilaginous meniscus removed from a knee joint affected by chronic pyrophosphate arthropathy. (Polarised light microscopy with polars partially crossed)

A diagnosis of pyrophosphate arthropathy, or the radiological demonstration of articular chondrocalcinosis, demand investigations to exclude hyperparathyroidism, haemochromatosis, true gout, and perhaps diabetes mellitus (although the evidence for an increased incidence of primary diabetes in pyrophosphate arthropathy is controversial). Occasionally, patients with chondrocalcinosis, while not suffering from one of the associated diseases mentioned above, have an isolated biochemical abnormality such as a raised serum alkaline phosphatase or plasma urate level. The significance of this is at present not clear.

PATHOGENESIS AND AETIOLOGY

Acute pyrophosphate arthropathy is regarded as being an example of *crystal synovitis* in which the CPPD microcrystals provoke inflammation by their physical presence, exactly as described above for urate crystals. It may well be that crystals reach the synovial fluid by rupture of superficial deposits in cartilage. In chronic pyrophosphate arthropathy it seems likely that the presence of CPPD crystals alters some property of the articular cartilage in which it is deposited, in a manner that leads to *secondary osteoarthrosis*. This would make it comparable to the joint disease in ochronosis (*see* p. 282).

Chemically, pyrophosphates are produced during intermediate metabolism, and appear in the urine in low concentrations. They have the property of inhibiting crystal formation, and it has been suggested that they may play a physiological role in the control of mineralisation of bone (alkaline phosphatase acting locally by lowering pyrophosphate concentration to allow crystallisation of hydroxyapatite). But what is entirely unexplained, at present, is why crystals of CPPD are laid down in cartilage.

Consideration of all the circumstances in which pyrophosphate may be deposited in cartilage suggests that this tissue is particularly liable to such deposition, which may be initiated by a variety of factors. The frequent occurrence of minor degrees of chondrocalcinosis in the very elderly suggests that senescence is one of the factors contributing to its appearance. This, or some other factor, is genetically determined to operate either much earlier in life, or more intensively, in the familial Czechoslovakian form of the disease. No real differences in the local joint pathology have emerged between what may be regarded as the 'primary' form of pyrophosphate deposition and the 'secondary' type associated with conditions such as haemochromatosis and hyperparathyroidism, although the identity of the crystalline material in the latter requires confirmation. Thus, it appears that a number of different causes may produce the same end-result; some may operate at the level of the cartilage, others at a general biochemical level. If so, pyrophosphate deposition may, like the hyperuricaemia of gout, be *multifactorial*, and the occurence of arthropathy may depend on the degree and duration of the deposition rather than the nature of the underlying cause.

TREATMENT

The most effective treatment of acute pyrophosphate arthropathy is aspiration of the synovial effusion and replacement with a corticosteroid preparation. This may dramatically cut short an attack.

Opinions vary about the value of colchicine during an acute attack. It is probably less effective than in gout. Likewise, neither phenylbutazone nor indomethacin are dramatically effective, although they are probably the drugs of choice. Recently it has been suggested that interval treatment with small doses of colchicine may help to reduce the frequency of acute attacks. Chronic pyrophosphate arthropathy is managed along the same lines as other forms of degenerative joint disease.

Lack of understanding about the underlying defect at present prevents the development of any more fundamental therapy. Further observation is needed to judge the effect on 'secondary' pyrophosphate arthropathy of treating either hyperparathyroidism or haemochromatosis. The few reports available are somewhat disappointing.

12

Joint Infections

J D Jessop

Suppurative arthritis results from bacterial invasion of joint tissues. The organisms most commonly responsible are staphylococci or haemolytic streptococci. However, joints may be infected by a wide range of bacteria including pneumococci, gonococci, meningococci, *E. coli*, *H. influenzae*, *Pseudomonas*, *Proteus vulgaris*, Salmonellae and Brucella. Tuberculous arthritis presents special features and will be discussed under a separate heading. Fungal joint infections such as coccidioidomycosis, are rarely seen in the United Kingdom. Arthritis complicating the course of viral infections is discussed in Chapter 17.

The widespread use of antibiotics has brought about a sharp decline in the incidence of joint infections. Nevertheless, septic arthritis does still occur, and its prompt diagnosis and adequate treatment remain a challenge to the clinician. Although it may appear spontaneously in an otherwise healthy person, certain groups of patients are particularly susceptible to this form of arthritis. Thus, the chronically ill or debilitated subject with lowered resistance to infection, may develop an intercurrent illness such as pneumonia from which infection may spread to a joint. Resistance to infection may also be lowered in those on long-term corticosteroid therapy and in those with blood dyscrasias, such as leukaemia or agranulocytosis. That joints damaged by other forms of arthritis are more vulnerable to superadded bacterial invasion is suggested by the occasional occurrence of septic arthritis in a rheumatoid joint. This may occur even in patients not receiving corticosteroids. Intra-articular injections and open operations on joints carry a slight but definite risk of introducing infection. This risk is greatest when a prosthesis is inserted. For reasons which are not clear, gonococcal arthritis has become very rare in the United Kingdom. In parts of North America it remains common among coloured females.

ROUTES OF INFECTION

The primary source from which infection reaches the joint is not always obvious, but there are three possible routes –

1. Most commonly the organisms are carried in the blood stream as metastatic infection from a source remote from the joint.
2. There may be direct entry of the organisms from penetrating wounds, following intra-articular injections or orthopaedic surgery, especially when this involves a prosthesis.
3. Infection may spread to the joint from an adjacent focus of infection such as osteomyelitis.

PATHOLOGY

Once the organisms reach the joint they multiply in the subsynovial tissues. The reaction of the joint to infection depends on several factors, including the resistance of the host, the severity of the infection, and the virulence of the organisms; it usually involves an outpouring of inflammatory exudate. The synovial membrane becomes heavily infiltrated with polymorphonuclear leucocytes and is subsequently replaced by granulation tissue. As the synovial membrane is destroyed, organisms enter the joint cavity. There is an accumulation of pus in the joint, and the granulation tissue erodes the intra- and extra-articular structures. Rapid loss of cartilage may occur in untreated cases, probably due to the enzymes released from bacteria and leucocytes. Thus, severe infective arthritis may lead to gross destruction of the joint with fibrous or bony ankylosis.

CLINICAL FEATURES

Patients of either sex and of all ages may develop septic arthritis, but it is more common in infants and children under fifteen and adults over sixty years of age. Although symptoms may occur spontaneously there is often a recent history of minor trauma to the joint. It is usually monarticular with a predilection for the larger joints such as the knee, hip or shoulder, although any joint may be involved, spinal or peripheral.

The onset of symptoms is usually abrupt. The joint is hot, red, swollen, exquisitely painful, and tender. The slightest movement is sometimes intolerable. There may be additional signs of infection such as cellulitis, lymphangitis, and tender enlargement of draining lymph nodes. Systemic manifestations of toxicity accompany, or precede by a day or two, the local signs and symptoms. These include malaise, fever, and rigors.

There is great variation in the severity of pyogenic arthritis, and certain organisms often show characteristic features. Thus, the haemolytic streptococcus may invade the skin and cause cellulitis. Gonococcal arthritis may remain a migrating polyarthralgia for some days before settling in one or a few joints.

The very rare occurrence of suppurative arthritis complicating rheumatoid arthritis may present great difficulty in diagnosis. It is necessary to appreciate that multiple joints may be involved and pus may be aspirated (with a positive culture) from joints lacking the classical signs of acute infection. This situation arises most commonly, but not exclusively, in patients receiving corticosteroid therapy.

INVESTIGATIONS

Synovial Fluid. The most important single investigation is the aspiration of joint fluid and isolation of the infecting organism. When septic arthritis is suspected it is mandatory to aspirate the joint before starting treatment with antibiotics. The clinician who first sees a patient with an acutely inflamed joint can do him no greater disservice than to temporise by prescribing an antibiotic. Even a single dose can interfere with the isolation of the responsible organism.

Immediate bacteriological examination is critical. A direct Gram's stain may show the organism, but in any case an appropriate range of cultures should be set up. Any organism isolated must be tested for antibiotic sensitivity. Unless examination of the direct smear clearly implicates a pyogenic organism, acid-fast bacilli must be sought, and it is advisable to consult with the bacteriologist about the question of examining for unusual agents such as fungi.

The synovial fluid is turbid, often blood-stained, and may be frankly purulent. Occasionally, it is so thick that a widebore needle is required for aspiration. The white cell count is invariably high, usually over 100,000 cells/mm^3 of which over 90 per cent are polymorphonuclear leucocytes. The protein content is high and the glucose content low.

Acute crystal synovitis (*see* Chapter 11) may mimic suppurative arthritis. Synovial fluid from an acutely inflamed joint in which the responsible organism is not clearly apparent on direct microscopy should therefore be examined by polarised light microscopy for the presence of crystals.

Blood. A neutrophil leucocytosis and elevated blood sedimentation rate are usual, but not invariable. Both may be seen also in crystal synovitis.

Blood cultures should always be performed. Positive results may indicate either invasion of the blood stream by an organism arising in the joint, or an underlying pyaemia, itself the cause of the arthritis.

Rising antistreptolysin 'O' titres may accompany streptococcal arthritis.

Genital Tract. A full urogenital investigation may be indicated to detect a gonococcal infection.

X-rays. Radiographs are unlikely to show changes before seven to ten days. A persistently active joint shows demineralisation of the neighbouring bones, followed by destruction of the cartilage and subchondral bone, and, finally, fibrous or bony ankylosis.

Finally, a thorough search must be made for possible sites from which the organism may have originated. Swabs should be taken from the throat and anterior nares, sputum and urine sent for culture, and swabs taken also from any infected leg ulcers or corns. If no growth is obtained from the synovial fluid, information from these sites may prove useful.

DIFFERENTIAL DIAGNOSIS

Septic arthritis may be confused with other forms of acute monarticular arthritis:

Acute Rheumatic Fever. Rheumatic fever in a child starting with one painful swollen joint may resemble septic arthritis. Unless other features of rheumatic fever make the diagnosis clear, joint aspiration is essential. This may require a general anaesthetic.

Haemarthrosis. Bleeding into a joint may produce extreme pain and swelling. In a first attack, and if the underlying coagulation defect is not known, differentiation from septic arthritis may require aspiration and haematological investigation.

Trauma. Patients with septic arthritis will often give a history of minor trauma to the joint. It follows that a diagnosis of 'traumatic synovitis' must be made with caution and, if necessary, the presence of infection excluded by bacteriological examination of synovial fluid.

Crystal Synovitis. Acute attacks of gout and pyrophosphate arthropathy may mimic septic arthritis. A positive diagnosis can be established immediately by examination of the joint fluid for crystals, using polarised light microscopy (*see* p. 168). A good screening test for pyrophosphate arthropathy is radiological examination of the knees for chondrocalcinosis (*see* p. 178).

Non-bacterial Inflammatory Arthropathy. Still's disease in children, palindromic rheumatism, acute rheumatoid arthritis, psoriatic arthropathy, and Reiter's disease may all simulate acute septic arthritis initially. Under these circumstances aspiration and bacteriological examination of the joint fluid is the only safe course.

Tuberculosis. Tuberculous arthritis should always be considered as a possible cause of any monarticular arthritis. It is discussed below.

COMPLICATIONS

Septicaemia. Spread of infection from the joint to the blood stream may lead to pyaemia or septicaemia, which may be fatal.

Osteomyelitis. Direct spread of infection from the joint to the neighbouring bone may produce osteomyelitis.

Chronic Synovitis. Sometimes, after an initial favourable response to treatment, recurrent painful effusions may occur. These are sterile.

Deformity. After recovery, the range of joint movement may be limited, particularly if the principles of splinting and mobilisation have been wrongly applied.

Ankylosis. Bony or fibrous ankylosis may be the final result of inadequately treated septic arthritis.

TREATMENT

Treatment will depend to some extent on the age of the patient and the site of infection, but the broad principles are as follows:

Diagnostic and therapeutic aspiration
Administration of antibiotics
Surgical drainage
Supportive care
Mobilisation

Aspiration. Joint aspiration is not only of diagnostic value, but also therapeutic, for it relieves pressure on neighbouring structures and reduces pain. In the early stages, effusions are usually large and may consist of thick pus. They often re-accumulate and may need daily aspiration during the first week of treatment. As the joint improves the effusion diminishes.

Antibiotics. Once fluid has been obtained for bacteriological studies, antibiotics should be prescribed. As the success of treatment depends largely on prompt and effective chemotherapy the choice of antibiotics is critical.

Initial examination of the fluid by Gram's stain can give useful guidance on chemotherapy while awaiting reports on culture and sensitivity. Thus, penicillin is effective against most Gram-positive organisms as well as Gram-negative cocci, while streptomycin is effective against many Gram-negative organisms. As it is preferable to use bactericidal rather than bacteriostatic drugs, treatment can be started with penicillin or streptomycin, or both, particularly if no organisms are seen on Gram's stain. If the patient is known to be allergic to penicillin, an alternative broad spectrum drug such as erythromycin or tetracycline can be used.

Organisms should be tested for sensitivity to the full range of antibiotics, and treatment changed, if necessary, to the appropriate drug once the sensitivities are known. However, most of these organisms are sensitive to penicillin and streptomycin, and by using these drugs in combination and in high dose the emergence of resistant strains is reduced to a minimum. The majority of antibiotics pass freely across the synovial membrane of inflamed joints, and the intra-articular administration of penicillin is therefore not essential. With severe infections 10 to 20 million units of crystalline penicillin may be required daily in divided doses at 4-hourly intervals. To ensure maximum blood levels and minimum discomfort to the patient this can be given intravenously. As the joint improves, the dose can be reduced to one million units 6 hourly, intramuscularly, and maintained at that level.

If streptomycin is also used, 0·5 G intramuscularly twice daily is usually effective, but the dose may have to be increased to 2·0 G daily in severe cases for seven to ten days. It is not a suitable drug for prolonged treatment because of its toxicity and the readiness with which resistant strains emerge. It must not be used in patients with impaired renal function.

Although antibiotics pass freely into inflamed joints, in severe infections it is probably useful to instil an antibiotic into the joint at the time of aspiration. Thus, 100,000 units of crystalline penicillin in 5·0 ml normal saline or 5·0 mg streptomycin in 5·0 ml normal saline can be injected into the joint following aspiration.

The response to antibiotics can be gauged by the clinical improvement and the return of laboratory tests to normal. A fall of temperature and increase in well-being is accompanied by less pain and swelling in the joint. The rate of re-accumulation of the effusion diminishes, and the fluid becomes clearer. Antibiotics should be continued for at least a week after the patient is apyrexial and the joint appears normal.

Failure of a joint to respond to treatment may be due to the wrong choice of drug, inadequate dosage, the development of resistance, or failure of the drug to penetrate the debris within a severely involved joint.

Surgical Drainage. Surgical drainage is seldom necessary. However, if a joint continues to deteriorate despite three to four days of intensive antibiotic treatment, open drainage should be considered. A particular case can be made for open drainage of the septic hip joint if difficulty is experienced in aspiration.

Supportive Care. In addition to antibiotics the limb should be immobilised in a splint in the form of a plaster of Paris half cast. This should maintain the joint in a good functional position. In the lower limb, if there is much muscle spasm, traction may be helpful.

Strong analgesics such as pethidine or morphia may be required for the first few days, but as improvement occurs, salicylates or phenylbutazone will probably be sufficient.

Mobilisation. Mobilisation should be started early to prevent the joint becoming fixed. As soon as pain decreases (usually during the first week) passive movements and static exercises should be started by the physiotherapist. As the inflammation is controlled, graded active exercises are started, but full ambulation with weight bearing should be delayed until all signs of inflammation have disappeared.

PROGNOSIS

With early diagnosis and prompt and effective chemotherapy the prognosis in an otherwise healthy patient is excellent. However, delay in diagnosis, inadequate antibiotic therapy, or poor general condition of the patient may result either in dissemination of the infection and, possibly, even death, or permanent joint damage. Gonococcal arthritis carries a particularly good prognosis, responding dramatically to penicillin therapy.

TUBERCULOUS ARTHRITIS

AETIOLOGY

Although tuberculous arthritis is now seen much less frequently in the United Kingdom than was the case twenty years ago, it nevertheless still provides a problem in both diagnosis and treatment. While the infecting organism was formerly nearly always of the bovine type, it is now usually the human variety that is responsible. The joint infection is always secondary to a focus elsewhere, usually in the mediastinal or mesenteric lymph nodes, and it is carried to the bone or joint in the blood stream. Predisposing factors include lowered resistance from chronic illness or from corticosteroid therapy. The role of trauma is unknown, but a history of recent injury to the site is certainly not uncommon.

PATHOLOGY

Tubercle bacilli are carried in the blood stream to bone. The joint then becomes infected by direct extension from this focus. More rarely, a focus may develop in the synovium, and for some reason this occurs particularly in the knee joint. Infection is followed by the formation of multiple tubercles with caseation, cavitation, and fibrosis but the outcome varies according to the site of infection.

The Spine. Infection most commonly occurs in the body of a lower thoracic vertebra, close to the intervertebral disc which also becomes infected. Cavitation plus the weight transmitted by the spine result in collapse of the vertebra with extension of the abscess under the anterior longitudinal ligament. The angular kyphus thus produced is known as a *gibbus.* The abscess may remain localised and press on neighbouring structures or track some distance from the site of infection.

Peripheral Joints. Although almost any peripheral joint may become involved, the hip and knee are the most common sites. The synovium is thickened, boggy, and covered with tubercles, while an effusion develops in the joint cavity.

Tendon Sheaths. Tuberculous tenosynovitis is uncommon, but tuberculous granulation tissue may remain localised to the flexor tendon sheath of a finger or of the wrist and palm to form a *compound palmar ganglion.*

CLINICAL FEATURES

Tuberculous arthritis, although more common in children, is being seen increasingly in the older age groups. It is very much more common among inhabitants of underdeveloped countries.

Although almost any joint may become infected, the commonest site is the spine. Here, early diagnosis may be difficult, the signs evolving very slowly after the first complaint of backache. Several months may elapse before definite tenderness of the affected vertebra can be elicited and before any general symptoms of tuberculous toxaemia appear.

Tuberculosis of a peripheral joint usually presents as a subacute or chronic monarticular arthritis, most frequently in the hip or knee, thus causing a limp. There is pain, swelling, limitation of movement, and marked muscle wasting. Usually, there is also some general malaise, weight loss, and fever. The onset is typically gradual with the signs and symptoms developing over a period of weeks or months, in contrast to the more acute evolution of a suppurative arthritis.

DIAGNOSIS

Synovial Biopsy. An absolute diagnosis of tuberculosis can be established only by the demonstration of tubercle bacilli in a smear, culture, or guinea-pig inoculation of the synovial fluid or synovial membrane.

Tuberculin Test. A positive Mantoux test is probably only significant in the first few years of life, after which 50 per cent of the population give a positive reaction. A negative test usually precludes the disease.

Radiology. Chest radiographs may reveal a pulmonary tuberculous lesion, but early X-rays of the joint are usually negative. The earliest signs are decalcification of bones near the joint, followed by irregularity of the joint surface. Later, there may be gross joint destruction and bony ankylosis.

Haematology. In the early stages there may be only elevation of the sedimentation rate. Later, a mild anaemia develops.

TREATMENT

Treatment consists of a combination of chemotherapy and local measures together with orthopaedic management.

Chemotherapy. Antituberculous chemotherapy follows conventional lines, using streptomycin, PAS, and isoniazid in the appropriate combinations for at least fifteen months.

Local Treatment. Immobilisation of the joint in a position of function is usually continued for some months. This is generally regarded as being an orthopaedic problem, and details of the specialised methods of splinting used will be found in orthopaedic textbooks.

Orthopaedic. Although the advent of chemotherapy has reduced the need for surgery, a number of cases still require operative procedures either to clear the infection, or to deal with the damaged joint. Again, details will be found in orthopaedic textbooks.

13

Rheumatic Fever

Anthony D M Jackson

Rheumatic fever is a generalised inflammatory disease with a tendency to recur. It affects mainly children and young adults, the principal clinical features being polyarthritis, carditis, and chorea, of which carditis is the most important in view of its liability to cause permanent damage to the heart.

INCIDENCE

The incidence of rheumatic fever has declined steadily over the past thirty years. Notifications in selected areas of England and Wales in recent years have indicated an annual incidence of about 1 per 10,000 children under the age of fifteen years. On this basis, the estimated number of new cases in children each year is 1,000 for England and Wales. Rheumatic fever is rare in children under the age of five years, and the highest incidence is between the ages of six and fifteen years.

AETIOLOGY

It is now established that rheumatic fever is a sequel of a previous infection with group A haemolytic streptococci. In epidemics of untreated streptococcal pharyngitis in closed communities, such as boarding schools or military training centres, the incidence of rheumatic fever may be as high as 3 per cent, but following untreated sporadic streptococcal infections less than 0·5 per cent of patients develop rheumatic fever. Treatment of streptococcal pharyngitis with a ten day course of penicillin considerably reduces the risk of subsequent rheumatic fever. The interval between streptococcal upper respiratory infections and the onset of rheumatic fever varies from one to six weeks, with an average of three weeks. The fact that rheumatic fever is commoner in children of school age and in individuals living in poor social conditions is probably related to the increased incidence of streptococcal infections in these groups.

It is not clear at present by what mechanism streptococcal infection causes rheumatic fever. The disease may be a hypersensitivity reaction to group A streptococci. It is also possible that there is an autoimmune mechanism at work by which antistreptococcal antibodies produced in the body act on heart muscle which is antigenically similar to the streptococcus. A cross-reacting antigen has actually been shown to be shared by streptococcal cell wall and heart muscle fibre.

CLINICAL FEATURES

The diagnosis of rheumatic fever is based on the presence of some or all of the following clinical features, which are termed 'major manifestations'–

1. Polyarthritis
2. Carditis
3. Chorea
4. Erythema marginatum
5. Subcutaneous nodules

In addition, there are some non-specific symptoms commonly associated with the disease and termed 'minor manifestations'–

1. Fever
2. Arthralgia
3. Abdominal pain

Polyarthritis

Polyarthritis is the commonest clinical feature of rheumatic fever, and is usually the presenting symptom. It occurs in some 75 per cent of initial attacks. The skin over the affected joints is hot and red, and the joints themselves are swollen and extremely painful and tender. The large joints of the limbs are most commonly affected, but the smaller joints in the feet and hands may be involved. The arthritis almost always affects more than one joint and proceeds from one joint to another. The acute stage lasts several days in each affected joint so that more than one joint may be affected at any one time.

Rheumatic fever does not produce radiological erosions or result in permanent joint damage. (Except in the rare curiosity known as *Jaccoud's arthritis*, in which recurrent attacks of rheumatic fever produce finger deformities and even radiological 'erosions': Eds.)

Carditis

The inflammatory process of rheumatic fever affects the endocardium, myocardium, and pericardium to varying degrees in about 50 per cent of initial attacks. This incidence of carditis becomes progressively lower beyond the age of eighteen years. The clinical features of the carditis usually appear following the arthritis in the first week or so of the disease and depend on the degree of endocarditis (mitral and aortic valvulitis), myocarditis, and pericarditis present. The physical signs of this carditis are –

Tachycardia
Murmurs
Cardiac enlargement
Congestive failure
Pericarditis
Prolonged atrio-ventricular conduction

Tachycardia is almost always present but is not diagnostic since it occurs in any child with a fever. In children, the pulse rate is easily raised by activity or anxiety and it is advisable to record the sleeping pulse rate. With active carditis the sleeping pulse rate is usually over 100 a minute.

Murmurs. The development of a murmur during the early stages of rheumatic fever is strongly suggestive of carditis. Three types of murmur may be heard –

Apical systolic
Apical diastolic
Aortic diastolic

The apical systolic murmur of mitral valvulitis is soft at first but may become louder. It is blowing in character and fills most or all of systole. It is maximal at the apex and is conducted towards the axilla. The first heart sound at the apex is soft and muffled. This apical systolic murmur must be distinguished from the common innocent systolic murmur of children which is best heard internal to the apex or at the left sternal edge and is short, mid systolic, not widely conducted and may vary in intensity with heart rate and posture.

The low-pitched apical mid-diastolic murmur is also due to mitral valvulitis. It is less common but of more serious significance. The aortic early diastolic murmur caused by aortic valvulitis is the least common of the three murmurs. It is best heard at the left sternal edge, and is soft and blowing.

Cardiac enlargement is present in at least 50 per cent of children with rheumatic carditis but may be difficult to detect on physical examination alone. Chest radiographs are helpful in determining the presence of cardiac enlargement.

Congestive heart failure and pericarditis are infrequent complications, occurring only in the most severe forms of rheumatic carditis. The two important findings in heart failure in children are oedema and enlargement of the liver, but distended neck veins and moist sounds in the lungs may also be present. Pericarditis without effusion is indicated by a pericardial friction rub and the presence of chest pain. In the presence of an effusion the diagnosis of pericarditis will depend largely on radiographic signs.

Prolonged A-V conduction is present in many cases of rheumatic fever but it is not specific. It is demonstrated by a prolonged PR interval (more than 0·2 second) in the ECG tracing. There may also be cycles of progressive lengthening of the PR interval, culminating in a dropped beat which can be detected at the pulse (Wenckebach phenomenon).

The severity of the carditis can be graded according to the physical signs—

1. Apical systolic murmur alone (least severe).
2. Apical systolic and diastolic murmurs.
3. Basal diastolic murmur with or without apical murmurs.
4. Congestive failure and/or pericarditis (most severe).

It is fortunate that the most common form of carditis seen in the United Kingdom at present is the least severe, especially since the incidence of residual rheumatic heart disease is directly related to the severity of the initial carditis (*see* Table 13.1, below). Nevertheless,

TABLE 13.1

Prognosis of Rheumatic Fever

Heart condition at onset	10-year follow-up	
	Heart Disease %	Deaths %
No carditis	6	0
Mild carditis	30	0
Severe carditis	64	4

severity of the initial carditis (*see* Table 13.1). Nevertheless, severe rheumatic heart disease may occasionally be identified in adults in whom previous acute rheumatic fever has never been recognised.

Chorea

Chorea is a disorder of the central nervous system that may occur alone ('pure chorea') or in association with other clinical features of rheumatic fever which it may precede, accompany or follow, although it rarely coincides with polyarthritis. Chorea is a self-limiting condition that subsides spontaneously after a period of weeks or months. Recurrences may occur but there are no permanent sequelae. It is commoner in females, and in older girls it is particularly liable to occur during pregnancy.

The clinical picture is characterised by abnormal purposeless jerking movements of the limbs and face. The onset is gradual. In the early stages the child becomes clumsy; she drops things easily and has difficulty in writing, doing up buttons, and tying laces. Fluids are spilt when drinking from a cup. When the disease is fully developed, the movements may affect the whole body and can be violent, but the severity is variable, and in some cases only one side of the body is affected (hemichorea). The movements of chorea are exaggerated by voluntary muscular effort but cease completely during sleep. The affected child is often emotionally labile with alternating bouts of laughing and crying.

On examination, the typical movements may be demonstrated, if they are not immediately obvious, by asking the patient to extend the arms and fingers and to protrude the tongue. The extended limbs show the typical writhing movements, and there is hyperextension at the metacarpophalangeal joints with hyperflexion at the wrists. The tongue is difficult to keep still and is constantly withdrawn and protruded so that the child tends to bite her tongue in an attempt to keep it still. Fine movements of the fingers such as picking up a pin are impossible. There are no specific neurological signs but the knee joint may remain extended for a brief period after elicitation of the knee jerk ('hung-up knee jerk').

Erythema Marginatum

Erythema marginatum, like many of the other clinical manifestations of rheumatic fever, is a suggestive but not specific finding. It is present in about 10 per cent of cases. The skin lesion is a non-irritating pink or red macule with a pale centre and a sharply defined but irregular margin. There may be many such lesions on the trunk and limbs, and several may join together. Erythema marginatum is transient but may recur during the course of the illness.

Subcutaneous nodules

These are less common than erythema marginatum and usually appear later in the disease than the other clinical features. The nodules are hard, mobile, non-tender swellings in the subcutaneous tissue. The common sites to find rheumatic nodules are the scalp and the extensor surfaces of joints, particularly the elbows, knees and ankles.

Other clinical features

Fever is a constant minor manifestation of rheumatic fever but is obviously not specific and has no special characteristics. In severe attacks in young children the fever tends to be greater and of longer duration than in mild cases in older children. There is no fever in children with pure chorea.

Arthralgia is pain in and around a joint with no objective signs. This mild form of joint involvement may occur in rheumatic fever but, in the absence of true arthritis, presents a problem in diagnosis since it is such a common symptom in a number of childhood illnesses.

Abdominal pain is sometimes the presenting symptom of rheumatic fever and may be severe enough to raise the possibility of appendicitis. In a sick child with fever, abdominal pain, and tender, possibly rigid, abdominal muscles it may be extremely difficult to exclude appendicitis if the polyarthritis or carditis are not yet evident.

LABORATORY INVESTIGATIONS

There is no diagnostic laboratory investigation for rheumatic fever. The following investigations may be helpful in making a diagnosis –

Antistreptolysin O (ASO) Titre

The presence of antistreptolysin O in the blood indicates some exposure to the streptococcal antigen, streptolysin O. The titre of antibodies is usually expressed as the reciprocal of the dilution and referred to as ASO units. Thus, an ASO titre of 1/100 is expressed as 100 units. In urban populations, healthy individuals have positive ASO titres which rise with age, presumably as a result of sub-clinical streptococcal infections. Thus, healthy children of school age may have titres up to 250 or even 300 units. In this age group, therefore, an ASO titre of 500 units or more is considered to be evidence of a recent overt streptococcal infection, although a titre below this level does not exclude such infection. About 80 per cent of children with rheumatic fever have ASO titres of 500 units or more, but it must be emphasised that titres of this level indicate no more than a recent streptococcal infection and are not diagnostic of rheumatic fever. Similarly, a single low ASO titre does not exclude rheumatic fever. In patients with rheumatic fever whose initial ASO titre is low the titre may rise in serial specimens of blood examined over a period.

Erythrocyte Sedimentation Rate (ESR)

The ESR is an entirely non-specific test which depends on the changes in the plasma associated with various disease processes. The upper limit of normal for children is about 20 mm/hour, and abnormally high ESRs are very common in children. It is exceptional, but not impossible, for children with rheumatic fever to have a normal ESR. However, a raised ESR is not diagnostic and does not distinguish between cases with and without carditis. In pure chorea the ESR is normal. It has been stated that the ESR is valuable as a guide to progress during the course of rheumatic fever. Changes in the severity of the disease, and the use of antiflammatory agents in treatment, have tended to limit the value of the ESR for this purpose.

C-reactive Protein

This is an abnormal protein found in the blood in many inflammatory conditions. Its significance is much the same as that of the ESR which is the more commonly used test.

Blood Count

The changes in the blood count in rheumatic fever are variable and non-specific. There is usually a mild or moderate anaemia and a polymorphonuclear leucocytosis.

Throat Swab

Throat swabs should be cultured in all cases of rheumatic fever, to determine the presence of haemolytic streptococci.

DIFFERENTIAL DIAGNOSIS

Rheumatic fever is a syndrome in which a collection of certain signs, symptoms, and investigations suggest the diagnosis, although there is no single pathognomonic finding. This is an extremely variable disease. Chorea or polyarthritis may be present alone. Polyarthritis may be mild but associated with severe carditis. Very mild attacks may pass unrecognised. In order to help with the diagnosis, a formula (the Jones criteria) has been devised using the major and minor clinical manifestations together with certain other criteria. According to this formula, which is set out at the top of page 201, the presence of two major criteria or one major and two minor criteria is strongly suggestive of rheumatic fever, especially if there is evidence of a preceding streptococcal infection. The Jones criteria, however, do not always settle the diagnosis in certain atypical or mild cases, and clinical experience and judgement have to be the final arbiters.

Major Criteria	*Minor Criteria*
Polyarthritis	Fever
Carditis	Arthralgia
Chorea	Prolonged P-R interval
Erythema Marginatum	Raised ESR
Subcutaneous Nodules	Evidence of a preceding group A streptococcal infection
	Previous rheumatic fever or inactive rheumatic heart disease

The following conditions commonly present problems in differential diagnosis –

Virus upper respiratory infections often present with fever, a rash and limb pains or even polyarthritis. In such cases the rash is maculo-papular and, unlike erythema marginatum, the arthritis is usually less acute and less painful than rheumatic arthritis and is less likely to pass from joint to joint.

Rheumatoid arthritis, although sometimes mimicking rheumatic fever in the acute stage, tends to affect small joints more often than the latter disease, and the arthritis is more persistent. Carditis of the type seen in rheumatic fever does not occur in rheumatoid arthritis. Adenopathy and splenomegaly are often present, and the appearance of the rash is different from erythema marginatum.

Anaphylactoid purpura (Henoch-Schonlein purpura) may present with painful swelling in the limbs but there is less acute inflammation of the joints and the swelling is often periarticular rather than articular. The typical maculo-papular-petechial rash of anaphylactoid purpura, though it may not be present at the onset of the disease, will settle the diagnosis when it appears. Abdominal pain is a common feature of anaphylactoid purpura and adds to the confusion between the two diseases.

Osteomyelitis may cause pain and swelling in more than one limb but it is unusual for a joint to be involved at more than one site. The maximum tenderness will usually be over the metaphysis even if there is some pain and tenderness of the neighbouring joint. In such cases of multiple osteomyelitis the accompanying septicaemia gives rise to a more severe swinging temperature than is usual in rheumatic fever. In doubtful cases repeated blood cultures are essential.

Non-specific limb pains. Acute pain in one or more than one limb, often presenting at night, is a common occurrence in children without any evidence of inflammatory disease. These are the so-called 'growing pains' of the older textbooks and are now thought to be muscle cramps, perhaps with a psychological overlay. In these cases the complete absence of local or systemic signs will exclude the diagnosis of rheumatic fever. There may be a history of previous pains of a similar type.

Sickle cell disease is often complicated by fever, abdominal pain, and painful swollen joints. The disease affects children of African races, and the diagnosis is established by haematological studies which reveal anaemia, red cell sickling, and the presence of an abnormal haemoglobin on electrophoresis. The joint symptoms are usually restricted to one joint.

Habit spasms or nervous tics are often confused with the symptoms of chorea, but careful study of the movements should distinguish the two conditions. Tics are repetitive purposeful movements which follow a set pattern, e.g. blinking the eyelids, clearing the throat, shrugging the shoulders etc. A child with a tic tends to repeat the same set of movements over and over again although, after a period of weeks or months, a different tic may arise which, in turn, is repeated for a time. The typical features of chorea are not seen in the child with tics.

TREATMENT

1. *Anti-inflammatory Drugs.* The role of salicylates and steroids in the treatment of rheumatic fever has been discussed and argued a great deal over the past ten years. There is still some controversy over this subject but the following is a summary of the main conclusions to date.

Both salicylates and steroids have a place in the treatment of rheumatic fever but neither has been shown to influence the eventual outcome as far as permanent heart damage is concerned. Both drugs suppress the acute signs and symptoms of the inflammatory process but it is doubtful whether they shorten the course of the disease. The use of these drugs is, therefore, symptomatic therapy. Steroids have a greater suppressive effect than salicylates but have more serious toxic effects. They are indicated, therefore, in the severe forms of the disease with moderate or severe carditis, especially if complicated by heart failure or pericarditis. Salicylates are indicated in the milder forms of the disease with either minimal signs of carditis or polyarthritis without carditis.

The dosage of these drugs is –

Steroids (prednisone):	2 mg/kg body weight/day in divided doses. Duration: 2–6 weeks (depending on severity and response)
Salicylates (soluble aspirin)	120 mg/kg body weight/day in divided doses. Duration: 1–4 weeks (depending on severity and response)

If anti-inflammatory drugs are withdrawn too soon or too abruptly there may be a 'rebound' with recurrence of signs and symptoms. This is less likely with the milder forms of the disease. It is usual to continue with either drug for 1 to 2 weeks after the acute signs and symptoms have subsided and the cardiac signs have stabilised. Steroids should be withdrawn gradually and the withdrawal period overlapped with salicylates which are continued for a further week or so.

It is very doubtful whether steroids have any effect on pure chorea, and salicylates do not. There is, therefore, no specific therapy for this condition.

2. *Antibiotics*. Antibiotics have no effect on the course of rheumatic fever. Nevertheless, in view of the close relationship between this disease and the haemolytic streptococcus, it is usually considered advisable to give a therapeutic 10-day course of penicillin to all cases whether or not haemolytic streptococci have been isolated from throat cultures. For this purpose phenoxymethyl penicillin (Penicillin V) given by mouth in a dose of 125–250 mg 6 to 8 hourly is satisfactory.

The value of prophylactic antibacterial therapy in preventing recurrences of rheumatic fever is unquestioned. It is obligatory to give such prophylaxis to all patients after an attack of rheumatic fever or pure chorea. There is some evidence that the risk of recurrences of rheumatic fever is slightly greater if oral penicillin or sulphonamides are used for prophylaxis than if monthly injections of long-acting benzathine penicillin are used. However, oral phenoxymethyl penicillin is the most popular prophylactic drug in the United Kingdom, at present. The dose is 125 mg or 250 mg twice daily according to age. Prophylaxis should be started on the completion of the ten-day therapeutic course and should be continued without interruption for at least five years or for the duration of school life, whichever is the longer. This will cover the period of maximum risk of recurrence, but in rare instances late recurrences develop, and some authorities continue prophylaxis into adult life. It would certainly seem advisable to continue to protect those adults with a past history of rheumatic fever who have a high risk of exposure to streptococcal infections, such as hospital workers, school teachers, and service personnel. It is sometimes argued that the child who throughout a first attack of rheumatic fever shows no evidence of carditis is statistically so unlikely to develop this complication in any subsequent attack, that antibacterial prophylaxis is unnecessary. This is not the view of the author.

An unusual but serious complication in patients with rheumatic heart disease is *bacterial endocarditis*. This complication may arise from the transient bacteraemia that follows dental extraction and similar manipulative procedures within the mouth. It is wise, therefore, to protect patients with rheumatic valvular disease by giving large doses of soluble penicillin to cover these procedures.

3. *Bed Rest.* The traditional value of prolonged bed rest in rheumatic fever must now be questioned. There is no clear evidence that bed rest has any specific value in preventing cardiac damage or in shortening the course of the disease, and the former practice of 'complete bed rest', with the child nursed flat on his back and not permitted even to feed himself, probably does more harm than good. The tendency nowadays is to keep the child in bed during the acute febrile phase of the illness. In patients with polyarthritis alone or with mild carditis this will usually mean 2 to 4 weeks in bed. In the more severe cases with moderate or severe carditis the duration of bed rest will need to be longer, possibly up to three months or more. It is usual to grade the return to full activity after getting up, and the duration of this progressive activity is roughly equal to the time spent in bed. Return to school is allowed when the child has reached the stage of full activity at home but strenuous physical activity at school is avoided for a further 4 to 8 weeks. Thus, mild cases of rheumatic fever may spend about 3 weeks in bed, 3 weeks in progressive activity out of bed, and a further 4 weeks in limited activity at school. Children with severe carditis may take 3 months, 3 months, and 2 months over these stages.

There need be no permanent restrictions of physical activity for those children who have recovered from rheumatic fever without heart damage. Even children with residual mitral or aortic valve disease probably do not need to be restricted, but this is a matter of opinion and some physicians would exclude such children from severe exertion and competitive sports. In general, it is better to err on the side of permissiveness than on the side of restriction for the young patient.

COURSE AND PROGNOSIS

The duration of an attack of rheumatic fever may be anything from a few weeks to many months. Joint symptoms last for only a week or two in most patients. Carditis varies greatly in severity and, therefore, in duration, lasting anything from six weeks to six months. Chorea is a benign self-limiting condition with an average duration of about two months though there may be recurrences for a year or so after the initial attack. Carditis may develop as much as ten years later in patients with pure chorea not given continuous prophylaxis.

In a combined United Kingdom–United States study of rheumatic fever completed in 1962, the figures for prognosis were as shown in Table 13.1

All the patients in this study were given antibacterial prophylaxis after the first attack. These results show that very few children with rheumatic fever develop rheumatic heart disease if there is no carditis in the initial attack. The incidence of rheumatic heart disease is directly related to the severity of the initial carditis, but even with severe carditis one third of the patients do not develop heart disease. The overall mortality of rheumatic fever is very low.

With the declining severity of the disease and with greater attention to adequate prophylaxis the prognosis for patients with rheumatic fever may be even better in years to come.

14

Osteoarthrosis

J D Jessop

Advancing age is accompanied by degenerative changes affecting all the tissues of the body to a varying extent, and at differing rates of progression. It is difficult to define these changes as physiological or pathological in the usual sense, even though (unless some disaster has overtaken the individual) they eventually terminate in some structural breakdown that causes death. Osteoarthrosis (OA) or degenerative joint disease (DJD) represents this degenerative process as it affects the joints. It normally begins in the third decade of life, but, since the degeneration of other tissues proceeds with it, the demands of the individual on the joints gradually diminish with ageing so that in the 'normal' no disparity develops between the anatomical state of the joint and the function it is required to perform. Thus, at autopsy in an elderly subject, gross degenerative change may be found in joints – 'osteoarthrosis' – which have been entirely symptomless in life, or at most have provoked the owner to remark that she 'feels her age' or that he 'is not as agile as he was'.

In the clinical sense, we talk of osteoarthrosis when the symptoms and signs in one or more joints seem to be disproportionate to their chronological age. Clearly, this disproportion will be determined by many factors. At one end of the scale are factors affecting the patient's capacity to adjust to advancing age, or to appreciate and react to painful stimuli, and at the other end there is gross mechanical distrubance of joints which has a profound effect on their function.

In order to give an account of such a wide spectrum of joint disease considerable over-simplification will be necessary, the various factors being dealt with somewhat in isolation. The reader will, therefore, have to bear constantly in mind that the clinical situation may be very much more complex.

PATHOLOGY

The pathological changes of OA are first seen in joint cartilage. They are most easily studied in the hyaline cartilage of synovial joints. The intervertebral disc, which presents similar pathological changes in a somewhat different setting, will be discussed separately. Normal articular hyaline cartilage covers the bearing surface of the bone, to which it is firmly attached by fibrous tissue. It averages about 3 mm in thickness. Like all connective tissue, cartilage consists of cells (*chondrocytes*), ground substance (*mucopolysaccharides*), and fibres (*collagen*).

Cartilage as a whole has no direct blood supply and derives its nutrition not from the underlying bone but from the synovial fluid. This bathing fluid is circulated over the cartilage by movements of the joint.

The function of joint cartilage is to provide a firm compressible, almost frictionless, cushion on which movement of the synovial joint can take place. Because of its poor blood supply, cartilage has little capacity for regeneration. No more than a limited growth of cells can take place in damaged cartilage, and these are mainly fibrocytes without the structure of normal cartilage.

The earliest lesion in OA is a softening of the matrix of the articular cartilage due to a loss of *chondroitin sulphate* in the superficial layer. It is not known what causes this – it may be due to an increased breakdown of mucopolysaccharides or to a slower rate of synthesis resulting from impaired chondrocyte function. Whatever the cause, the result is a separation of superficial fibrils, often but not necessarily, starting in the areas of greatest stress. Flakes of cartilage break away into the joint space and are phagocytosed by synovial cells. This activity may give rise to a low-grade synovitis. The deeper chondrocytes may for a time react by producing more chondroitin sulphate.

As the separation of fibres, *fibrillation*, becomes more extensive, bone change begins to occur. This is characterised by proliferation of bone with increased vascularity, the subchondral bone becoming thickened as if it were attempting to carry the extra stress that follows the loss of cartilage. New bone also forms at the joint margins forming *osteophytes*. These changes, by altering the stresses within the bone produce a situation in which trabecular fracture is likely to occur. Cysts form, which may communicate with the joint through these *microfractures*. Joint movements produce pressure changes (greatly increased where an effusion is present) that are transmitted to the cysts through these microfractures and cause them to become distended and enlarged.

Physical changes can be seen to accompany these developments. A disappearance of the normal glistening surface of the cartilage occurs first. This is followed by patchy development of a soft roughened surface which advances slowly and irregularly, producing ulcerated areas with exposed bone. These areas of bone become smooth and eburnated through constant wear. As the bone, in its turn, fails to sustain the stresses applied to it, it becomes increasingly roughened, cysts collapse, osteophytes continue to develop, and remodelling occurs. The final result, with perhaps all these changes taking place concurrently, or at least overlapping, is complete loss of the normal joint structure, and gross anatomical deformity.

AETIOLOGY

Many factors can be responsible for the changes described above. If we accept that these develop as a result of a disparity between the mechanical properties of the joint itself and the forces imposed on it, then we have to consider, on the one hand, the variability of the cartilage itself (its 'quality'), and, on the other, the factors determining the total forces applied during the life of the joint. In the clinical situation many aetiological factors may affect both of these variables.

A simplification is to divide all OA into two broad categories. Firstly, that in which degeneration occurs in an otherwise apparently normal joint—*primary osteoarthrosis*—and secondly, that which occurs as a result of a clearly recognisable abnormality within the articulation; for example, anatomical changes producing increased wear, or clear-cut biochemical abnormality affecting the physical properties of the joint structure—*secondary osteoarthrosis*.

Genetic Factors

An inherited predisposition is an important factor in certain forms of OA. Where this takes the form of a simple generalised arthropathy it may be termed *primary generalised osteoarthrosis*. The clinical hallmark of this is involvement of the terminal interphalangeal joints of the fingers, producing the Heberden's node and we therefore prefer to call this *nodal multiple osteoarthrosis*. Inheritance of this common form of OA suggests determination by a single autosomal gene, dominant in the female, and recessive in the male. A second type of generalised OA, in which Heberden's nodes are absent, also occurs. This is due to a variety of inherited disorders that may produce damage to joints, disturbing their integrity, and rendering them liable to *secondary* osteoarthrosis. Obvious examples are the developmental disorders of the musculo-skeletal system such as chondro-osteodystrophy (Morquio-Brailsford) and multiple epiphyseal dysplasia. Other examples include the hypermobility syndrome and Marfan's syndrome. Inherited metabolic anomalies may also alter the quality of articular cartilage, rendering it more vulnerable to wear and tear, e.g. homogentisic acid in ochronosis or urate crystals in gout.

Metabolic Factors

Metabolic abnormalities of inherited type have already been mentioned above. The metabolic abnormality underlying osteoarthrosis remains unknown in the majority of cases. It is tempting to speculate that there may be a relatively simple, but unrecognised, metabolic disturbance causing primary generalised osteoarthrosis. The characterisation of *Kashin-Beck's syndrome* in Russia, in which multiple OA develops as a result of eating cereals infected with a fungus (Fusaria) or the widespread changes in cartilage produced by eating the sweet pea (*Lathyrism*), are examples of rare, but recognised, acquired metabolic abnormalities producing osteoarthrosis.

Endocrine Abnormalities

Acromegalic arthropathy (p. 274) is an example of one known endocrine abnormality leading to OA. There may be others.

Inflammatory Arthropathies

The joint damage of any inflammatory arthropathy may itself produce secondary OA. In the more advanced case of rheumatoid arthritis, for example, the joint changes will represent a combination of both inflammatory and degenerative processes. It follows that an attack of rheumatoid arthritis that remits may be the cause of osteoarthrosis in later years. If the original attack was overlooked, the final clinical picture may present considerable diagnostic difficulty.

Anatomical Abnormalities

Any congenital or acquired anatomical deformity of a joint may render it liable to secondary OA. Thus, congenital dislocation of the hip, Perthes' disease, osteochondritis, slipped epiphysis, avascular necrosis, or fractures involving a joint may all be responsible for the later development of secondary OA.

Neuropathic Causes

Where there is impairment of sensory appreciation of articular pain the normal protective mechanisms cease to operate. In this situation gross secondary osteoarthritic changes may develop. This is the Charcot joint described on page 282.

Trauma

Major trauma is likely to produce anatomical change and is discussed above. But minor trauma, if repeated regularly, can have a similar effect. This may occur typically in certain occupations causing osteoarthrosis, of the knees in colliery workers, in the elbows of workers using pneumatic drills, and in the lumbar spine of those engaged in heavy lifting. Traditionally, OA of weight-bearing joints such as the knees is thought to be aggravated by obesity, and this may be regarded as a form of trauma. Internal derangements of joints may also provide a sufficient source of trauma to cause secondary OA.

CLINICAL FEATURES

Clinically, osteoarthrosis usually involves one, or only a small number of joints. It commonly affects subjects aged fifty years or over, but there are variations in the incidence of joint involvement, depending upon the factors already mentioned, as well as age, sex, obesity, and occupational hazards. Symptoms often bear little relation to radiographic appearances or, indeed, to pathological changes in cartilage, except where major weight-bearing joints such as the hip or knee are involved. The presenting symptoms are usually pain in the region of the joint, with a slowly progressive loss of movement, and development of deformity, but there is considerable variation in the rate of progress in any one individual. The cause of the pain is not precisely known, since the factors governing bone pain are not understood. Pain may be caused by trabecular micro-fractures or soft tissue strains. Nocturnal aggravation is probably due to hyperaemia. It is known that capsular traction causes pain, and stresses on the fibrotic capsule almost certainly contribute to the symptoms. Pain may also arise from the low grade synovitis that results from phagocytosis of particles of cartilage.

Pattern of Joint Involvement

The pattern of joint involvement in secondary osteoarthrosis will be essentially that of the underlying cause, to which the reader is referred. It is only necessary here to draw attention to the characteristic distribution of nodal multiple osteoarthrosis. This condition affects the distal interphalangeal joints—the Heberden's nodes—the first carpo-metacarpal joints, the first metatarso-phalangeal joints (but not the lateral metatarso-phalangeal joints), the acromio-clavicular, the knee, and the apophyseal joints of the spine, but virtually all the joints in the body may be affected, with the possible exception of the wrists and the temporo-mandibular joints.

The general clinical picture of osteoarthritic joints is described in Appendix A, to which the reader should refer. There follows here some selected examples of important features of OA in commonly affected joints.

The Hand

Heberden's Nodes. These have already been mentioned. They are very

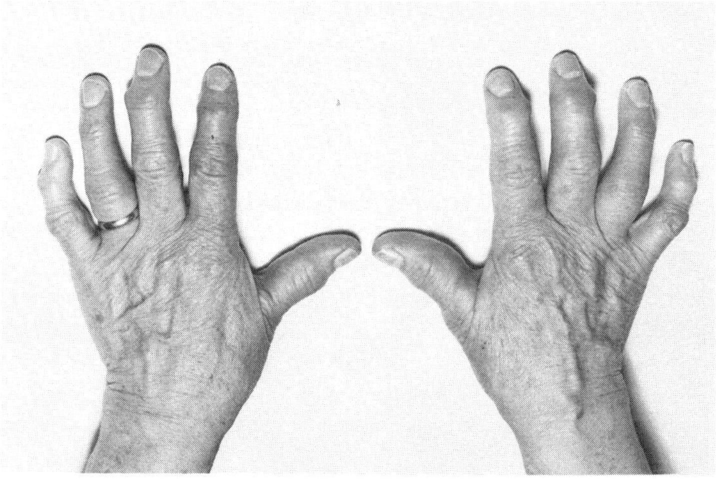

(*a*) The bulbous swellings at the terminal interphalangeal joints are Heberden's nodes, while the 'square' appearance of the hands is due to involvement of the first carpometacarpal joint producing adduction of the first metacarpal and wasting of the nearby small muscles

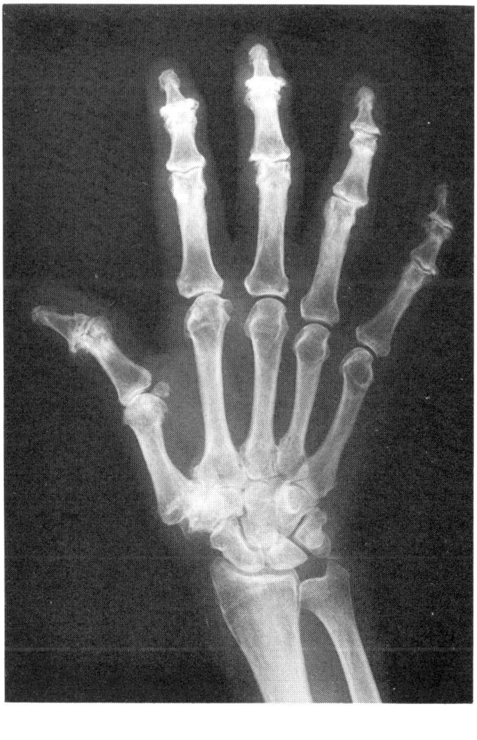

(*b*) The radiograph confirms the pattern of joint involvement (emphasis on the terminal interphalangeal joints and the first carpometacarpal joint)

FIGURE 14.1 The hands in nodal multiple osteoarthrosis

common and highly characteristic protuberances consisting of pea-sized marginal osteophytes situated at the base of the distal phalanx. The mode of inheritance that accounts for their frequent occurrence in middle-aged women has already been described. They usually develop slowly with varying degrees of pain and are commonly associated with generalised osteoarthrosis. They gradually become symptomless. Rarely, they develop acutely as painful, red, tender, cystic swellings. The appearances may then closely mimic the distal interphalangeal joint involvement of psoriatic arthropathy (and, occasionally, even suggest gout).

Osteoarthrosis of proximal interphalangeal and metacarpo-phalangeal joints may occur with or without Heberden's nodes. In the latter case it is sometimes secondary to an earlier inflammatory arthropathy.

First Carpo-metacarpal Joint. Involvement of the joint between the trapezium and the first metacarpal is a common and highly characteristic feature of nodal multiple osteoarthrosis. Severe involvement is associated with swelling, and a deformity in which the thumb becomes adducted and the base of the metacarpal subluxed to produce the deformity of the 'square hand'. There is often simultaneous involvement of the joint between the trapezium and the scaphoid, but symptoms from this are usually overshadowed by those from the trapezio-metacarpal joint. Together, Heberden's nodes and the 'square hand' present an unmistakable picture (Fig. 14.1). This is the clinical hallmark of *nodal multiple osteoarthrosis*.

The Wrist

Primary osteoarthrosis rarely involves the wrist; secondary OA may, however, develop following an ununited fracture of the scaphoid, an imperfectly reduced Colles' fracture, or a previous inflammatory arthropathy.

The Elbow

Osteoarthrosis of this joint is seldom severe unless there has been a predisposing cause such as fracture or repeated occupational trauma. One important result may be an 'entrapment neuropathy' with a neurological deficit in the distribution of the ulnar nerve.

The Shoulder

While primary osteoarthrosis of the glenohumeral joint is rare, degenerative changes in the acromio-clavicular and sterno-clavicular joints are common and produce visible prominences. This is usually unimportant. Lesions of the periarticular structures in the region of the shoulder joint are dealt with in Chapter 15.

The Foot

First Metatarso-phalangeal Joint. No joint in the body receives more weight than this. Like the first carpo-metacarpal it is also commonly affected in nodal multiple OA. It is, also, the site of hallux rigidus or valgus discussed in Chapter 16. As already pointed out, the lateral metatarso-phalangeal joints are not commonly affected in osteoarthrosis.

The Knee

Together with the hip, osteoarthrosis of the knee is an important cause of disability. Although the cause of the pain is not understood, careful observation suggests that early disability results from repeated abnormal stresses resulting in minor fibrous tears. These can be identified as localised areas of tenderness that are often relieved by local infiltration with hydrocortisone. Sometimes, but surprisingly rarely, OA of the knee joint progresses to the later stages with the development of varus or valgus deformity, with increasing distortion of the direction of weight-bearing and progressive degenerative changes inevitably taking place. These usually involve collapse of one or other tibial (rarely femoral) condyle.

Involvement of the patello-femoral compartment is occasionally the predominant feature. When this occurs prematurely it is known as chondromalacia patellae (*see* p. 234).

The Hip

Osteoarthrosis of this important weight-bearing joint usually appears in middle age. If it occurs at a younger age there is often a predisposing cause; for example, trauma, inflammatory arthropathy, slipped femoral epiphysis, congenital dislocation, avascular necrosis of the femoral head, or Paget's disease of bone.

The first symptom is usually in one hip. Pain on weight-bearing may be felt in the groin, buttock, or thigh. However, a particularly misleading situation may arise if the pain is felt exclusively in the knee. This common clinical trap is due to pain being referred through the articular branch, derived from the obturator nerve, which supplies both joints. There is wasting and weakness of the glutei and quadriceps muscles. An important physical sign is the downward tilting of the pelvis when the patient stands on the affected leg. This, the *Trendelenberg sign*, is described in Appendix A (p. 307).

The condition is usually progressive, although there is considerable individual variation. Deformity gradually develops, with upward subluxation of the head of the femur into the superior margin of the acetabulum (Fig. 14.2), and further deformity may occur as the juxta-articular cysts in the acetabulum collapse. The joint becomes externally rotated with a flexion and adduction deformity. At this stage, pain and deformity usually cause severe limitation of functional capacity.

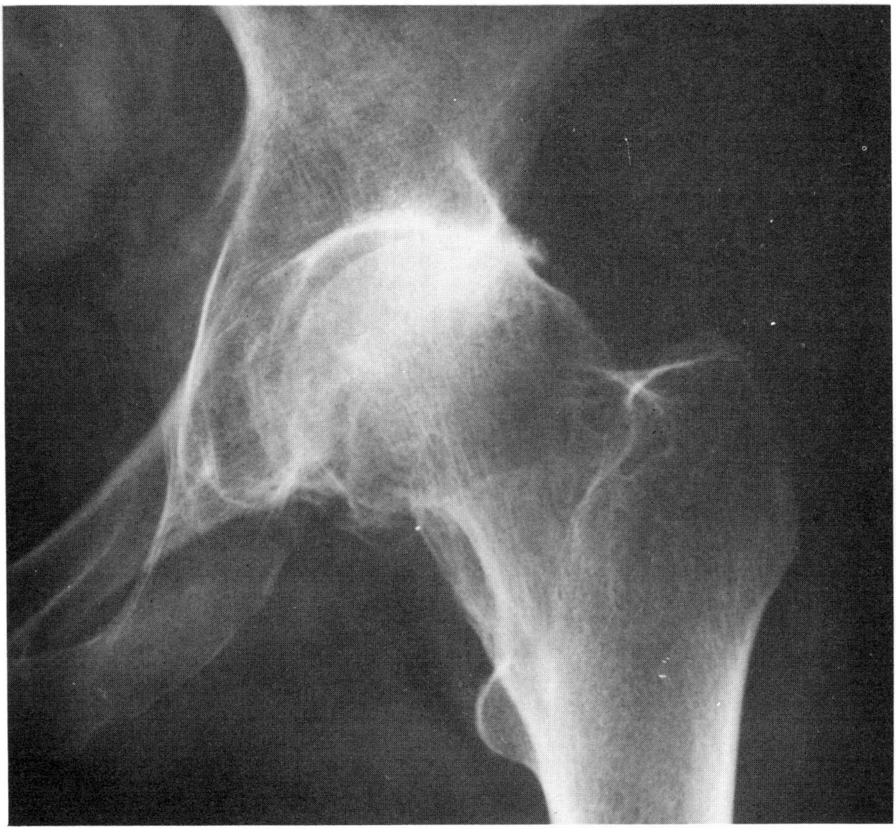

FIGURE 14.2 Osteoarthrosis of the hip joint. The head of the femur is tending to move upwards into the roof of the acetabulum. The secondary bony overgrowth represents attempts at buttressing both at the upper margin of the acetabulum and along the neck of the femur

THE SPINE

The joints of the spine consist of the posterior apophyseal articulations, which are lined with synovium, and the intervertebral, non-synovial joints composed of fibrocartilagenous discs. Degenerative changes may occur at either site. OA occurring in the spine is known as *spondylosis* (in contrast to inflammatory spinal joint disease, or *spondylitis*).

The fibrocartilagenous discs which separate the vertebrae are composed of an annulus fibrosus and a central nucleus pulposus. The strong annulus is firmly attached to the adjacent bones and ligaments. The nucleus pulposus, placed slightly posteriorly within the annulus, is composed of mucopolysaccharide and collagen fibres and has an affinity for water, which causes it to remain distended under pressure within the confines of the annulus. With advancing age the water content diminishes and the disc shrinks.

The classification of spinal disease becomes very confusing when applied to the extremely common mechanical derangement in which an intervertebral disc protrudes outwards to produce pressure on nerve roots or other structures. This – the 'slipped disc' of the layman – may occur in a young adult as a direct result of trauma, in which case it represents a primary internal derangement of the joint, unrelated to degenerative changes; or it may occur in an elderly subject without obvious trauma, in which case it is due to disc degeneration, or spondylosis. Between these two extremes there are all gradations, and clinically it is often difficult to assess the relative contributions of trauma and degeneration. This chapter is concerned with degenerative joint disease, not with traumatic internal derangements of joints, but in the spine the two cannot clearly be separated, and no attempt has been made here to draw a sharp distinction.

Disc degeneration occurs normally with age. Changes in the annulus fibrosus are analogous to osteoarthrosis in synovial joints; minor strains and tears allow the margin of the annulus to bulge outwards. When this is postero-lateral it may compress nerve roots.

Disc prolapse implies rupture of the nucleus pulposus through the annulus. Postero-lateral protrusion is the commonest form of rupture to give rise to symptoms. Protrusion in this direction is dictated by the slightly posterior position of the nucleus and the strong posterior longitudinal ligament which is in the midline. Anterior and lateral protrusions rarely cause symptoms. Vertical prolapse through the hyaline cartilaginous plate into the cancellous bone of the adjacent vertebral body produces a characteristic radiological change known as the *Schmorl's node*.

Cervical Spine (cervical spondylosis)

Apophyseal Joints. Involvement of these joints is particularly common in middle-aged women and is part of the picture of multiple osteoarthrosis. There is usually pain, stiffness, and some limitation of neck movements which may be accompanied by crepitus. Symptoms are aggravated by movements of the neck, in particular by lateral flexion and rotation. These movements are usually restricted.

Intervertebral Joints. Disc degeneration usually gives rise to symptoms around middle age. The commonest level to be affected is C5-C7 (Fig. 14.3) (in contradistinction to rheumatoid arthritis which affects mainly the upper cervical region). Symptoms vary from a dull ache to severe attacks of pain in the neck, with limitation of movement.

If there is compression of nerve roots, there may be pain radiating down

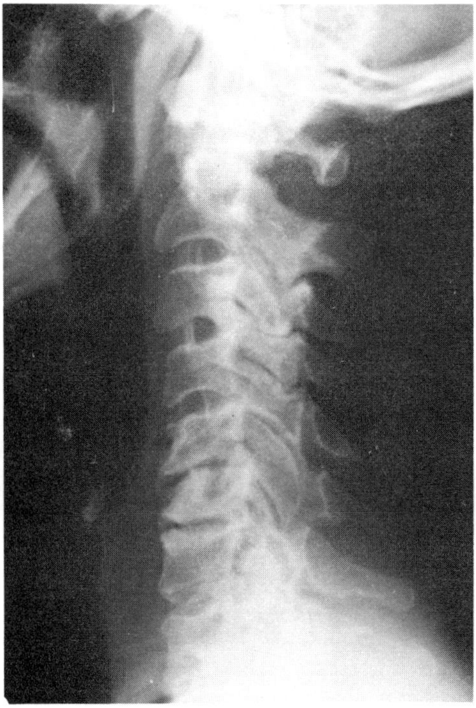

FIGURE 14.3 Osteoarthrosis (spondylosis) of the cervical spine. Characteristically the sclerosis, osteophyte formation, and narrowing of disc spaces are prominent in the lower cervical region (C.5–7)

the arm, paraesthesiae in the finger tips, and reflex and motor changes in the distribution of the compressed nerve root.

If new bone, or a cartilaginous bar, compresses the spinal cord posteriorly, there may be signs of upper motor neurone or other long tract lesions affecting the legs. An additional complication of cervical spondylosis is interference with the blood supply to the brain, by kinking of the vertebral arteries as they run upwards through the foramina before entering the foramen magnum to form the basilar artery. Transient blackouts and visual disturbances may then be precipitated by neck movements.

The usual course of cervical spondylosis is one of intermittent attacks of pain, stiffness, and limitation of movement of varying degrees of severity, but in general the tendency is for attacks to become less severe and less frequent in later years.

Prolapsed Disc. Prolapse usually affects the 5th or 6th intervertebral disc. Disc degeneration is an important predisposing cause, while trauma is usually the precipitating factor. A small herniation compressing a nerve root in the intervertebral foramen can cause pain radiating down the arm. Because the roots in the cervical region have a short horizontal course, passing over the intervertebral disc before entering the foramen, a lateral protrusion is likely to compress only one nerve root against the ligamentum flavum, pedicle, or articular facet (in contrast to the situation in the lumbar region).

The characteristic features are pain, paraesthesiae, and slight muscular weakness in the distribution of the nerve root. The motor, sensory, and reflex signs will be determined by the distribution of the compressed nerve root, and the completeness of the lesion. There is often an acute onset of painful stiff neck, followed a few days later by pain radiating to the shoulder and down the arm. The continuous aching pain is often exacerbated by coughing, sneezing, and neck movements, especially by lateral flexion towards the side of the lesion, and by rotation to the opposite side; the former movements compressing and the latter stretching the root.

Dorsal Spine

Symptoms arising from the dorsal spine are much less common than those from the cervical or lumbar spines, unless there is an obvious predisposing cause such as longstanding scoliosis, or osteochondritis (Scheuermann's disease). Usually, there is pain in the lower dorsal region with limitation of extension and rotation, and with tenderness on percussion of the affected area. Pain may radiate through the trunk to the chest or abdomen or round the chest wall in girdle distribution. Acute disc lesions in the dorsal region are rare.

Lumbar Spine (lumbar spondylosis)

A common cause of low back pain is degenerative change in the lumbar discs and, perhaps, in the apophyseal joints.

Intervertebral Discs. Lumbar disc protrusions are the commonest cause of low back pain with sciatica. This usually occurs against a background of degenerative joint disease. As mentioned above, the disc protrusion of the young adult is likely to be traumatic and should not be classified as OA.

The precipitating trauma is usually slight. The annulus fibrosus characteristically ruptures posteriorly, and a fragment of torn annulus is extruded into the vertebral canal. In more severe cases there may be frank prolapse of the nucleus pulposus through the tear. If there is concomitant rupture of the posterior longitudinal ligament the protrusion may be in the midline posteriorly instead of in the more usual postero-lateral position. The fibro-cartilage or nucleus pulposus may impinge on the related nerve root or compress it against the lamina and ligamentum flavum. As the rupture is usually to one side of the midline, only one nerve root is affected in its extra-thecal course; but because the roots of the cauda equina run nearly vertically within the theca, one or more of those passing caudally may also be compressed. If the rupture is in the midline, roots on both sides may be involved. If it is large enough, the protrusion may also compress the cauda equina. The majority of disc lesions are at the L4/5 or L5/S1 level (Fig. 14.4), and it is only here that a disc

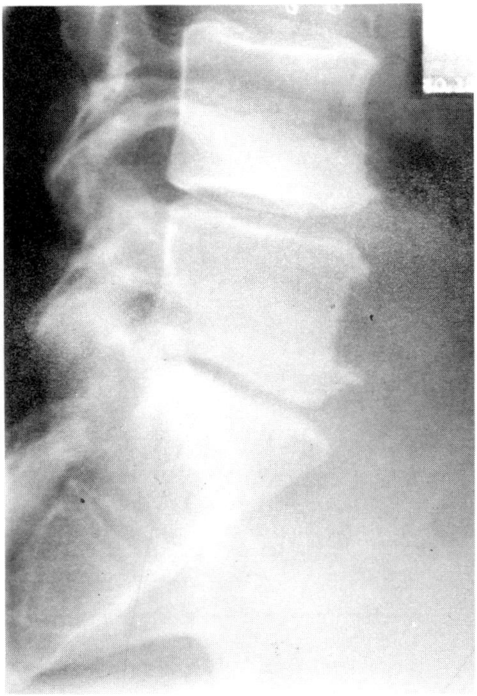

FIGURE 14.4 Osteoarthrosis (spondylosis) of the lumbar spine. Sclerosis, osteophyte formation, and narrowing of the disc spaces are most prominent at the L.5–S.1 level, but are also present at L.4–5

lesion produces the syndrome of low backache with sciatica. Unlike the situation in the cervical spine, cord compression is not a feature of lumbar disc lesions since the spinal cord ends opposite the lower border of L1.

Apophyseal Joints. Radiologically these joints are usually involved *pari passu* with disc degeneration of the intervertebral joints. They are also part of the pattern of joint involvement in multiple OA. On anatomical grounds it seems likely that they contribute to the symptomatology.

Clinical Features. The initial complaint is usually one of pain in the lower lumbar or lumbosacral region. Less often, back pain may be absent, and the initial complaint is one of sciatic pain alone. The onset may be gradual with no particular relationship to injury, or it may be acute with severe pain fixing the spine in a particular attitude, usually forward flexion.

In the acute case, sciatic pain often accompanies the initial low back pain, while with a gradual onset it may be delayed. In severe cases, sciatic pain radiates into the buttock, the posterior aspect of the thigh and calf, and the lateral aspect of the ankle and foot. In less severe cases pain may be limited to the thigh.

Pain is aggravated by movement of the spine, such as rolling over in bed, and by any manoeuvre (such as coughing, sneezing, or straining at stool) that causes elevation of the cerebrospinal fluid pressure within the theca. This increases the pressure from within on a nerve root already compressed by the disc. In Naffziger's test, digital pressure on both jugular veins in the neck increases the pressure of cerebrospinal fluid and causes pain or paraesthesiae in the distribution of the affected nerve root. Pain is more constantly aggravated by manoeuvres that put the sciatic nerve on the stretch. Thus, forward flexion of the lumbar spine or straight leg raising with the patient supine produces pain, and if the patient sits up in bed the knee and hip on the affected side are flexed to avoid stretching the sciatic nerve. Because of these features that increase pain, the back is usually held rigid and movements are limited by muscle spasm which results in scoliosis to one or other side and flattening of the normal lumbar lordosis. Forward flexion is usually more limited than lateral bending.

Neurological Picture. Although the only symptom of a lumbar disc lesion may be pain, there is frequently an associated neurological deficit due to compression of one or more nerve roots forming the sciatic nerve. The sciatic nerve is formed from the 4th and 5th lumbar and the upper three sacral roots, and compression may cause paraesthesiae or numbness in the distribution of the involved root. Thus, an L4 and L5 lesion causes sensory changes mainly over the dorso-medial aspect of the foot and great toe, while in S1 compression sensory changes may extend over the lateral margin of the foot, toes, ankle, and lateral aspect of the leg. If several sacral roots are involved, sensation may be lost up the back of the thigh into the buttocks and perineum.

Motor weakness, if present, is usually slight; occasionally it is sufficiently severe to produce a foot drop. L4/5 lesions produce wasting and weakness mainly of dorsiflexion of the foot, L5/S1 mainly of the great toe and everters of the foot, while an S1 lesion mainly involves flexors of the foot and toes. The motor signs are usually accompanied by diminution or absence of tendon reflexes; with L4 involvement the knee jerk is diminished, and with an S1 lesion the Achilles tendon reflex may be diminished or absent. L5 lesions do not produce reflex changes.

Cauda Equina Paralysis. The above neurological lesions represent a partial or complete nerve root lesion on one side. Rarely, a massive protrusion may compress part or whole of the cauda equina and produce bilateral paralysis or sensory loss. This syndrome usually starts with back pain radiating into both legs, producing bilateral sciatica progressing to a paralytic lesion.

In less acute cases it may start as unilateral sciatica but an additional strain may precipitate sudden severe exacerbations of back pain, bilateral sciatica, numbness, and weakness of both legs. Pain may then be abolished because of complete interruption of the sensory pathway. There is a flaccid paralysis of feet and legs, absent ankle jerks and sensory loss extending from the feet up the back of both legs to the buttocks and perineum. There will also be paralysis of the rectal and vesical sphincters.

Upper Lumbar Lesions. Protrusions of the second and third discs are less common than those of the fourth and fifth, but rarely they may even cause a cauda equina paralysis. Small lateral protrusions may cause back pain with anterior crural pain, but never sciatica. Sensory impairment may extend over the anteromedial aspect of the shin and there may be diminution or abolition of the knee jerk.

RADIOLOGY

The single most useful investigation in the diagnosis of OA is radiology. Although pain may appear before there are any changes apparent on X-ray, and the radiological severity may not always correspond with the clinical disability, nevertheless the X-ray appearances usually enable OA to be clearly differentiated from the inflammatory arthropathies, and provide a reliable method of assessing the extent of damage to a joint

The characteristic radiological signs of OA are the following:

1. *Narrowing of the joint space.* As the (radiolucent) cartilage is worn away, the clear space between the adjacent bone cortices becomes narrowed.
2. *Marginal osteophyte formation.* New bone formation results in bony projections growing outwards around the joint and inwards into the joint cavity.
3. *Subchondral sclerosis.* New bone is also laid down in adjacent subchondral bone ends. The affected bone end thus becomes more densely radio-opaque.
4. *Bone cyst formation.* The probable mechanism for the formation of bone cysts has been discussed. Radiologically these cysts appear as rounded translucences in the periarticular bone. They vary in size from or 2 mm up to a few centimetres, and differ from the erosions of inflammatory arthropathy in not having an obvious opening into the joint space.
5. *Deformity.* In the latter stages there is increasing deformity due to collapse of subchondral bone and cysts, subluxation, gross bone overgrowth, and the presence of loose bodies within the joint.

RADIOLOGY – RA *v.* OA

	RA	OA
Bone density	Porotic	Sclerotic
Erosions	Characteristic	Absent
Cysts	Sometimes	Common
Osteophytes	Absent	Characteristic
Loss of joint space	Yes	Yes
Late deformity	Yes	Yes

N.B. The late stages of RA may show features of (secondary) OA.

OTHER INVESTIGATIONS

Unlike rheumatoid arthritis, which is a systemic inflammatory disease, primary OA is a degenerative disorder limited to the joints. This is reflected in the results of laboratory investigations. Characteristically, the ESR and other routine blood tests are all normal, and rheumatoid factor is absent from the serum. Synovial fluid aspirated from OA joints tends to be clear, with a low cell count, normal (high) viscosity, and a relatively low protein content (*see* p. 322).

TREATMENT

Osteoarthrosis occurs at an age when other senescent changes may tend to exaggerate any personality defect, difficulties in interpersonal relationships, or general dissatisfaction with a life situation. This sometimes leads to psychological disturbances such as depression and anxiety becoming expressed as the symptoms of degenerative joint disease.

Inevitably, the clinician caring for patients with degenerative locomotor disorders has his attitude towards osteoarthrosis coloured because his patients with organic rheumatological complaints are diluted by patients whose basic problems are psychological or social. The competent doctor will feel that these non-organic factors require diagnosis, explanation, and treatment in the same way as organic disease. However, whether or not this attitude is adopted, there is a very real danger that interest in the problem of managing actual articular symptoms will be blunted to the point where the management of OA becomes an uncritical routine of prescribing analgesics and placebo physiotherapy.

It must be said at once that much can be done to help the patient with OA; but this requires a clear understanding on the part of the clinician of the natural history of the disease, the mechanism by which symptoms are produced, and the methods by which they can be relieved. The various aspects of management are discussed below. Perhaps the two most important points to emphasise are, firstly, that analgesic therapy is generally disappointing and is unlikely to solve any real problems, and secondly, that most *pain in OA is due to trauma* (using this word in a very broad sense). This forms the basis of logical non-operative treatment.

DIAGNOSIS AND EXPLANATION

In milder cases this may be the most important aspect of management. The man with cervical spondylosis or the woman with Heberden's nodes is often more worried that the 'rheumatism' will lead to a crippling polyarthritis, than by actual symptoms from the lesion. And, as with cancerophobia, these fears are often concealed. So the first objective is to establish the diagnosis firmly, and the second, to explain the disease carefully to the patient. The man with cervical spondylosis can be reassured that this condition almost invariably remits spontaneously after a time; while the women with Heberden's nodes can be guaranteed that her hands will not become crippled. Finally, the aims and limitations of therapy need to be stressed. Many patients (and even some doctors) are convinced that these conditions can be cured if only the right analgesic tablet or technique of physiotherapy is discovered. This leads, in extreme cases, to the patient going from doctor to doctor, then exploring the less orthodox methods of treatment.

REST AND PROTECTION

Rest, in the sense of protection from trauma, is the sheet anchor of conservative therapy in OA. To apply this principle successfully it is necessary to understand the mechanism by which symptoms are produced. Pain seldom arises spontaneously from the rested OA joint; it is usually due to some form of trauma, typically minor, to which the joint is particularly vulnerable. This may be a stretching or 'strain' of some soft tissue joint component, a subchondral bone trabecular fracture nipping of structures between the articular bearing surfaces, or capsular tension when the range of movement exceeds certain limits. The summation of all these minor episodes may suggest a continuous process, but careful history-taking will usually reveal the episodic nature of the symptoms. An additional factor is introduced when spondylosis is complicated by pressure of an intervertebral disc on a nerve root, but similar general principles of non-operative treatment are, in fact, applicable in this situation too.

The principle of treating degenerative joint disease by rest and avoidance of trauma can, with a little imagination, be applied to most joint in the body. The principle is more important than the details of it application, so only a few examples have been selected to illustrate this approach.

The Hip and Knee. Pain due to osteoarthrosis of the large weight-bearing joints may respond dramatically to a reduction in daily wear-and-tear trauma. In the first place this involves adjusting the patient's way of life both at home and at work so as to *reduce the time during which the affected joint is weight-bearing.* A change from a standing to a sedentary job, for example, may enable him to live within his painfree limits. The previously athletic man who develops OA of a weight-bearing joint will sometimes want to 'walk it off' by strenuous exercise. He will, however, usually be convinced by the argument that a worn bearing is an indication to conserve the life of a machine by using it sparingly, and that exercise is helpful, therefore, only when the weight is off the joint.

Improvement in posture and gait reduces trauma by allowing weight-bearing to be mechanically more efficient. Useful means of achieving this are walking aids and footwear adjustments. Osteoarthrosis of either the hip or the knee may produce deformity and painful limitation of the joint, leading to a grossly abnormal gait with altered weight-transmission mechanics, so that walking produces a destructive grinding away of the joint-bearing surfaces. Outstandingly effective in this regard is the humble *walking stick.* Used in the hand on the side *opposite* to the affected joint, it can restore gait-posture to an extent that greatly reduces abnormal forces acting on the joint. Other walking devices include tripods, crutches, and frames. Selection of the correct walking aid of the right size, and training in its use is best arranged by consultation between physician and physiotherapist. When shortening of a leg complicates osteoarthrosis of a weight-bearing joint, *built-up footwear* can similarly reduce trauma by restoring mechanical efficiency.

In theory, *correction of obesity* is a highly effective method of reducing trauma in a weight-bearing joint. Not only does it reduce the load, but it allows a better alignment of the legs. It is often difficult to achieve.

Another approach to the avoidance of trauma is the principle of *splinting* applied in various ways. Actual mechanical splints have little application in the case of the hip joint, but the severely affected knee may sometimes require a hinged, metal caliper (the locking hinge allows flexion on sitting). No splint is available that can control gross varus or valgus knee deformity; this demands surgery. In practice, the most important application of the principle of splinting is that which improves the joint's natural stabilising mechanism—the muscles. The stability of a large weight-bearing joint depends, to a large extent, on the co-ordinated pull of the muscles acting across it. Therefore, the wasting and weakness of these muscles that results from disease of a weight-bearing joint will reduce stability and allow increased trauma during walking. Striking improvement in muscle power and function can be achieved by correct training and exercising. This is the responsibility of the physiotherapist.

Cervical Spondylosis. The majority of patients experiencing symptoms from cervical spondylosis will recover spontaneously. It is customary to treat this condition by applying the same principles of avoiding trauma. Occasionally, an obvious postural defect can be corrected, for example, by adjusting working conditions. Usually a neck splint is prescribed—either a soft (felt) or firm (plastic) collar that is worn, if necessary, both by day and by night.

Lumbar Spondylosis. Nowhere is the principle of treatment by rest and avoidance of trauma more important than in lumbar spondylosis, particularly if there is associated nerve root pressure. The first line of treatment of an acute attack is bed rest, in whatever position the patient finds comfortable. If the symptoms subside, he is then mobilised gradually, doing no more than can be managed within the pain-free range. Pain persisting for a few weeks despite complete bed rest, particularly if associated with localising neurological signs, is regarded as an indication for myelography and consideration of surgery (laminectomy).

In milder cases, or in patients who have recovered from an acute attack, the objective is to avoid, as far as possible, the circumstances likely to produce a recurrence. Such patients require to be taught a discipline of never extending the back against resistance, from a flexed position. This involves using the legs rather than the back when straightening up with a load. Occupations involving heavy lifting should, if possible, be avoided by subjects with a tendency to develop lumbar disc lesions.

If symptoms are only partly relieved by strict bed rest, a useful measure may be to allow the patient to get about with the lumbar spine protected by a plaster of Paris cast round the trunk. Similarly, the patient liable to recurrent episodes of lumbar disc disorder may benefit from wearing a lumbosacral (Goldthwaite) surgical corset. Essentially, this appliance makes forward flexion of the lumbar spine uncomfortable (thus encouraging the maintenance of lumbar lordosis), and may provide some protection against recurrences.

ANALGESIC DRUGS

Analgesic therapy plays a part in the treatment of OA, and the discussion of the role of the various analgesic drugs in rheumatoid arthritis (page 44) provides a guide also to their use in OA. Stronger, habit-forming, drugs may be required for the initial treatment of acute lumbar disc lesions.

It must be pointed out that analgesic drugs are always a supplementary form of treatment in OA and never, in themselves, provide the solution to a problem. In degenerative joint disease there is no drug available with effects comparable to those of salicylates in rheumatic fever, phenylbutazone in ankylosing spondylitis, or indomethacin in acute gout.

PHYSIOTHERAPY

The role of the physiotherapist in treating OA is to improve the strength of muscles acting across the affected joint and to train the patient in matters such as gait, posture, and the use of walking aids.

Physiotherapy departments are usually equipped also to provide symptomatic analgesia (counter-irritation) by the application of heat in various forms. Traditionally, this is prescribed to facilitate the execution of muscle-strengthening exercises. This is acceptable only if the main purpose of treatment is not obscured. Experience shows that electrical gadgetry and the detailed techniques of applying heat can so mesmerise patient, physiotherapist, and doctor that these procedures become an end in themselves. While there is clearly no harm in teaching patients with painful nodal multiple OA of the hands how to obtain temporary relief by immersing the hands in warm molten wax prepared at home, the prescription of short-wave diathermy by itself for degenerative disease of the hip, knee, or spine indicates a complete failure to grasp the principles of treating OA.

The techniques for improving the strength of muscles acting across affected joints (and thus of providing the physiological splinting and protection mentioned above) involve the use of exercises. Neither electrical stimulation nor massage play any part. The joint need not necessarily be moved during the exercise, and static muscle contractions, such as the familiar quadriceps drill in OA of the knee, can be effective. An additional benefit from this type of exercise may be an increase in the range of movement in the joint. The detailed application of these techniques is the province of the physiotherapist. Much the most effective method in managing OA of weight-bearing joints involves the use of exercise in a *deep pool* in which the body weight is supported by water.

The other role of the physiotherapist in OA, that of training and education, requires little comment. The selection of the right type of walking aid, and instruction in its use, is one example; another is instruction in how to raise a load without precipitating a lumbar disc lesion. Useful advice to patients includes such matters as periods of prone lying for patients with OA of the hip (to avoid flexion deformity) and, similarly, avoidance of pillows placed under an affected knee while in bed.

MANIPULATION

It is clear that large numbers of patients seek manipulative treatment from both qualified and unqualified practitioners, and it is essential that the physician should provide himself with an objective and unbiased philosophy in order to be able to prescribe for, and advise, his patient rationally.

Manipulation, a passive mobilisation of joints, is a procedure used most commonly in OA of the spinal joints. It is either carried out as a manipulation under anaesthesia (MUA) by the orthopaedic surgeon, or without an anaesthetic by the osteopath. Physiotherapists may make use of 'osteopathic' techniques. It is essentially a technique of treatment, and not a 'science' or a system of medicine. (Unfortunately it tends to develop into a fashionable cult.)

The justification for this form of treatment rests on the claim (or belief) that passive mobilisation of osteoarthritic joints results in the rapid relief of symptoms, a belief widely held but unsubstantiated by data. It finds its usual application in the attempted relief of pain arising from trivial degenerative changes giving rise to pain related to the spinal joints, but which are insufficient to cause significant neurological signs. When these are present, manipulation is contra-indicated. In the absence of adequate clinico-pathological studies the means whereby these procedures sometimes produce relief remains speculative. That manipulation itself, with the belief that 'something has been put back in place', has a profound placebo effect is certain.

In practice, when pain in the neck or back has failed to respond to conventional treatment (and in the absence of any clinical or radiological evidence of significant disease other than mild OA) treatment by longitudinal stretching, passive mobilisation, or MUA may provide symptomatic relief. Such a view should not be extrapolated to the belief that the natural history of the osteoarthrosis has been altered. The problem remains of preventing subsequent morbidity, along the lines discussed elsewhere in this chapter.

LOCAL INJECTIONS

Intra-articular injections or hydrocortisone are seldom of value in OA. They are occasionally tried in a particularly irritable knee or the carpometacarpal joint of the thumb.

Sometimes a tender point may be discovered in the soft tissue beside a joint affected by OA. Such a tender area may be the site of a tear or strain, and thus be the source of the discomfort in that particular exacerbation. Local infiltration of the area with a mixture of local anaesthetic and hydrocortisone is sometimes very effective.

Surgery is discussed in Chapter 16.

15

Medical Orthopaedics

H L F Currey

Collected together in this chapter is a variety of conditions that fall somewhere between the provinces of the orthopaedic surgeon and the rheumatologist. Many of these conditions are relatively trivial, and indeed should seldom be seen in hospital, for both diagnosis and effective treatment are often within the scope of the general practitioner. However, most of them may at times mimic (and may be mistaken for) inflammatory joint disease, and it is largely for this reason that we have selected them for discussion here.

SHOULDER LESIONS

The very wide range of movements of which the shoulder joint is capable is made possible by the anatomical arrangement of this articulation. In contrast to the situation in the hip joint, the shallow glenoid cavity offers little resistance to free humeral movement in all directions, and, of course, the scapula itself is also mobile. The stability of the gleno-humeral joint is maintained, not by a 'ball-and-socket' arrangement, but by the presence of the tendons that surround it. Thus, the long head of biceps tends to hold the humeral head into the glenoid cavity, while the joint capsule is strengthened by the incorporation into it of the flattened expansions of four tendons: subscapularis and supraspinatus anteriorly, infraspinatus and teres minor posteriorly. Together these constitute the 'rotator cuff'. Upward movement of the humeral head is also limited by a fibro-osseous arch between the acromion and coracoid processes. Between this arch and the rotator cuff lies the subacromial bursa, which often communicates with the main joint cavity.

The unique anatomical arrangement of the shoulder may account for the frequency with which this joint becomes involved in a variety of ill-understood pathological conditions in which pain and stiffness are the outstanding features. It is not known to what extent these conditions represent varying expressions of a single underlying pathology, or whether different disease processes may produce the same end result. The most likely aetiological factor seems to be repeated mechanical traumata to one or more components of the rotator cuff, leading to inflammatory and degenerative changes. Such changes may then spread by contiguity to involve other structures around the joint. Disuse of the joint may itself lead to stiffness, so that pain and immobility become self-perpetuating.

A number of descriptive terms are now accepted for classifying these conditions clinically. Unfortunately, some of these terms imply a pathological and anatomical exactness of diagnosis that is often not justified. But, until the underlying pathological changes are better understood, they will continue to be used.

Rotator Cuff Lesions. This general term is used to describe those painful conditions of the shoulder in which pain and limitation of movement is apparent during the execution, actively, of movements produced by one of the rotator cuff muscles. What at first may appear to be a generally painful and stiff shoulder can, on careful examination, prove to have a relatively free and painless range of motion, except for one particular movement, the execution of which (especially against resistance) produces sharp pain. This finding is regarded as evidence of 'tendinitis' of the muscle tendon in question. Observed over a period, such a process may spread to involve other tendons of the rotator cuff, until there is painful limitation of all movements. The condition is then referred to as *capsulitis* (of the whole rotator cuff and joint capsule). If this progresses to complete loss of movement at the gleno-humeral joint, then the descriptive term *frozen shoulder* (*see* below) is appropriate.

Rotator cuff lesions are usually seen in young or middle-aged adults; the onset may be apparently spontaneous or may follow a recognised, often minor, traumatic incident. Involvement of a particular tendon is recognised by sharp pain when those movements served by the tendon are attempted against resistance. If other movements are full and painless, this clearly differentiates the condition from arthritis of the joint. However, if the lesion has extended to become a *capsulitis*, it is necessary to differentiate it from an inflammatory arthropathy (primary degenerative disease of the shoulder joint is uncommon). If other joints are unaffected, if morning stiffness is not a feature, and if the sedimentation rate is normal, then it is very unlikely that a stiff painful shoulder is due to an inflammatory arthropathy. When the supraspinatus tendon is involved (*see* below) X-rays may reveal local calcification.

Rotator cuff lesions vary in severity from those that produce only mild discomfort, to others that are extremely painful and seriously interfere with sleep. They last for weeks, or months, and may follow a fluctuating course, with relapses provoked by minor strains or trauma but with eventual complete recovery. Treatment is discussed below.

Supraspinatus Tendinitis. This is very much the most commonly recognised rotator cuff lesion. Adults of all ages are affected, and there is usually a history of a minor 'sprain' or trauma. The symptoms are often somewhat vague, and the pain is often localised (as in other shoulder lesions) to the point of insertion of the deltoid. Examination, however, reveals tenderness over the greater tuberosity and over the upper part of the joint. Movement is seldom grossly limited, but active abduction of the arm is painful through the intermediate range (60° to 120°). This 'painful arc' is very characteristic of supraspinatus tendinitis, and it probably indicates the range through which the inflamed tendon rubs against the acromion above. A very characteristic sign is abolition of the painful arc by externally rotating the arm before carrying out abduction (which places the greater tuberosity behind, and away from, the acromion).

Radiographs of patients suffering from this condition may reveal *suspraspinatus tendon calcification.* Pathologically, this probably represents a late change following degeneration in a relatively avascular structure. Its relationship to symptoms is variable. It may be present in cases of otherwise typical supraspinatus tendinitis, and it is occasionally seen in asymptomatic shoulders. On the other hand, it may rarely be associated with attacks of extremely acute and severe pain which may well represent attacks of 'crystal synovitis' following rupture of the calcific material into the tendon sheath, bursa, or joint cavity. Chemically, the calcific material is known to be apatite (not calcium pyrophosphate, the offending microcrystal in pseudo-gout attacks).

Treatment of Rotator Cuff Lesions. The natural history of rotator cuff lesions is towards eventual complete resolution after a period of weeks or months. Information is sadly lacking about the effectiveness of therapeutic measures in influencing the course of this condition. However, experience confirms that, as one might expect, local injections of corticosteroids may sometimes abort the attack. The injection consists of 2 to 5 ml either of corticosteroid suspension alone, or of corticosteroid mixed with local anaesthetic. This is infiltrated in the region of the affected tendon sheath or, with more general capsulitis, into the subacromial bursa.

If one or more injections fail to cure the condition, it is customary to prescribe physiotherapy in the form of counter-irritation (such as some type of heat) combined with active and passive movements of the joint through the pain-free range, on the basis that this may prevent contraction of the joint capsule. In obstinate cases of supraspinatus tendinitis associated with radiological calcification, the calcific mass may be evacuated surgically. This is usually curative.

Subacromial Bursitis. Because of its situation, this structure is probably frequently involved in lesions of the rotator cuff; occasionally, it may become distended with an effusion to become apparent as a cystic swelling bulging out from beneath the acromion. If calcific material from the supraspinatus tendon ruptures into the bursa, it may become acutely inflamed. However, primary inflammation of the bursa must be a rare event and 'subacromial bursitis', unqualified, is an incomplete diagnosis. A needle passed under the acromion readily enters the bursa and, unless a more specific target is sought, this is a satisfactory site for depositing corticosteroids in the injection treatment of painful shoulders. Such injected material can be expected to enter the main joint cavity if, as is usual, the two cavities communicate.

Frozen Shoulder. In this common and seriously incapacitating condition all movements of the shoulder are painful and grossly limited. It may occur as the end-result of a number of different processes, the common factor probably being a self-perpetuating cycle of stiffness and pain. The mean age group of these patients is significantly higher than in other painful shoulder conditions, and senescent changes may play an important role.

A frozen shoulder may arise without any obvious predisposing cause; more often it appears in one of the following circumstances:

1. Following an injury to the shoulder, or as a late result of a rotator cuff lesion.
2. In association with ischaemic heart disease or chronic pulmonary disease.
3. Following a neurological lesion, particularly hemiplegia or herpes zoster.
4. Following intrathoracic surgery or operations on the breast.

In the fully developed condition, spontaneous pain, especially at night, is added to the pain on any movement. Fortunately, it is usually unilateral; even so, these elderly patients tend to become very distressed and severely incapacitated. The condition tends to drag on for weeks or months, and although the pain may disappear, the patient may be left with considerable restriction of the shoulder joint.

The best treatment is prophylactic. Pain and immobility of a shoulder joint in an elderly subject require active mobilisation to prevent the development of a frozen shoulder. Once the condition is established, treatment seems to achieve much less. Regular analgesics are often needed, and it is certainly worth trying the effect of one or more injections of a corticosteroid preparation into the joint cavity. Physiotherapy in the form of heat and active exercises within the pain-free range often gives these patients some immediate relief, and may possibly speed their eventual recovery. More certainly, forcing the joint beyond the painless range by over-enthusiastic treatment will delay recovery.

The Shoulder-hand Syndrome. This term is applied to a rare disorder in which a 'frozen shoulder' is associated with a stiff, painful condition in the hand on the same side. To some extent it is an extension to the hand of the process that occurs in the shoulder, and the same aetiological factors may be involved. In its most severe form it is an extremely incapacitating condition in which the arm, with the elbow flexed, is held to the side and protected against trauma in a manner reminiscent of causalgia. All hand movements are limited by pain and stiffness, and there is usually considerable swelling of the extremity. Vasomotor and trophic changes may occur, and X-rays may show patchy osteoporosis. The condition has some features in common both with Sudeck's atrophy, and with causalgia. All three conditions tend to occur in patients who (at least by the time the diagnosis is made) appear to have a psychological disturbance, and all three may be helped by interruption of the sympathetic nerve pathway to the limb.

Treatment consists of the administration of analgesic drugs (perhaps combined with a phenothiazine derivative) and physiotherapy aimed at mobilising the limb. Results tend to be disappointing. If symptoms persist, temporary (followed, if necessary, by permanent) interruption of sympathetic nerve pathways to the limb should be tried. Improvement has been claimed to occur with systemically administered corticosteroids.

TENNIS ELBOW (lateral humeral epicondylitis)

This common minor disorder is seen in adults of all ages. The patient notices the gradual onset of an ache in the region of the lateral humeral epicondyle at the point of attachment of the common extensor origin. Sharp exacerbations of the pain may be provoked by the execution of particular movements, such as lifting objects in a certain way, or by placing the forearm and wrist in a particular position. In mild cases it may even be difficult for the patient to reproduce the circumstances which bring on pain. Physical examination reveals an elbow joint that is normal, with a full range of movement, but with localised tenderness in the region of the lateral humeral epicondyle (careful probing may be needed to discover this tender point). Manoeuvres that either put the wrist extensors on stretch (such as passive flexing of the pronated wrist) or cause these muscles to contract (such as active wrist extension against resistance) may reproduce the pain.

The pathogenesis is unknown, although there is much to suggest that a minor tear of the common extensor origin at its point of attachment may initiate the process. Patients will often recall a particular wrenching manoeuvre involving the forearm occurring at the onset of the complaint, and such actions may precipitate relapses after apparent recovery. Despite the name, actually playing tennis is a relatively uncommon cause, usually due to some fault in technique, and especially difficult to treat successfully if the patient continues to play tennis.

Untreated, the condition tends to wax and wane until it finally disappears spontaneously after a period of months. Treatment consists of injecting 2–4 ml of a corticosteroid preparation mixed with local anaesthetic into the site of maximum tenderness. Use of a Hypospray gun eliminates the immediate pain produced by the conventional needle injection. Both methods, however, are sometimes followed by a painful period 12 to 24 hours later. Single injections by either method will cure about 60 per cent of patients; so repeated injections may be required. Following injections, patients are advised to avoid manoeuvres that were previously painful for at least two weeks. The occasional obstinate case fails to respond to repeated injections; such patients are usually cured by one of a variety of open operations on the affected site. Physiotherapy is probably of no value.

Golfer's elbow (Medial humeral epicondylitis). An exactly comparable condition to tennis elbow may occur on the opposite side of the joint. In this instance, the tender site is at the point of origin of the common flexor tendon from the medial epicondyle. It is the less common form of epicondylitis and is not especially associated with golf. Prognosis and treatment are exactly the same as for tennis elbow, but injection techniques must take into account the position of the nearby ulnar nerve.

DE QUERVAIN'S SYNDROME (tenosynovitis of abductor pollicis longus)

At the point where the tendon of the long thumb abductor runs over the radial styloid process, it is contained within a synovial-lined fibrous tunnel. This arrangement apparently makes it particularly vulnerable to wear-and-tear damage. Nearby tendons, e.g. extensor pollicis brevis, may be similarly affected.

The condition is most commonly seen among people who regularly use their thumbs a great deal. They will usually complain of pain (often poorly localised) in the region of a wrist joint; this tends to be aggravated by repetitive movements employing the thumb. Physical examination reveals a wrist joint that can be put through a full range of movement painlessly, but in which there may be tenderness in the region of the radial styloid process. Extension of the thumb in abduction reproduces the pain and, pathognomically, there is sharp aggravation of the pain if this movement is executed while the examiner exerts pressure over the tendon of abductor pollicis longus at the point where it runs over the radial styloid process. Continued use of the thumb at work produces progressively more incapacitating pain, which may become neuralgic in character.

Treatment, in the first instance, is by injection of the tendon sheath with a mixture of a corticosteroid suspension mixed with local anaesthetic. This can be repeated. If it fails, immobilisation of the tendon by a plaster cast that includes the forearm and reaches to the distal skin crease of the thumb may be tried for six weeks. If this also fails, then open surgical exploration of the tendon is indicated. Slitting of the tendon sheath over the affected segment is curative.

CARPAL TUNNEL SYNDROME

This common and important disorder results from compression of the median nerve as it passes through the tunnel formed by the bones of the wrist and the transverse ligament. It occurs in adults of all ages, is commoner in women, and tends to be seen in association with a wide variety of general conditions, in which the common predisposing factor is assumed to be a tendency for tissues within the carpal tunnel to increase in volume. These conditions include obesity, pregnancy, myxoedema, systemic sclerosis, and rheumatoid arthritis. In rheumatoid arthritis the condition may be missed because both patient and doctor ascribe the pain, muscle-wasting and weakness to the arthritis, and overlook the neurological lesion. This is a particularly serious mistake for, in a rheumatoid hand, function may be achieved by compensating for mechanical derangements. Such a hand is almost certainly particularly vulnerable to a superadded motor and sensory neurological deficit.

The patient will often give a history that is absolutely characteristic and diagnostic. She will have noticed the gradual onset of a dull 'numb' pain in the hand associated with tingling in the fingers. This wakes her at night, and she will try to get relief by hanging her arms down and wringing the hands. The pain and numbness is poorly localised to the distribution of the median nerve in the hand, and it may spread up the arm. In severe cases, the motor and sensory loss may interfere particularly with the finer functions of the fingers.

In the mildest cases there may be very little to find clinically (and positive signs are not necessary to establish the diagnosis if the history is typical). A useful sign is that of Tinel, in which tapping over the median nerve at the wrist (i.e. over the middle of the joint, or over the palmaris longus tendon if present) produces momentary tingling in the median nerve distribution. More advanced cases may show obvious signs of a median nerve lesion, with sensory impairment in the appropriate distribution and wasting and weakness of the thenar muscles. Particularly affected are abductor pollicis brevis (which moves the thumb from beside the palm, forward in a plane at right angles to the hand), and opponens pollicis (tested by getting the subject to pinch together the tips of the thumb and little fingers). In doubtful cases, electro-diagnostic testing may be very helpful (although some mild but definite cases may show no electrical abnormality). Typical findings are delay in median nerve motor conduction between wrist and abductor pollicis brevis, signs of denervation in this muscle, and impaired sensory conduction between the index finger and wrist.

The course of the disorder is unpredictable. In some, there is a steady progression until a more or less complete median nerve lesion is present; in others, the symptoms may fluctuate and sometimes disappear completely. For obvious reasons, in pregnancy the symptoms may clear after delivery.

This is an eminently satisfactory condition to treat. Mild cases may obtain dramatic relief by wearing a wrist splint at night, or by injection into the carpal tunnel of a soluble corticosteroid preparation. (These methods may be of value also in establishing the diagnosis.) For more severe cases, and those in which simple measures fail, surgical decompression of the nerve by division of the transverse ligament (a relatively minor procedure) cures the pain, although severely wasted muscles may not recover.

TRIGGER FINGER (stenosing tenovaginitis)

In this minor disorder, a thickened section of a digital flexor tendon tends to jam as it passes through a narrowed segment of its tendon sheath. The result is that either flexion or extension of the digit proceeds fully up to a certain point, at which it sticks. If greater force is applied, the resistance is overcome, and the digit completes the movement as a sharp 'snap'. Careful palpation of the tendon sheath during this manoeuvre will usually reveal the site of obstruction to be opposite the metacarpophalangeal joint. Presumably the condition represents a reaction to repeated minor frictional trauma. It is most common in the dominant hand of middle-aged women. Rheumatoid arthritis is an important predisposing cause.

Treatment is, initially, by injection of hydrocortisone into the tendon sheath. If this fails, it is a simple matter to free the constriction surgically.

CHONDROMALACIA PATELLAE

The same senescent changes of hyaline cartilage that are the basic lesion of osteoarthrosis may sometimes develop prematurely in the patella. The aetiology is unknown, although there is some evidence that abnormally mobile patellae may be particularly at risk. The condition is not uncommon, and may be very troublesome.

The patient, usually a young adult and often athletic, complains of the insidious onset of discomfort, poorly localised, within the knee joint. This ache tends to appear during periods of activity, and afterwards subsides slowly. Symptoms are typically intermittent, with complete freedom from pain for weeks at a time. In the occasional more severe case, the pain becomes constant and a synovial effusion develops. The knee may 'catch', but does not lock.

Physical examination reveals a joint in which there may be an excess of fluid, but in which passive movement is full and relatively painless. Rubbing the patella against the underlying femoral condyle is painful. A useful test is to get the patient, lying supine, to contract the quadriceps ('press the knee on to the couch') while fixing the patella firmly against the femoral condyles so as to resist upward sliding. In the presence of chondromalacia patellae this produces sharp pain.

The prognosis is less gloomy than might be anticipated from experience based on osteoarthrosis in later life. Generally, the tendency is towards eventual remission, without the development of progressive degenerative changes. Nevertheless, the individual case may present a very difficult problem in management. On the whole, treatment is less than satisfactory. It certainly seems advisable to avoid all vigorous exercise and all activities that provoke the pain, for a period of weeks or months. If, after such a period, activities are restarted and the pain returns, a plaster cast may be applied to immobilise the knee for a period of weeks. It is probably worth aspirating synovial effusions only if they become very large. Intra-articular injection of corticosteroids and physiotherapy are not of proven value. There is considerable divergence of opinion about the value of surgical measures such as shaving off hyaline cartilage from the undersurface of the patella, or actual patellectomy. It remains to be proven that these operations produce better results than perseverance with conservative measures.

'PAINFUL HEEL'

Among patients attending a rheumatology clinic, a symptom encountered from time to time is that of pain in a heel on walking. This may occur as an isolated complaint, or as part of the symptom complex of some seronegative arthropathies. It thus has some diagnostic value.

Painful heels tend to occur at two sites. The one is in the centre of the plantar (weight bearing) surface of the heel, the other posteriorly at the point of insertion of the Achilles tendon. Both cause tiresome discomfort on walking, and clinically both are associated with tenderness locally at the affected site.

Both types of painful heel are thought to represent an inflammatory reaction at the site of insertion of a ligamentous structure into the calcaneal bone. Inferiorly, this is the posterior attachment of the plantar fascia; posteriorly, the insertion of the Achilles tendon; hence the alternative terms *plantar fasciitis* and *Achilles tendinitis*. One bursa is always present at the site of insertion of the Achilles tendon, and another (adventitious) bursa may develop nearby. To what extent *bursitis* contributes to local pain at this site is difficult to assess clinically.

Occasionally, the cause of these two types of heel pain is obvious; for example, contusion due to direct trauma, or pressure from an ill-fitting shoe. More often, no local cause is apparent, and the condition probably results either from minute traumatic tears at the fibro-osseous junction, or from inflammation in this site due to an underlying inflammatory arthropathy.

When the condition occurs in isolation, without any evidence of a general disorder, the patient is often a middle-aged woman, and the plantar site is involved. Examination reveals pain only on pressure over the central part of the plantar surface of the heel. Special investigations are negative, unless X-rays show ossification around the posterior part of the plantar fascia. This appears as a tapered *calcaneal spur*. In contrast to the type to be described below, such a spur has clear, smooth edges without erosions. It may be due to elevation of the periosteum by small fascial tears. At any rate, it is the result of the primary lesion, not the cause of it. Treatment consists of the local injection into the painful area of a corticosteroid preparation mixed with local anaesthetic (2 to 3 ml). Use of the Hypospray technique avoids the pain of injection. Repeated injections may be necessary. Modifications to shoes to provide heel cushioning may be helpful. The occasional resistant case finishes up by having the spur resected surgically. Even this may fail.

Painful heels of similar character may be experienced by patients suffering from one of the 'seronegative inflammatory arthropathies': ankylosing spondylitis, Reiter's disease, psoriatic arthropathy, and colitic arthropathy. The features these conditions have in common, and the ways in which they differ from rheumatoid arthritis have been discussed in Chapter 5. Painful heels (Achilles or plantar) may occur early in the course of any of them, and will then be a useful diagnostic pointer. The radiological features differ in that any spurs tend to be fuzzy in outline, and eroded rather than smooth. This appearance is probably a local manifestation of the more general radiological 'periostitis' seen in these subjects. Treatment is by injection (*see* above) if general measures directed at the underlying disease are not effective.

VIRUS MYALGIA

Most people have at some time or another experienced an episode of pain and stiffness affecting a group of muscles, and lasting one or a few days. The common sites are the muscles of the neck, shoulder girdle, or lumbar region. The cause of such episodes is often difficult to determine. Undoubtedly some are due to intervertebral disc lesions; many remain undiagnosed. However, it is sometimes not appreciated that virus infections can produce just this clinical picture, and for such cases, *virus myalgia* would seem to be the appropriate description.

Typically, such patients present with a short history of a painful and stiff neck or lower spine, and examination reveals movements in the affected area to be limited by pain. Careful enquiry, however, may reveal that the patient also has more general symptoms, such as mild general malaise, perhaps coryza, and fever. The diagnosis is usually made clear by the occurrence of a similar disorder in other members of the family or other occupants of an institution. A number of different viruses are probably involved, and some cases may be mild variants of Bornholm disease.

Typical virus myalgia settles spontaneously over a few days, leaving no sequelae. This differentiates it from another condition, *neuralgic amyotrophy*, also encountered in rheumatology clinics. In this, a myalgia-like pain in the neck, shoulder, and arm is shortly followed by a lower motor neurone paralysis of one of the muscles in the region of the shoulder joint. There may be slight sensory changes too.

METATARSALGIA

Subjects with anatomical abnormalities of the feet, such as claw-toes or equinus deformity, are liable to develop pain in the region of the metatarsal heads on walking. Such pain is correctly referred to as *metatarsalgia*. Pain in this site may also occur in the condition known as *Morton's metatarsalgia*. This develops in feet that are not obviously deformed, and is probably due to pinching of the superficial branch of the lateral plantar nerve as it runs between the heads of the fourth and fifth metatarsals. It produces, on walking, episodes of sharp pain which may be eliminated by the use of properly fitting shoes with or without a metatarsal bar. Continued pressure on the nerve leads to the formation of a 'neuroma' which may require excision.

The importance of these conditions to the rheumatologists is that pain in the region of the metatarsal heads is one mode of presentation of rheumatoid arthritis. Not infrequently patients will recall an episode of metatarsal pain, on walking, that occurred months (sometimes even years) before the disease showed itself as a polyarthritis. Often this initial episode will have been labelled 'metatarsalgia', but radiological erosions of the metatarsal heads in question may establish, in retrospect, the true diagnosis. It is clear, therefore, that the diagnosis of metatarsalgia should be made only after the presence of an inflammatory arthropathy has been excluded.

TIETZE'S SYNDROME

This is an uncommon and benign condition in which one or more painful swellings appear on the upper costal cartilages. The aetiology is unknown, although violent coughing and direct trauma are suspected of playing a role.

The patient notices the gradual appearance, over the upper costal cartilages, of one or more tender lumps. Deep breathing and coughing may produce local pain. On examination, the lumps are firm and somewhat tender, but not warm. Special investigations show no evidence of a generalised disorder. The course is variable. There may be spontaneous remission, or the lumps may persist for years, although becoming painless. If the pain is troublesome, local injections of a corticosteroid preparation may give temporary relief.

16

Operative Surgery in the Rheumatic Diseases

M A R Freeman

Operative surgical treatment in the rheumatic diseases is never curative: rarely, the pathological process may be arrested or even reversed, more commonly its existence and progression has to be accepted and surgery offered to provide palliation of the patient's disability – pain, stiffness, and deformity. Unfortunately, even the causation of this disability is obscure but an attempt must be made to explain it if the rationale of operative surgery is to be understood.

This chapter is, therefore, divided into two parts. In the first part the general principles of the surgery of the rheumatic diseases are outlined in relation to the probable causation of pain, stiffness, and deformity. In the second part the application of these principles is discussed in relation to the joints involved in rheumatoid arthritis (RA), ankylosing spondylitis, and osteoarthrosis (OA).

The discussion concerns solely the operative treatment of the rheumatic diseases. It should be stressed that non-operative treatment invariably precedes, and forms an adjunct to, operative surgery.

Part I: General Principles

THE AETIOLOGY OF PAIN, STIFFNESS, AND DEFORMITY

Pain (Table 16.1) in the rheumatic diseases appears to arise mainly in three tissues: the capsule of the involved joint, the bones of the joint, and the muscles acting on it. Cartilage is not innervated and, accordingly, is insensitive to pain. Synovial membrane is poorly innervated, and experiments with human volunteers have shown that it is almost insensitive to pain arising from mechanical stimulation. No doubt active inflammation of the synovial membrane, as of the capsule, is painful, but active inflammation of these tissues in the rheumatic diseases is not treated surgically.

TABLE 16.1

The Causes and Surgical Treatment of Pain in the Rheumatic Diseases

Disability		Tissue of origin		Pathological process		Available surgical procedure
Pain	may arise in	→ synovial membrane	→ where it may be due to	→ inflammation	→ and may be relieved by	→ synovectomy
		capsule and ligaments →	,,	→ inflammation and distension	→ ,,	→ synovectomy
		bone →	,,	→ collapse and ? load carriage in the presence of diseased cartilage	→ ,,	→ arthrodesis, arthroplasty, osteotomy (drilling and shaving of cartilage)
		muscle and tendon →	,,	→ spasm	→ ,,	→ ? any operation producing analgesia

The fibrous capsule and ligaments of all joints are well innervated both with mechanoreceptor afferents subserving perceptual and reflex proprioception, and with pain afferents. The effective mechanical stimulus for the provocation of capsular pain appears to be excessive tension in the capsule. In the context of the rheumatic diseases, excessive capsular tension may be brought about by two pathological events: firstly, an increase in the volume of material within the capsule, that is to say by an increase in the bulk of the synovial membrane or by an accumulation of intra-articular fluid; and secondly, by capsular fibrosis leading to shortening and tethering of the capsule. Joint movement and position affect the severity of this pain in two ways. In all joints some position within the normal range draws the capsule most tightly against the synovial contents, and it is this position that provokes pain when the bulk of the intracapsular tissues is increased. Secondly, the pain arising from capsular fibrosis is provoked only or chiefly when the capsule has shortened to such an extent that it limits movement: when this limited movement is attempted by the patient with sufficient force to apply tension to the capsule, pain is produced. Thus, capsular pain interferes with movement, and in an attempt to avoid it the patient tends to hold the joint immobile in a position of capsular relaxation.

Although, histologically, nerve fibres which might be pain afferents have been described in bone, the effective stimulus for the provocation of pain in bone is unknown. Traction on the periosteum is painful, but this is not relevant to pain induction in intra-articular bone where the true periosteum is replaced by cartilage or synovium. Indeed, it is not certain that pain in the rheumatic diseases arises from bone at all, but it seems to be a fair assumption (based upon a variety of clinical observations) that some of the pain of which patients complain is bony in origin and that such pain is provoked when bone underlying softened or eroded cartilage is subjected to load. It may be speculated that this is due to the generation of abnormal mechanical stresses in the bone, possibly leading to trabecular micro-fractures or to some alteration in bone blood flow. For the moment such speculations, although fundamental to an understanding of arthritic pain, remain almost entirely unsubstantiated. Pain of this type might be expected to be exacerbated by load carriage rather than by movement.

Muscular pain is probably provoked by local anoxia or by the accumulation of metabolic end-products, arising from abnormally sustained muscular contractions. Such contractions—known clinically as muscle spasm—have not been convincingly demonstrated electromyographically but their existence may be inferred from the fact that the passive range of movement in a diseased joint is often increased by a general anaesthetic producing muscle relaxation. Muscle spasm of this type appears to be a

TABLE 16.2

The Causes and Surgical Treatment of Stiffness and Limitation of Movement in the Rheumatic Diseases

Disability			Tissue of origin				Pathological process				Available surgical procedure
Stiffness and limitation of movement	may arise in	→	articular cartilage	→	where it may be due to	→	ulceration	→	and may be relieved by	→	nothing
			synovial membrane	→	,,	→	increased intra-capsular bulk and adhesion formation	→	,,	→	synovectomy
			capsule and ligaments	→	,,	→	adhesion formation, oedema and fibrosis	→	,,	→	division and removal of the capsule as part of the operation of arthroplasty
			bone	→	,,	→	collapse, osteophytosis	→	,,	→	arthroplasty, ? osteotomy, ? debridement
			muscle and tendon	→	,,	→	spasm, adhesion formation (fibrosis), tendon rupture, tendon sheath adhesion and stenosis	→	,,	→	? any analgesic operation on joints tenotomy, tendon suture, division of sheaths } ? + synovectomy

reflex consequence of joint disease and imposes immobility on the affected joint.

Joint stiffness (Table 16.2) is a loose term covering two disturbances of function—a sense of added resistance encountered by the patient when he attempts to move the affected joint, and a total inability to move the joint through some part of its normal range. The first factor is perhaps, in part, due to a rise in intra-articular friction caused by disruption of the normal cartilaginous bearing surface, but seems mainly attributable to soft tissue thickening, oedema and, probably, over-contraction ('spasm') of the antagonist muscles.

A reduction in the passive range of movement may be due to pain and muscle spasm, in which case the range will return under anaesthesia, or to such mechanical factors as capsular and peri-capsular fibrosis, osteophyte formation, and collapse of the articulating bony surfaces.

Deformity (Table 16.3) in its early stages may be regarded simply as a loss of part of the normal range of movement: thus, for example, a patient who is unable fully to extend his knee may be said to have a flexion deformity or contracture of that joint. Deformity may, however, progress to a point at which the two joint surfaces start to take up a position in relation to each other which does not occur anywhere in the normal range of movement: in other words the joint becomes subluxated and, finally, dislocated.

Advancing dislocation implies a mechanical derangement of the tissues which normally regulate the co-aption of the articulating bones, and the presence of a deforming force. Of these two factors, the first is the most important in the rheumatic diseases: ligaments become stretched by synovial swelling and effusion, bones become deformed by progressive collapse and by osteophyte formation. The deforming forces at work consist of the body weight and the play across the joint of muscles of normally unequal power (such, for example, as the finger flexors and extensors), muscles in 'spasm', or muscles suffering progressive fibrosis. In the leg, the position of a joint may be normal until weight-bearing is attempted. The deforming force of the body weight may then be sufficient to subluxate the diseased joint. Subluxation or dislocation of this kind affects particularly the hip and the knee, and is referred to as *instability*.

THE ROLE OF SURGERY (*see* Tables 16.1, 16.2 and 16.3)

Surgical intervention has as its objective the relief of pain, stiffness, and deformity, and may be directed towards six tissues: synovial membrane, articular cartilage, capsule, bone, nerves, and muscles and their tendons.

1. *Synovial Membrane*. Removal of the synovial membrane—synovectomy—is employed in RA in those joints in which the synovium is extensive and accessible. The joints that fall into this category and which are most commonly treated by synovectomy are the knee and the metacarpo-

TABLE 16.3

The Causes and Surgical Treatment of Deformity in the Rheumatic Diseases

Disability		Tissue of origin		Pathological process		Available surgical procedure
Deformity	may arise in	→ capsule and ligaments	→ where, in the presence of a deforming force, it may be due to	→ distension leading to laxity of capsule and ligaments	→ and may be relieved by	→ capsular reefing
		bone	→ ,,	→ collapse	→ ,,	→ arthrodesis, arthroplasty, osteotomy

phalangeal joints of the fingers. Since the synovial membrane is the tissue primarily involved in RA (*see* Chapter 3), it would seem theoretically possible to arrest the disease in an involved joint, or even in the patient as a whole, by synovectomy. There is controversy as to whether or not this theoretical objective can be realised in practice, but in the author's opinion this outcome occurs rarely, if ever, and the benefits of synovectomy are entirely symptomatic. The operation relieves *pain* by removing inflamed synovium and by reducing the bulk of the intra-capsular contents and, hence, the tension on the capsule. It also retards the capsular stretching which precedes *deformity*. It might be expected that by reducing intracapsular bulk the operation would also reduce *stiffness*, but in practice any such possible increase in the range of movement is usually more than offset by a decrease due to postoperative adhesion formation.

2. *Articular Cartilage*. Healing by regeneration does not occur in articular cartilage and, hence, surgical intervention cannot produce a new cartilage surface once the original has been destroyed by disease. Drilling and shaving of fibrillated cartilage on the patella has, however, been employed for osteoarthrosis of the patellofemoral joint and may lead to the formation of some fibro-cartilage on the articular surface. Osteotomy may have the same result. Cartilage grafting is being studied experimentally.

3. *The Capsule*. Removal of a fibrotic capsule would theoretically be an attractive procedure to relieve *pain* and *stiffness*. In practice, capsulectomy alone is rarely employed but the procedure represents an important step in various forms of arthroplasty. Capsular reefing may be undertaken as part of the reconstruction of joints in RA to reduce *instability*.

4. *Bone*. Three types of operation may be undertaken on bone: arthrodesis, arthroplasty, or osteotomy.

In *arthrodesis* the joint is excised and the originally articulating bones are brought into apposition so that they unite with each other. *Pain* is relieved since the diseased joint is obliterated. The bones may be fixed in a better functional position than that taken up by the diseased joint so as to reduce *deformity*, and in the legs *instability* is eliminated. These advantages are achieved, however, at the cost of a total loss of movement.

The operation of *arthroplasty* aims ideally to reconstruct a joint so that pain, stiffness, and deformity are relieved. At its simplest, this may be achieved by excision of one or both of the articulating bone surfaces without a subsequent attempt to obtain fusion. This procedure, excision arthroplasty, relieves *pain* by reducing capsular tension and, probably, by the removal of painful bone. It may also reduce *deformity* by allowing, for example, realignment of the dislocated toes or fingers in RA. Movement may be retained at the new false joint, but the range is never full, it is not always painless, and the joint, if loaded, is likely to be unstable.

In an attempt to reduce *stiffness* and increase *stability* following excision arthroplasty, various materials have been placed between the freshly resected bone ends in the hope of reducing the degree of adhesion formation between the excised joint surfaces. Since separation of the joint surfaces now depends upon the interposed implant rather than upon the creation of a broad gap between the bone ends, the bone resection can be more limited. As a consequence, the normal architecture is more nearly retained and, hence, the final joint is more stable. Unfortunately, the anatomy of only a few joints lends itself to interposition arthroplasty, and for practical purposes the only example of the procedure in current use is cup arthroplasty at the hip.

As an alternative method of improving the *stability* of joints such as the hip after excision arthroplasty, the excised component may be replaced with a prosthesis fashioned from one of the implantable metals. Although improving the stability of the joint, such procedures often produce relatively poor pain-relief—perhaps because one of the diseased bony articulating surfaces is still loaded and the tension in the capsule remains unchanged.

Theoretically, the most effective arthroplasty would be the replacement of both components of the joint with a prosthetic implant. Appropriate implants are now available for the hip—where the early results appear good—and on a much smaller scale for the knee, elbow, and fingers. Ideally, total replacement arthroplasty should bring *pain relief* since both bone surfaces would be removed, while the capsule could be relaxed or excised; *stiffness* post-operatively would be due only to muscle shortening and scar formation; and *stability* would be conferred by an appropriately designed device. In practice, a final evaluation of this procedure at the hip must await the results over the next ten to twenty years since only in this period of time can the function of the prosthesis and of the bone-prosthesis bond be adequately assessed. At the other joints, the surgical and biomechanical problems posed by the procedure are in the early stages of solution.

The final type of bony procedure available in the rheumatic diseases is *osteotomy*. In this operation the bone adjacent to the joint is divided surgically and then allowed to unite. Mere division of the bone appears to relieve *pain* but why this is so is not understood: possibly the blood flow to the bone between the osteotomy site and the joint is altered or conceivably, the articular bone is partially denervated. Following division, the bone may be angulated so as to compensate for fixed *deformity* at the joint, and it was with this objective in mind that the operation was originally introduced. Such displacement, besides correcting the overall deformity, may relieve pain by bringing cartilage-covered bone into the weight-bearing area, by redistributing load (for example in the osteoarthrosic knock-knee), or by transposing the range of movement so that the everyday range does not impose traction on the capsule. It has been suggested that osteotomy may sometimes reverse the pathological process in osteoarthrosis.

5. *Nerves.* Articular neurectomy has been attempted to relieve joint *pain.* The procedure is not useful in practice since joints are supplied by numerous irregular small nerves that cannot be displayed surgically. Theoretically, a neurectomy sufficiently complete to relieve joint pain effectively would expose the patient to the risk of neuropathic changes.

In certain places in the body, peripheral nerves traverse tunnels whose walls are inelastic: for example, the carpal tunnel contains the median nerve and is bounded by the transverse carpal ligament and the carpal bones with their intervening articulations. If such a tunnel also contains synovial tissue, the nerve may become compressed in the tunnel if the bulk of synovial membrane increases; for example, in RA, the synovial sheaths of the flexor muscles of the digits and to a lesser extent the synovial membrane of the carpal joints may proliferate and compress the median nerve in the carpal tunnel. Such compression can be relieved surgically by dividing the transverse carpal ligament, an operation that may be combined with the removal of involved synovium.

6. *Muscles and Tendons.* Muscles may become permanently shortened in a position of *deformity* so that the deformity cannot be corrected unless the affected muscles are divided. Such divisions are usually carried out by tenotomy: besides helping to relieve deformity, tenotomy may temporarily bring *pain-relief*, perhaps by reducing muscle spasm.

In RA, tendons may rupture and require repair. Proliferation of their synovial sheaths may necessitate synovectomy or the incision of the retinacula retaining the tendons.

Part IIA: Surgery of the Inflammatory Arthropathies

Of the inflammatory arthropathies by far the commonest requiring surgical relif is RA, and it is with this disease that this section is largely concerned. During the active phase of RA, the joint surfaces may become partially or totally destroyed. Even if the active phase of the disease then remits, symptomatic progression in the involved joint is common as a consequence of secondary degenerative changes. Thus, the surgery and pathology of chronic, 'burned-out', RA merges into that of OA.

Of the other inflammatory arthropathies, ankylosing spondylitis affecting the spine and hips, and Reiter's disease affecting the feet may require surgical relief.

Still's disease does not lend itself to the surgical procedures available in the adult: operations on bones are avoided if possible because they may interfere with growth, and soft tissue procedures are rarely indicated.

TABLE 16.4

Orthopaedic Surgery in the Treatment of Rheumatoid Arthritis of the Upper Limb

	Tissue operated upon and nature of operation									
	Synovial membrane:	Articular cartilage:	Capsule and ligaments:	Bone:						Muscles, tendons:
	Synovectomy		Reefing and capsulectomy	Arthrodesis	Arthroplasty:				Osteotomy	Tendon suture and realignment
Joint involved					Excision	Inter-position	Partial replacement	Total replacement		
Inter-phalangeal	Rare	—	—	Yes	—	—	—	—	—	—
Metacarpo-phalangeal	Yes (and of extensor tendon sheaths)	—	Yes	—	Yes (of head of metacarpal)	—	—	Experimental	—	Tendon suture and realignment
Radio-carpal	Occasional	—	—	Yes	—	—	—	—	—	(Division of flexor retinaculum for carpal tunnel syndrome)
Radio-ulnar	Occasional	—	—	—	Yes (of head of radius or distal ulna)	—	—	—	—	—
Elbow (humero-ulnar and humero-radial)	Occasional	—	—	Rare	Rare	—	—	Experimental	—	—
Shoulder	—	—	—	Occasional	Rare (of head of humerus)	—	Rare (of head of humerus)	Experimental	—	—

THE UPPER LIMB (*see* Table 16.4)

THE HAND AND WRIST

Synovectomy (Fig. 16.1) is widely employed at the metacarpo-phalangeal joints of the fingers, the radio-carpal and inferior radio-ulnar joints, and for the extensor (and, less commonly, flexor) tendon sheaths.

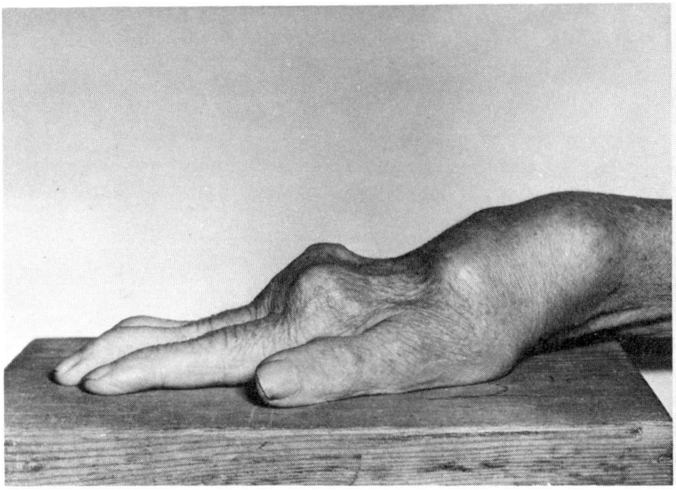

FIGURE 16.1 The appearance of the rheumatoid hand showing gross thickening of the synovial membranes of the metacarpophalangeal and wrist joints and of the extensor tendon sheaths

At the metacarpo-phalangeal joints of the fingers, increasing synovial bulk progressively distends the capsule, and erodes the cartilage and bone. As a consequence, the joints become free to subluxate and, finally, to dislocate. Since the finger flexors are stronger than the extensors, dislocation takes the form of palmar and then proximal displacement of the phalanx on the metacarpal. A similar mechanism produces anterior dislocation of the wrist, and disruption of the inferior radio-ulnar joint. The extensor tendons may rupture as a consequence of a nutritional disturbance, combined with abrasion over the prominent dorsum of the distal ulna. As the fingers deviate ulnarwards the extensor tendons come to lie to the ulnar side of the metacarpal head so that their line of pull tends to increase this deviation.

By removing bulky synovium before subluxation has taken place this evolving deformity may be arrested. At this stage, however, marked pain from capsular distension is not a feature, so that the surgical decision is a difficult one: probable slowing of the progression of deformity and some pain-relief have to be set against the loss of movement that often follows this procedure.

At the time of synovectomy the capsule may be incised and reefed so as to stabilise the joints and re-align the extensor tendons. The tendons themselves may be repaired if they have ruptured and their synovial sheaths may be excised if their bulk interferes with the function of the hand.

Once deformity has occurred, and especially when the metacarpo-phalangeal and wrist joints have subluxated, operations on the bones of the hand are indicated.

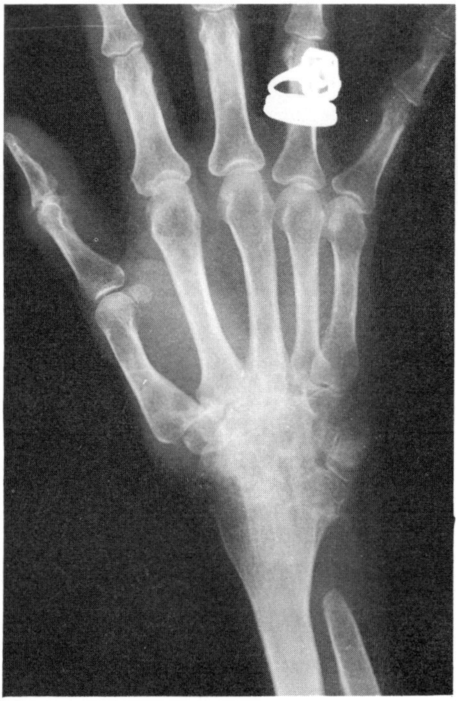

FIGURE 16.2 An antero-posterior radiograph showing the final result following arthrodesis of the wrist and excision of the distal ulna

Arthrodesis (Fig. 16.2) of the radio-carpal joint is an excellent procedure and is one of the mainstays in the surgical treatment of the rheumatoid hand. The wrist can be rendered stable and pain-free so that the power of the grip is much improved. The loss of movement compared with that occurring in the normal wrist impairs function very little; compared with the pre-operative state of the wrist any loss is insignificant.

Excision arthroplasty of the metacarpal heads from dislocated metacarpo-phalangeal joints makes it possible to re-align the fingers with the metacarpus. The consequent improvement of function is limited by stiffness at the false joint due to adhesion formation. In an attempt to improve motion, *total replacement arthroplasty* (Fig. 16.3) has been attempted using prostheses constructed of cobalt-chrome, polypropylene or silastic, but at present these procedures are not in general clinical use. Excision of the dorsally dislocated distal ulna from the inferior radio-ulna joint (a

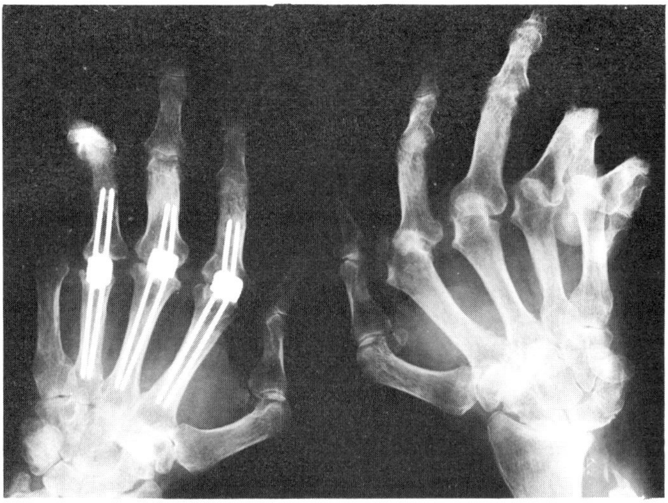

FIGURE 16.3 A postoperative radiograph showing total replacement of 2nd, 3rd, and 4th metacarpo-phalangeal joints by Flatt prostheses

second example of *excision arthroplasty*), usually combined with fusion of the radio-carpal joint, produces a useful increase in the range of painless supination and pronation.

THE ELBOW

Synovectomy is occasionally useful at the elbow when the joint is painful, the synovial membrane thickened, but the bone intact.

Arthrodesis is occasionally indicated to confer painless stability, but the objections to this procedure in RA—that fusion is difficult to obtain and that the presence of other involved joints makes loss of movement functionally objectionable—usually outweigh the advantages.

Excision arthroplasty of the radial head may increase the range of painless motion—especially of pronation and supination. Excision of the entire joint may provide a good range of painless movement but the associated instability is such that little increased function is obtained. *Total replacement arthroplasty* of the humero-ulnar joint, using a hinge combined with excision of the head of the radius, is feasible but is still in the experimental stage.

TABLE 16.5

Orthopaedic Surgery of Rheumatoid Arthritis of the Lower Limb and the Spine

	Tissue operated upon and nature of operation									
	Synovial membrane:	Articular cartilage:	Capsule and ligaments:	Bone:						Muscles, tendon:
	Synovectomy		Reefing and capsulectomy	Arthrodesis	Arthroplasty:				Osteotomy	Tendon suture and realignment
Joint involved					Excision	Inter-position	Partial replacement	Total replacement		
Inter-phalangeal	—	—	—	Yes, occasion-ally	Yes	—	—	—	—	Yes (extensor)
Metacarpo-phalangeal	—	—	—	—	Yes	—	—	—	—	—
Joints of foot	—	—	—	Occasional	—	—	—	—	—	—
Ankle	Rare	—	—	Rare	—	—	—	—	—	—
Knee	Yes	—	—	Yes	Yes (of patella)	Rare	Yes (of tibial con-dyles and, rarely, femoral condyles)	Occasional (of tibio-femoral joint)	Yes	—
Hip	—	—	—	Rare	Yes (of head of femur)	Yes (cup arthro-plasty)	Rare (of head of femur)	Yes	Occasional	Occasional (adductor tenotomy)
Spine	—	—	—	Yes (of atlanto-axial joint in RA)	—	—	—	—	Occasional (of cervical and lumbar spine in ankylosing spondylitis)	—

THE SHOULDER

Synovectomy is not undertaken at this joint since the membrane is relatively inaccessible surgically and its bulk is hard to assess clinically.

Arthrodesis is hard to secure in RA, but it is occasionally indicated in a severely painful joint. The loss of total shoulder movement is not as severe as might be expected since scapulo-thoracic motion is unaffected and by itself provides a useful range of shoulder movement.

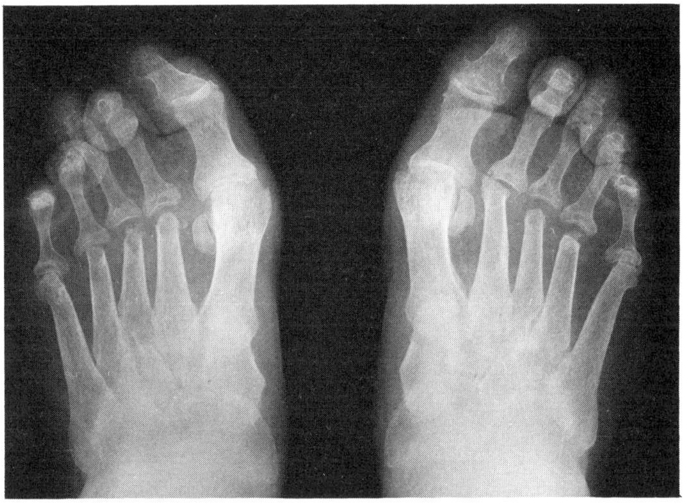

FIGURE 16.4 A postoperative radiograph following excision of the 2nd, 3rd, and 4th metatarsal heads. This operation is usually extended to include the 1st and 5th metatarsals

Excision arthroplasty of the humeral head may be undertaken as an alternative to arthrodesis: the operation and the after-care are less arduous than for arthrodesis, and the pain relief is comparable. However, the false joint is too unstable to allow effective abduction so that the functional result is worse than that following arthrodesis. *Partial replacement arthroplasty* using a prosthetic replacement for the humeral head (the Neer prosthesis) has not proved useful in RA. *Total replacement arthroplasty* is being studied experimentally.

THE LOWER LIMB (*see* Table 16.5)

THE TOES

The commonest consequence of RA requiring surgical relief in the feet is a claw-toe deformity. As a result of this deformity, which consists of dorsal dislocation of the phalanges on the metacarpal heads and flexion contractures of the proximal interphalangeal joints, the dorsum of the involved toe rubs on the upper of the shoe while the head of the metatarsal is driven painfully downwards through the sole on weight-bearing.

Synovectomy has not been used extensively in an attempt to prevent this deformity in the foot in the way in which it has been used in the hand. However, *excision arthroplasty* of the metatarsal heads (Fowler's operation), together occasionally with excision of the base of the proximal phalanx, is used commonly (Fig. 16.4). At the time of excision arthroplasty, the extensor tendons may be divided. This procedure allows the toes to be brought into line with the fore-foot and very successfully relieves pain under the metatarsal heads. Postoperatively the gait lacks the 'toe-off' spring of a normal gait, but such a spring has already disappeared by the time the operation becomes indicated. At the metatarso-phalangeal joint of the great toe the deformity is that of a hallux valgus rather than a claw toe but, again, the operative treatment is *excision arthoplasty*.

As an alternative to excision arthroplasty, grossly deformed toes may be amputated through the metacarpo-phalangeal joints.

THE MIDTARSAL AND ANKLE JOINTS

Pain arising from the midtarsal and ankle joints is best treated by well-fitting shoes or boots with appropriate insoles. Occasionally, isolated involvement of one of these joints may merit arthrodesis, and, rarely, the indications appropriate for synovectomy at the knee may exist at the ankle.

THE KNEE

As in the hand, *synovectomy* is a useful procedure in the knee. The operation is indicated for a joint in which there has not been gross destruction of bone but in which marked, chronic synovial thickening is causing pain. The systemic state of the patient's disease is not affected by the operation, nor does it affect the decision to operate.

Through a medial parapatellar incision all the synovium save that in the posterior recesses of the joint is removed. Recently it has been suggested that an additional incision should be made to gain access to the posterior synovium in order to make the synovectomy complete. Active movement of the knee is started as soon postoperatively as pain allows, to reduce the chances of postoperative joint stiffness, but even so, a manipulation under anaesthesia is commonly required early in the postoperative course.

Analysis of the results of this operation suggests that, in the short term, it usually relieves pain without altering the range of movement. A long-term controlled trial will be necessary to answer the important question of whether synovectomy influences the subsequent progression of destructive changes in the operated joint.

As the disease advances, increasing pain, stiffness and deformity may necessitate *arthrodesis*, *arthroplasty*, or *osteotomy*.

Arthrodesis offers the patient a stable painless knee but at the price of absolute stiffness (*see* Fig. 16.15). This disadvantage is particularly serious in polyarthritic disease such as RA, for with a stiff knee patients need good hand, hip, and spine function in order to reach their feet and dress themselves. With two stiff knees it is possible to rise from an ordinary chair only by using the arms, which may be impossible if the arms are involved in the disease, while if the patient falls she cannot get up from the floor unaided. These disadvantages make bilateral arthrodesis of the knee very rarely appropriate in RA. Even for bilateral involvement of the knees, however, arthrodesis of one knee is often worthwhile since it allows the patient to take less weight on the other knee, at which movement can, if necessary, be retained by some form of arthroplasty.

Excision arthroplasty is confined to the patello-femoral joint, where it is represented by excision of the patella. This operation may be indicated in isolation if the tibio-femoral joint is relatively satisfactory or, more

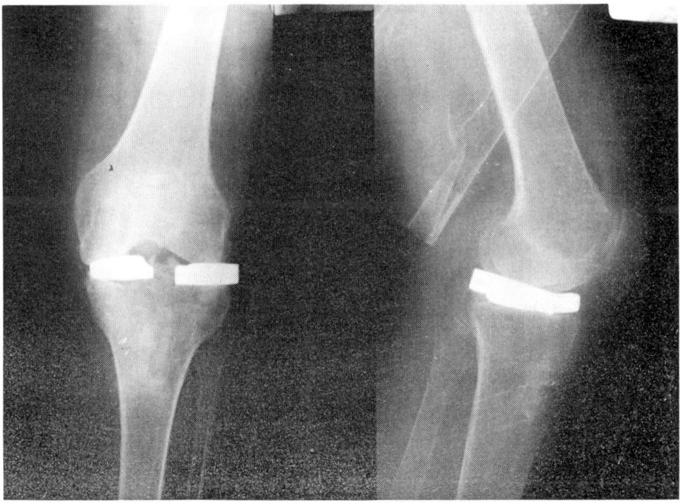

FIGURE 16.5 A postoperative antero-posterior and lateral radiograph showing MacIntosh prostheses in the medial and lateral compartments of the knee

commonly, it is carried out at the same time as synovectomy or some other form of arthroplasty at the tibio-femoral joint. Postoperatively, extension of the knee is possible through the reconstituted patellar tendon. Pain-relief is moderately good but some reduction in the range of movement and the development of an extensor lag are not uncommon disadvantages of the procedure.

Partial replacement arthroplasty is useful at the tibio-femoral joint (Fig. 16.5). This most commonly takes the form of excision of the tibial condyles followed by their replacement with cobalt-chrome prostheses (the MacIntosh operation). At the same time the femoral condyles are smoothed off. This procedure is especially indicated if the tibial condyles have collapsed: it may then be used not only as a means of replacing diseased, painful bone but also of correcting the valgus or varus angulation at the knee caused by the collapse of the tibial condyle.

A prosthesis is also available for the replacement of the femoral condyles but this has as yet hardly been used outside its place of origin (the Massachusetts General Hospital, Boston).

Total replacement of the tibio-femoral joint is possible using a prosthesis in the form of a hinge. Appropriate devices have been described by Walldius in Scandinavia, Shiers in England, and Young in the USA, but to date they have not been widely used. A few experimental attempts have been made to replace the femoral and tibial condyles with separate prostheses.

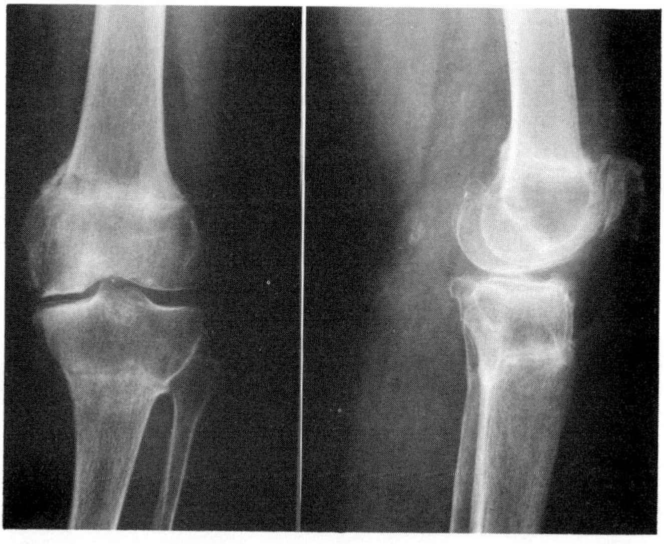

FIGURE 16.6 A postoperative antero-posterior and lateral radiograph following a Benjamin osteotomy at the knee. The lines of sclerosis in the tibia and femur indicate the united osteotomies

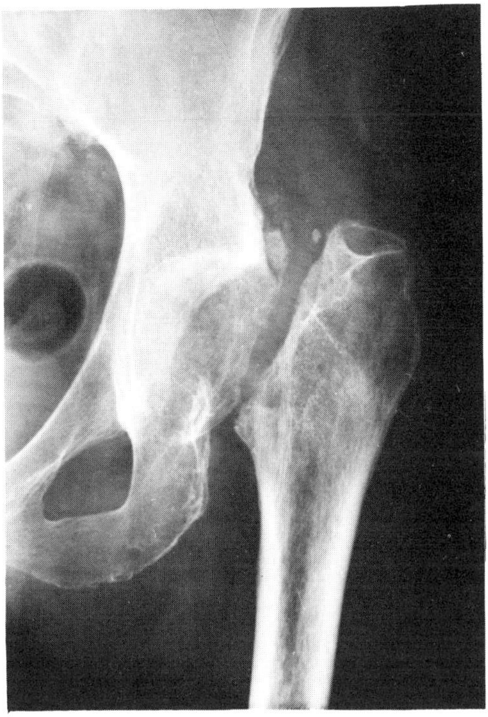

FIGURE 16.7 A postoperative radiograph following a Girdlestone excision arthroplasty of the hip

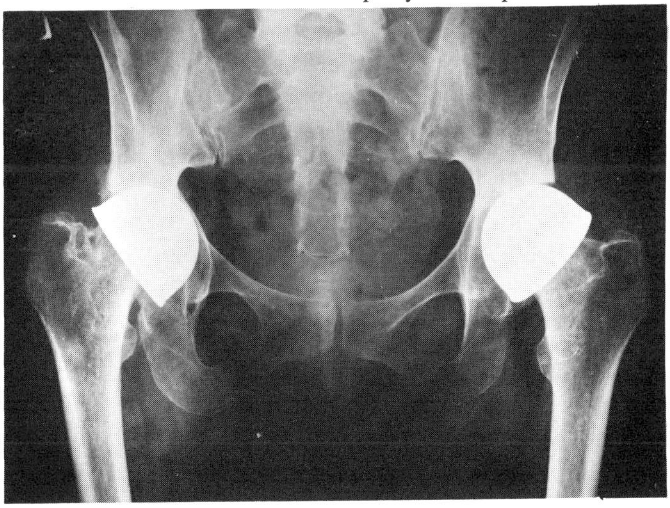

FIGURE 16.8 A postoperative radiograph following bilateral cup arthroplasty at the hip: an example of interposition arthroplasty (Courtesy Mr W. A. Law, FRCS)

Interposition arthroplasty using an appropriately shaped cobalt-chrome insert (the Platt prosthesis) to separate the re-fashioned tibial and femoral joint surfaces has been performed but has not proved to be generally successful.

Osteotomy may be undertaken distal to the tibial condyles, proximal to the femoral condyles, or at both levels simultaneously (the Benjamin operation) (Fig. 16.6). The operation brings pain-relief for reasons discussed in Part I of this chapter and permits the correction of flexion, valgus, or varus deformities. It is indicated, particularly, for a painful knee that is too deformed to be suitable for synovectomy, but in which the range of movement is too good to necessitate arthroplasty.

THE HIP

Synovectomy is not undertaken at the hip for the same reasons as those that apply to the shoulder.

Arthrodesis is never indicated in inflammatory polyarthropathy since it suffers from the same objections as those that apply to arthrodesis of the elbow and knee. Furthermore, joints in addition to the involved hip have to be immobilised in plaster-of-Paris to obtain fusion, and in RA this risks disastrous stiffness affecting several joints.

Excision arthroplasty is a useful procedure and takes the form of removal of the femoral head and proximal femoral neck (the Girdlestone operation) (Fig. 16.7). This operation relieves pain and permits a sufficient range of movement to enable the patient to lie and sit comfortably. The hip, however, is unstable so that walking is difficult and usually requires the aid of at least two sticks. The operation is particularly indicated for patients with a significantly painful hip who lead a wheel-chair existence not merely because of their hip but because of multiple joint involvement. Postoperatively, such patients are still mainly chair-bound but they can now sit and lie down in comfort, while, if the state of their other joints permits, they can walk about the house with the aid of sticks or crutches.

Interposition arthroplasty using one of a number of moulded metal cups to separate the reshaped femoral head and acetabulum is one of the procedures commonly employed for RA and also for involvement of the hip in ankylosing spondylitis (Fig. 16.8). At its best, the operation produces a comfortable, stable and mobile hip, but to obtain results of this calibre the surgeon and the team providing the postoperative physiotherapy must be performing the operation repeatedly; the occasional cup arthroplasty tends to give a poor result. Even in experienced hands cup arthroplasties may need to be revised.

Partial replacement arthroplasty, in which the head and neck of the femur are replaced by a prosthesis, is rarely indicated since the prosthesis tends to intrude into the porotic acetabulum, producing pain and further limitation of movement.

Total replacement arthroplasty using a prosthesis replacing the acetabulum as well as the head of the femur is gaining increasingly widespread acceptance in Great Britain (Fig. 16.9). Two devices have been most frequently employed, one constructed entirely of cobalt-chrome

(a)

(b)

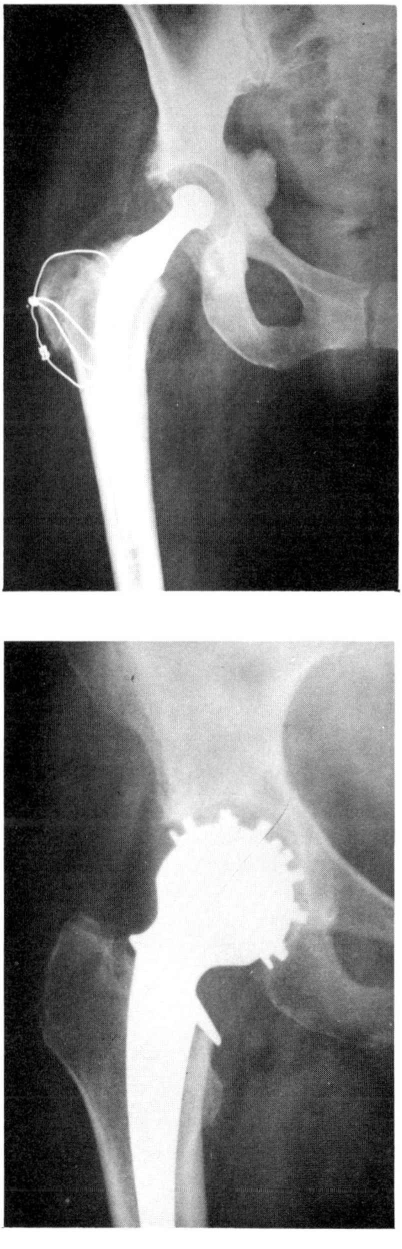

FIGURE 16.9 Postoperative radiographs following total replacement of the hip with (*a*) Charnley's Low Friction arthroplasty and (*b*) the McKee-Farrar prosthesis (Courtesy Mr M. Heywood-Waddington, FRCS)

(the McKee-Farrar prosthesis) and one in which the acetabulum is constructed of high density polyethylene and the head of the femur of stainless steel (the Charnley prosthesis). Both devices are attached to the bone with a cold-curing acrylic cement. It is still too early to give a definitive assessment of this operation since it has been progressively introduced on a limited scale over the past ten years and is only now receiving widespread acceptance in Great Britain. The short-term results, however, have been extremely encouraging; pain is relieved, a useful range of motion is regained, and the hip is stable. Postoperatively, the convalescence is short, weight-bearing may be allowed within two weeks of operation, and the prolonged, tedious, and sometimes painful physiotherapy that some other procedures require is unnecessary. If these results continue in the long-term and are maintained when the procedure is in general use, the operation may well be indicated for most cases of advanced RA of the hip; at the present time, because of uncertainty surrounding the long-term results, the operation is avoided in patients under the age of sixty unless the prognosis for life is shortened by intercurrent disease.

Osteotomy gives far less satisfactory results in RA than in OA, and so for the former it is rarely employed at the hip.

THE SPINE (*see* Table 16.5)

Rheumatoid arthritis may affect all the facet joints of the spine but surgery is indicated only at the atlanto-axial joints where the disease may lead to instability of the atlas on the axis, with consequent potential danger to the spinal cord. This complication of RA is treated by *arthrodesis* (in the spine called 'fusion') of the axis to the atlas and, sometimes, for greater security, to the occiput and to C3 (Fig. 16.10).

Ankylosing spondylitis produces progressive, rigid, flexion contractures, particularly at the cervical and lumbar levels. Arthrodesis has not been attempted to arrest the progress of the deformity, but lumbar and, more hazardously, cervical spinal *osteotomy* is used to correct the deformity, followed by a fusion at the osteotomy site (Fig. 16.11)

Part IIB: The Surgery of Osteoarthrosis

Primary osteoarthrosis affects certain joints such as the hip, knee and carpo-metacarpal joint of the thumb much more commonly than it affects others such as the shoulder and wrist. Secondary OA following injury or another primary disease process may affect any joint.

Articular cartilage appears to be the tissue primarily affected in OA. Bone and capsular changes are marked but probably secondary.

(a)

(b)

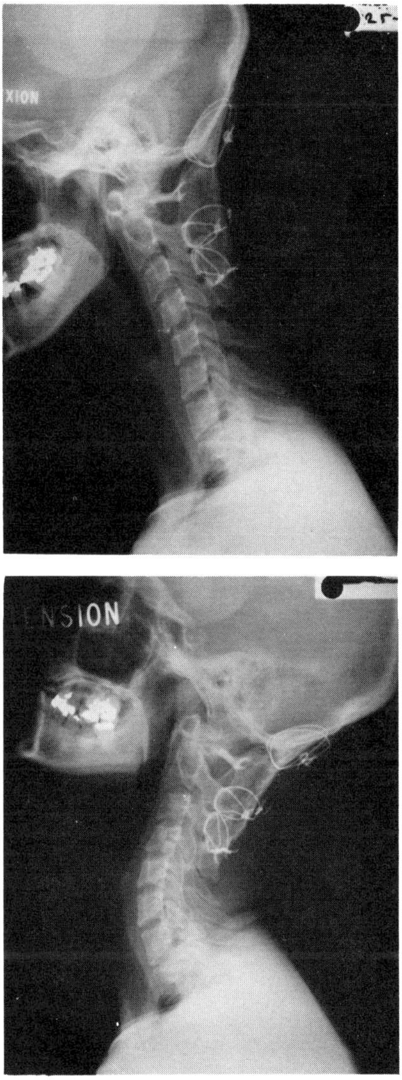

FIGURE 16.10 Lateral postoperative radiographs showing successful fusion of the occiput, C1 and C2. It will be seen that no movement occurs at the arthrodesed levels during (*a*) flexion, and (*b*) extension

Changes in the synovial membrane are insignificant. Hence, operations designed to affect bone and capsule play a large part in the surgery of OA; operations on the synovial membrane (*synovectomy*) play none.

THE UPPER LIMB (*see* Table 16.6)

THE HAND

The only joint in the hand commonly requiring surgical treatment for primary OA is the carpo-metacarpal joint of the thumb. Here the disease

TABLE 16.6

Orthopaedic Surgery in Osteoarthrosis of the Upper Limb

	Tissue operated upon and nature of operation									
	Synovial membrane:	Articular cartilage:	Capsule and ligaments:	Bone:						Muscles, tendon:
	Synovectomy	—	Reefing and capsulectomy	Arthrodesis	Arthroplasty:				Osteotomy	Tendon suture and realignment
Joint involved					Excision	Inter-position	Partial replacement	Total replacement		
Inter-phalangeal	—	—	—	Rare	—	—	—	—	—	—
Carpo-metacarpal (thumb)	—	—	—	Yes	Yes (of trapezium)	—	—	—	—	—
Wrist	—	—	—	—	—	—	—	—	—	—
Radio-ulnar	—	—	—	—	Yes (of head of radius)	—	—	—	—	—
Elbow	—	—	—	Yes	—	—	—	Experimental	—	—
Shoulder	—	—	—	Yes	Rare (of head of humerus)	—	Rare (of head of humerus)	Experimental	—	—

(a)

(b)

(c)

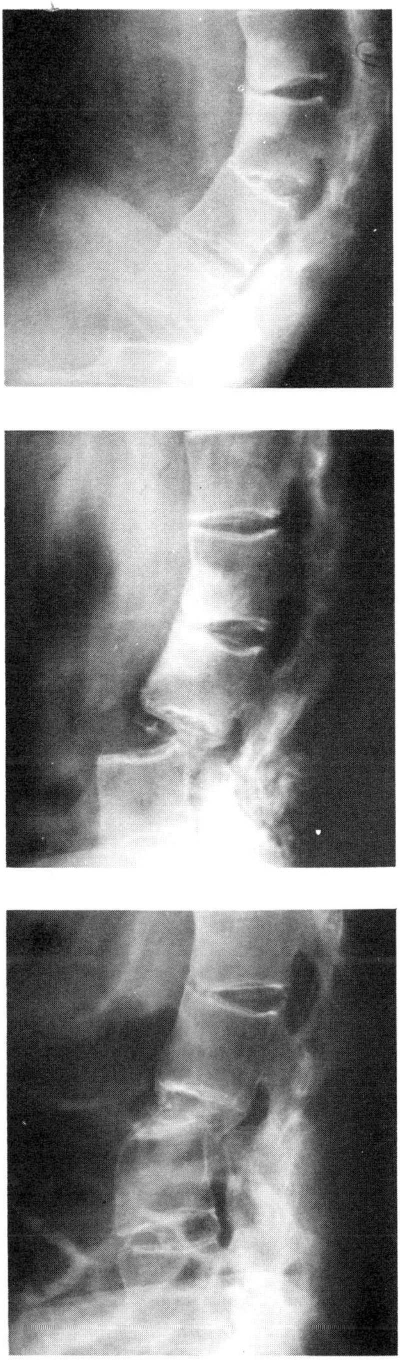

FIGURE 16.11 Lateral radiographs of the spine in ankylosing spondylitis showing (*a*) the pre-operative state (*b*) the condition soon after osteotomy, and (*c*) the final state when the osteotomy has united (Courtesy Mr W. A. Law, FRCS)

Table 16.7

Orthopaedic Surgery in the Treatment of Osteoarthrosis of the Lower Limb and the Spine

	Tissue operated upon and nature of operation									
	Synovial membrane:	Articular cartilage:	Capsule and ligaments:	Bone:						Muscles, tendon:
	Synovectomy	Drilling and shaving	Capsulotomy, capsulectomy as part of an arthroplasty	Arthrodesis	Arthroplasty:				Osteotomy	Tenotomy
Joint involved					Excision	Inter-position	Partial replacement	Total replacement		
Inter-phalangeal	—	—	—	Yes	Yes	—	—	—	—	—
Metatarso-phalangeal	—	—	Yes	Yes (of 1st M-P joint)	Yes (of head of M-T or base of prox phalanx)	—	—	—	—	Yes (extensor tenotomy)
Joints of foot	—	—	—	Yes	—	—	—	—	—	—
Ankle	—	—	—	Yes	—	—	—	—	—	—
Knee patello-femoral	—	Rare	—	—	Yes (of patella)	—	—	—	—	—
tibio-femoral	—	—	—	Yes	—	Rare	Rare	Yes (experimental)	Yes	—
Hip	—	—	Yes	Yes	Yes (of head of femur)	Yes	Yes	Yes	Yes	Yes (adductor and psoas tenotomy)
Lumbar and cervical spine	—	—	—	Yes	—	—	—	—	—	—

may be treated by *arthrodesis* of the diseased joint or by *excision arthroplasty* of the trapezium. At their best, these operations give indistinguishable results with an excellent return of painless function.

THE RADIO-ULNAR JOINTS

The distal radio-ulnar joint may be affected by secondary OA following fractures adjacent to the joint, such as Colles' fracture. The proximal radio-ulnar joint is similarly affected following fractures of the head of the radius. In both cases the treatment of choice is *excision arthroplasty*: in the distal joint by excision of one to two inches of the distal ulna; in the proximal joint by excision of the head of the radius.

THE ELBOW JOINT

Primary osteoarthrosis may affect all components of the joint. Should the joint be so painful as to require surgery, which is rare, the most commonly employed procedure is *arthrodesis* of the humero-ulnar joint in sufficient flexion to allow the patient to feed himself and wash, together with excision of the head of radius.

THE SHOULDER

The shoulder is rarely affected by OA, primary or secondary, but when it is, it is well treated by *arthrodesis*. Although fusion is not easy to secure, it is easier than in RA because the bone is hypertrophic rather than porotic. The functional results of a sound arthrodesis in the position of function (i.e. approximately the position taken up by the shoulder when the hand is brought to the mouth) are good.

THE LOWER LIMB (*see* Table 16.7)

THE TOES

Certain conditions commonly affect the toes which, although they cannot confidently be regarded as examples of primary OA, may nevertheless be considered here as non-inflammatory arthropathies akin to OA, requiring surgical relief. These conditions are hallux rigidus, hallux valgus, claw toes, and hammer toes. Hallux valgus and claw toes commonly occur together as a primary entity, but they may, as has already been mentioned, be seen in RA.

Hallux rigidus is a condition causing pain and stiffness of the first metatarso-phalangeal joint of young adults. The aetiology is unknown but it is possibly an example of premature primary OA analagous to chondromalacia patellae. By the time the patient presents for surgical treatment, hyperextension has often developed at the interphalangeal joint of the great toe to compensate for the stiffness at the metatarso-phalangeal joint. Thus, the therapeutic need is to relieve pain rather than

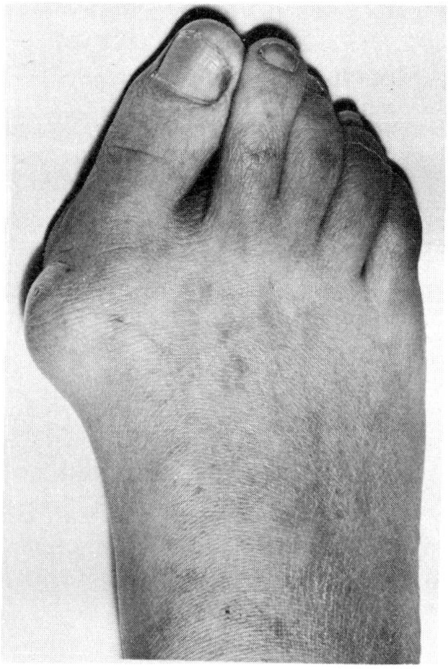

(a)

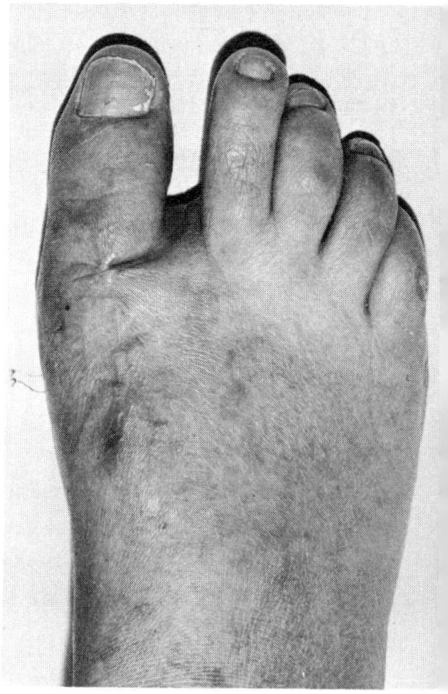

(b)

(c)

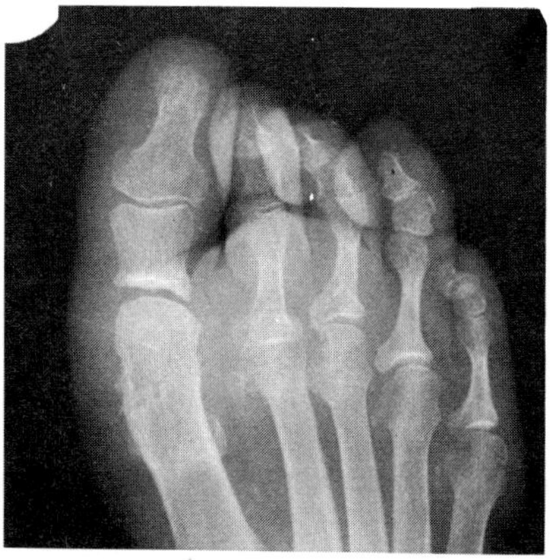

FIGURE 16.12 The appearance of the foot with hallux valgus (*a*) pre-operatively, and (*b*) following a Keller's operation. (*c*) The radiological appearance of the foot following excision of the medial exostosis on the head of the first metatarsal and excision of the base of the proximal phalanx of the great toe (Keller's operation)

to reduce stiffness and, since the patients are young adults, a permanent result is required. *Arthrodesis* of the involved joint meets these requirements and is the treatment of choice.

Hallux valgus occurs commonly in middle-aged women and is almost certainly initiated by the wearing of shoes that force the great toe to deviate laterally (i.e. into valgus) at the metatarso-phalangeal joint (Fig. 16.12). Once this deviation is initiated, it is exacerbated by bowstringing of the extensor and flexor tendons across the lateral side of the joint. The condition occasionally occurs in adolescents and young adults but here the primary pathology is the presence of an unusually broad forefoot due to a varus position of the first metatarsal.

Possibly because the toes cannot function in restrictive footwear, the intrinsic muscles of the foot appear to weaken. As a consequence, the transverse anterior metatarsal arch collapses, causing broadening of the forefoot. The second to fifth toes develop extension contractures at the metatarso-phalangeal joints which may eventually dislocate dorsally. The proximal and distal interphalangeal joints are flexed. This set of deformities is described as clawing of the toes (Fig. 16.13).

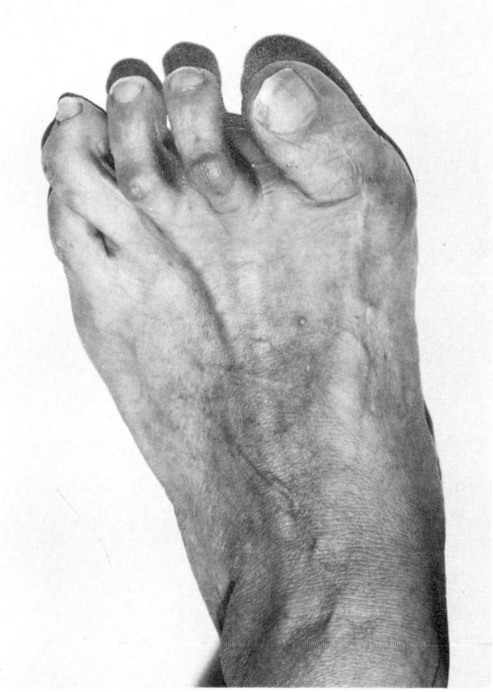

FIGURE 16.13 The appearance of claw toes

Occasionally, a solitary toe may develop an acute flexion contracture at the proximal interphalangeal joint, with compensatory extension contractures at the distal interphalangeal joints. This deformity is described as a hammer toe (Fig. 16.14).

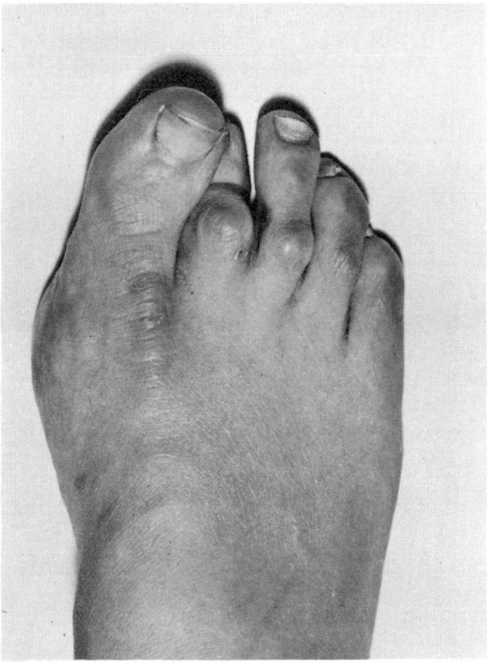

FIGURE 16.14 The appearance of hammer toe—in this case the 2nd toe

Callosities develop where the skin of the foot is exposed to abnormally severe friction and pressure against the shoe: over the medial aspect of the head of the first metatarsal where the bone itself develops an exostosis (a 'bunion'); over the dorsum of the proximal interphalangeal joints of the second to fifth toes; under the second to fourth metatarsal heads; and over the lateral aspect of the fifth metatarsal head (a 'bunionette'). The involved joints develop secondary OA changes and become stiff and painful.

Hallux valgus is treated by *excision arthroplasty* of the first metatarsophalangeal joint either by removing the base of the phalanx (Keller's operation) or the head of the first metatarsal (Mayo's operation) (*see* Fig. 16.12). Medial exostoses remaining after these procedures are excised and, if necessary, the capsule may be incised laterally to re-align the toe.

Claw toes may be treated by *dorsal capsulotomy and extensor tenotomy* at the metatarso-phalangeal joint together with spike *arthrodesis* of the proximal interphalangeal joint in an extended position.

THE FOOT AND ANKLE

Osteoarthrosis, primary or secondary, occasionally affects any of the tarsal (especially the subtalar) joints or the ankle. If surgical treatment is necessary, arthrodesis of the involved joint is the only procedure available.

THE KNEE

A condition which is probably primary OA affects the patello-femoral joint of young adults and is known as chondromalacia patellae (*see* p. 234). In this disease the articular cartilage covering the patella and, subsequently, that covering the patellar articular surface of the femur becomes softened, fibrillated, and finally ulcerated, a sequence of events identical with that seen in primary osteoarthrosis elsewhere. Uniquely in this joint, however, the condition has been treated by various surgical procedures aimed directly at the cartilage. Thus, the cartilage and subchondral bone have been *drilled* and the fibrillated cartilage *shaved.* It is doubtful if these procedures are beneficial, although the regeneration of fibrocartilage following drilling of the patella in advanced OA of the knee has been described. Unable as we are to explain and reverse the pathological process in the cartilage, operative surgical treatment must usually take the form of *excision arthroplasty* of the patella. Fortunately, in only a minority of patients is the condition severe enough or persistent enough to merit this procedure.

Chondromalacia patellae apart, the knee, after the hip, is the joint most commonly affected by OA.

Arthrodesis is the treatment of choice provided the state of the other joints makes a stiff knee tolerable, and provided the patient has already lost all but a few degrees of joint motion as a consequence of the disease process. Several methods of arthrodesis have been described but the Charnley arthrodesis is perhaps the most reliable and most widely used (Fig. 16.15).

Arthroplasty, save for *excision arthroplasty of the patella*, has little part to play in OA of the knee. Excision arthroplasty of the tibio-femoral joint would obviously lead to intolerable instability. *Interposition and partial replacement arthroplasty*, the Platt and MacIntosh operations, respectively (*see* p. 256), give poor results in OA, and *total replacement arthroplasty* is scarcely out of the experimental stage.

Thus, if pain demands surgical relief while the range of movement is

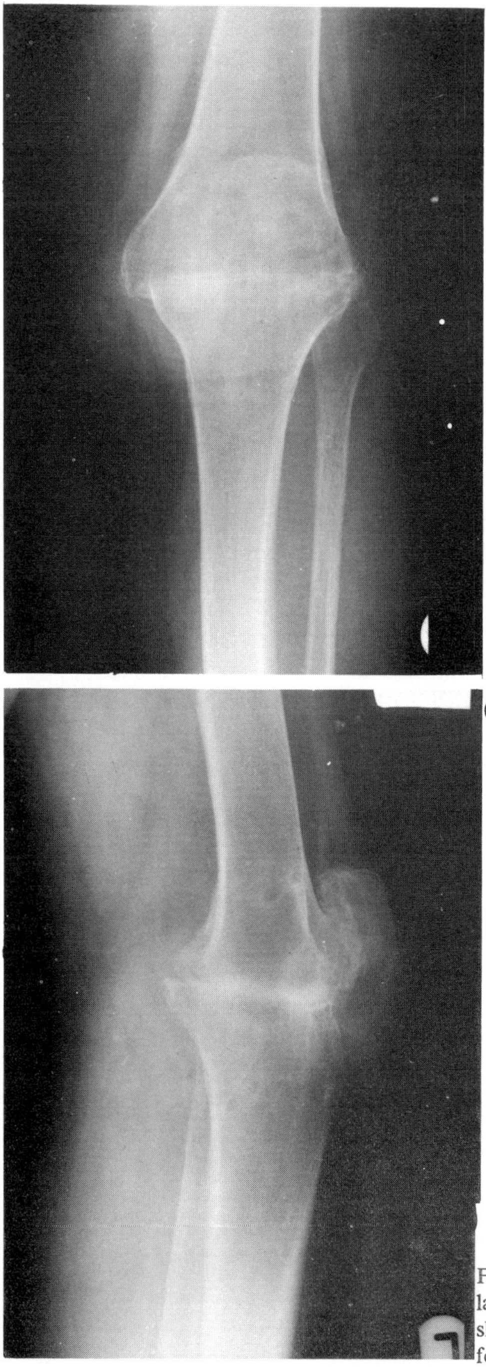

(a)

(b)

FIGURE 16.15 Antero-posterior and lateral postoperative radiographs showing the appearance of the knee following arthrodesis too good to make arthrodesis acceptable or if arthrodesis is contra-indicated because of the state of the other joints, *osteotomy* is the only available procedure. The operation is particularly indicated if there is significant tibia vara or valga since the opportunity can then be taken to re-align the knee and thus improve weight-transmission through it. The varieties of osteotomy used in RA are also applicable to OA.

THE HIP

Osteoarthrosis of the hip requires surgical treatment more commonly than does any other rheumatic disease in any other joint.

Arthrodesis is mainly applicable to secondary OA following trauma in young adults (Fig. 16.16). The soundly arthrodesed hip is secure for

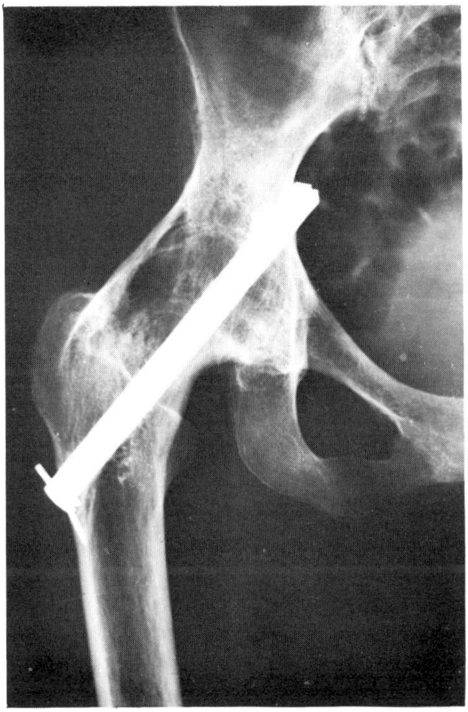

FIGURE 16.16 An antero-posterior postoperative radiograph of the hip following a Watson-Jones arthrodesis

a life-time, and function may be so good that the gait is almost indistinguishable from normal provided that the spine, the other hip, and the knees are fully mobile.

Excision arthroplasty is used chiefly as a salvage procedure if other operations have failed, or, occasionally, primarily for patients whose general condition is such that their life is in any event sedentary and they seek only a comfortable hip (*see* Rheumatoid Arthritis, p. 258 and Fig. 16.7).

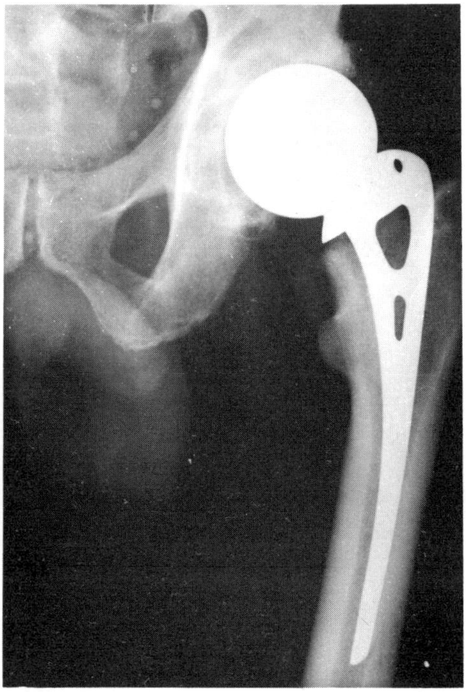

FIGURE 16.17 A postoperative radiograph of the hip showing replacement of the femoral head with a Moore's prosthesis

Interposition arthroplasty, using one of the variety of cup-shaped implants available to separate the refashioned femoral head and acetabulum (*see* Fig. 16.8), gives good results in experienced hands.

Partial replacement arthroplasty, using a Moore (Fig. 16.17) or Thompson prosthesis to replace the femoral head, has been widely used but is going out of favour since the results are poor: pain and stiffness both commonly persist postoperatively.

Total replacement arthroplasty using the implants already described (*see* Rheumatoid Arthritis, p. 259 and Fig. 16.9) is proving as successful in the short-term as it is in RA; at its best the operation results in almost normal hip function.

Capsulectomy and tenotomy, especially of the adductor muscles and, occasionally, of the ilio-psoas muscle, may form one step in all forms of arthroplasty.

Osteotomy is employed—at the intertrochanteric level using internal fixation of the osteotomy site—when pain, especially night pain, demands surgical relief but the range of movement is still good, the presence of 70 degrees of active flexion being taken as a rough dividing line between a hip suitable for osteotomy and one suitable for arthroplasty (Fig. 16.18). Since total replacement arthroplasty is avoided in patients under the age

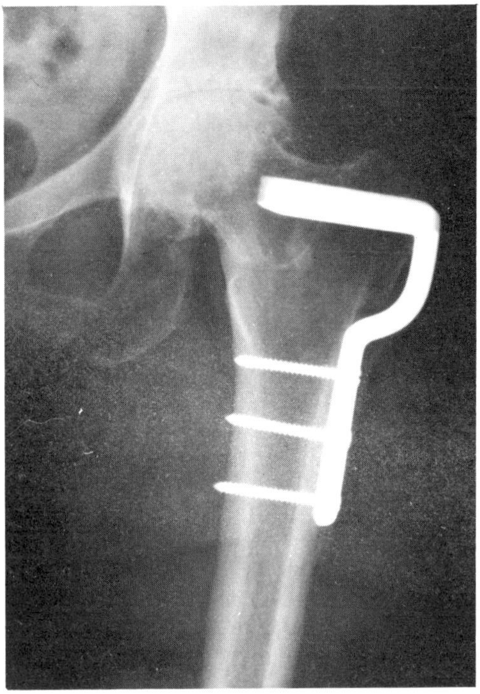

FIGURE 16.18 A postoperative antero-posterior radiograph of the hip following intertrochanteric osteotomy using a Müller Harris spline to provide internal fixation. The line of sclerosis crossing the femur at the intertrochanteric level represents the site of the united osteotomy

of sixty (*see* Rheumatoid Arthritis, p. 260), osteotomy is employed particularly in this age group; over the age of sixty it is being supplanted by total replacement arthroplasty.

Correction of deformity now forms a secondary objective of osteotomy, though the procedure was originally introduced for this purpose. There is some clinical evidence to suggest that osteotomy performed early in the disease may reverse the pathological process. If this is so, osteotomy represents the only operation capable of producing this result. It has additionally been argued that osteotomy can be used to improve the stability of a subluxing hip and to bring relatively healthy cartilage into the line of maximum weight-transmission.

Whatever may be the reason, osteotomy brings significant relief of pain, especially of night pain, to about 80 per cent of patients who have the operation. Stiffness is often not relieved, however, so that in terms of the return of function osteotomy is by no means an entirely satisfactory procedure.

17

Less Common Rheumatic Conditions

Colin G Barnes

This chapter includes a variety of less common conditions, some of them true arthropathies, others masquerading as such. Since no systematic review of these is possible they are briefly outlined in alphabetical order for ease of reference.

ACROMEGALY

Recurrent pain and swelling of small and medium-sized joints sometimes occurs in association with acromegaly. Clinically, this may resemble an inflammatory arthropathy, but it appears to be related to widespread periosteal new bone formation which, later in the disease, gives way to osteoporosis.

Premature osteoarthrosis may develop in many joints, with a combination of periosteal new bone formation, cystic changes in the juxta-articular bone, and osteophyte formation. In distinction from inflammatory arthropathies the joint spaces in the apparently affected small joints of the hands are preserved, and may even be widened.

ANAPHYLACTOID (HENOCH-SCHOENLEIN) PURPURA

Anaphylactoid non-thrombocytopenic purpura, due to an acute diffuse angiitis, is associated with urticaria, angio-neurotic oedema, abdominal colic, and transient synovitis. The condition develops characteristically in children with a peak age incidence at three years; more than half the patients are under six years, and there is a slight preponderance of males. Preceding streptococcal infection is sometimes identifiable as providing the allergen which, however, in many cases remains unknown.

The eponymous title Henoch-Schoenlein purpura derives from Henoch's original description of the colicky abdominal pain attributable to bleeding into, and oedema of, the intestinal wall, and to the description of the articular manifestations by Schoenlein. These consist of attacks of transient synovitis, leaving no residua, usually affecting the knee joints.

The development of the rash may be diagnostic, the papules being some 5 mm or more in diameter, distributed symmetrically over the buttocks and legs and, occasionally, more widespread. When the angiitis is sufficiently severe the lesions may become discoloured due to the deposition of blood pigments. This is the typical allergic purpura. The disease is usually self-limiting but an important complication is an acute proliferative glomerulo-nephritis with proteinuria and haematuria—indistinguishable from acute "Ellis type 1" glomerulo-nephritis. Intussusception may rarely occur from the gastro-intestinal tract involvement; vomiting or even haematemesis are less uncommon. Gut manifestations provide the only absolute indication for corticosteroid therapy.

ATRIAL MYXOMA

The presence of a myxomatous tumour in the heart will produce obvious cardiovascular manifestations of embolisation and valvular obstruction. Rarely, this may be associated with systemic symptoms with which the patient may present—malaise, weight loss, fever, Raynaud's phenomenon, and arthralgia. The latter is usually of limb girdle and peripheral distribution but without soft tissue swelling, effusion, joint tenderness, or erosive change. Tests for rheumatoid serum factor are negative but there may be anaemia, a raised ESR, and elevation of alpha-2 and gamma globulins. Symptoms resolve on surgical removal of the myxoma.

AVASCULAR NECROSIS

Avascular, or aseptic necrosis most commonly involves the femoral heads, though the humeral head, and probably the femoral condyles, may also be affected.

A quadrant of the upper surface of the femoral head becomes ischaemic and collapses, producing deformity. This leads either to remodelling or, more commonly, to severe degenerative changes.

Clinically there is a rapid onset of pain and limitation of movement, although characteristically in the hip it is flexion, rotation, and abduction that are limited while extension is preserved.

Radiological changes are absent in the early stages, and it is only later that the characteristic appearance develops. A slightly depressed area on the upper surface of the femoral head is seen first, usually associated with a zone of subcortical translucency. Later, the infarcted quadrant becomes increasingly dense and collapses inwards, leading to flattening of the femoral head. Secondary degenerative changes may develop rapidly.

While this condition sometimes develops *de novo*, it may also occur during the course of rheumatoid arthritis or other inflammatory arthropathies, or in association with corticosteroid therapy, decompression (caisson) disease, hepatic cirrhosis, alcoholism, or after minor trauma. Infarction of the affected segment of bone is thought to be the common mechanism.

Surgical treatment is often required. Early osteotomy to re-align the weight-bearing area of the femoral head may lead to effective re-modelling. Alternatively, an arthroplasty involving the replacement of the femoral head is required.

BEHCET'S SYNDROME

This syndrome's eponymous title is derived from the description of a 'triple symptom complex', of buccal (Fig. 17.1) and genital ulceration and iritis, by Hulusi Behcet in 1937. However, many systems may be involved and the clinical features are widely distributed. The various manifestations may be grouped into major and minor diagnostic criteria as follows –

Major criteria –

buccal ulceration	
genital ulceration	
skin lesions –	ulceration
	erythema nodosum
	erythema multiforme
	sepsis
eye lesions –	uveitis
	corneal ulceration
	retrobulbar neuritis

Minor criteria –

thrombophlebitis –	superficial veins, deep veins and venae cavae
inflammatory arthropathy	
gastro-intestinal lesions –	peptic ulceration
	'ulcerative colitis'
central nervous system – lesions	mental changes
	mid-brain lesions
	transverse myelitis of the cord
cardiovascular lesions –	pericarditis
a positive family history	

Since there is no specific pathological abnormality, it is suggested that the diagnosis requires three major criteria, or two major and at least two minor criteria to be present.

Although inflammatory, the arthropathy is non-erosive and leaves no

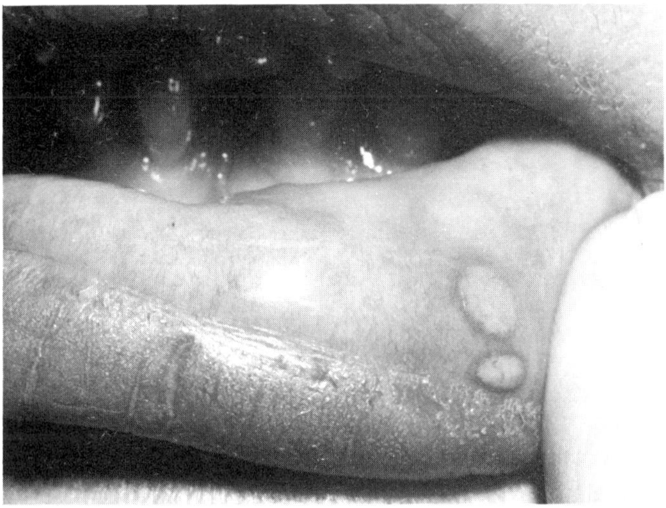

FIGURE 17.1 Buccal ulceration in Behcet's syndrome

residua. The knees are the most commonly affected joints. Tests for serum rheumatoid factor are negative.

Treatment is symptomatic, and neither gold nor corticosteroids have been shown to have any effect on the arthritis. Corticosteroid therapy, however, may be needed to control the uveitis which, if left untreated, can lead to blindness.

CLUTTON'S JOINTS

A painful and symmetrical synovitis of the knees is one of the many manifestations of congenital syphilis. The elbows occasionally may be similarly affected. The onset is usually insidious but occasionally acute. The arthropathy pursues a benign self-limiting course without residua. Because the age of onset is in the same range as that of Still's disease the differential diagnosis may be difficult, and other features of congenital syphilis should always be sought.

ERYTHEMA NODOSUM

Joint involvement occurs in up to 75 per cent of patients with erythema nodosum whatever the aetiology. Arthralgia, without joint swelling, but associated with morning stiffness is usual, although synovial swelling, tenderness and joint effusion may develop in up to one-third of patients. The arthropathy not infrequently precedes the appearance of the skin lesions and may persist for a very variable time ranging from a few weeks to as long as several years. It always runs a benign course, and joint deformity or destructive change does not develop. The knees and ankles are most frequently affected but the wrists and small joints of the hands may also be involved. Tests for rheumatoid factor are usually negative, and radiographs of the affected joints do not reveal erosive changes. The ESR is usually elevated. Treatment of the arthropathy is by the administration of salicylates in full dosage. In the rare persistent case, corticosteroids may be required, and usually bring about dramatic improvement. It goes without saying that any underlying cause requires investigation and treatment on its own merits.

FAMILIAL MEDITERRANEAN FEVER

Familial Mediterranean fever (FMF) is an inherited condition almost entirely restricted to Sephardic Jews originating in the region of the Eastern Mediterranean. Isolated cases in other parts of the world occur exclusively in those whose ancestors originate from this region. Transmission is by an autosomal recessive gene but males are more frequently affected.

While the disease may present in childhood, the maximum age of onset is in the second decade of life. Intermittent high fever and abdominal pain occur in most patients, lasting from 12 to 72 hours. The essential feature is a serositis commonly causing abdominal pain, but pleurisy and arthritis are also features.

In practice, the diagnosis of the abdominal pain may be difficult – this is continuous during an attack and may be localised or generalised. Because of this, acute intra-abdominal emergencies such as peritonitis, a perforated peptic ulcer, appendicitis, cholecystitis, or acute pyelonephritis are frequently suspected. Laparotomy then reveals only an inflamed peritoneum with a small amount of turbid exudate.

Joints are similarly affected with acute pain, swelling, tenderness, and limitation. The swelling is due to a combination of synovial hypertrophy and effusion. The knees are most commonly affected, occasionally the hips.

An impressive feature of the disease is the astonishing propensity to complete recovery of the joints after what appears to have been a potentially damaging arthritis. Occasionally, this does become chronic but erosive change does not develop although periarticular osteoporosis and narrowing of the joint space may occur in longstanding cases. Secondary degenerative change may result. Tests for serum rheumatoid factor are negative.

Amyloidosis is a common complication. This may occur in the course of typical FMF or as an isolated phenomenon in members of susceptible families, presumably as a partial expression of the syndrome. Renal amyloidosis is the usual cause of death.

HAEMOGLOBINOPATHIES

Involvement of the locomotor system in the haemoglobinopathies is of four types –

1. Synovitis
2. Infarction
3. Haemorrhage
4. Periosteal reaction.

Synovitis. Arthralgia is the most common articular manifestation although there may also be joint swelling and effusion. It usually occurs in sickle-cell disease during crises, and the cause is uncertain.

Infarction. Bone infarction with resultant avascular necrosis is a prominent feature of sickle-cell (SS) disease and thalassaemia. This may present with local bone pain, or features of necrosis of the femoral or humeral heads (rarely a patella).

Haemorrhage. Haemorrhage into a joint, or into subchondral bone, may result in destruction of articular cartilage.

Periosteal reaction. A true dactylitis with associated pain and swelling may occur in sickle-cell disease with marked periosteal reaction of the phalanges, the metacarpal and the metatarsal bones.

HAEMOPHILIA

The articular manifestations of haemophilia and Christmas disease result from the haemarthroses that punctuate the lives of these patients.

Acute Haemarthrosis. An acute bleed into a joint may occur spontaneously but more commonly follows minor trauma. The affected joint becomes hot, swollen, and exceedingly painful. The presence of blood in the joint produces an inflammatory reaction with multiplication of synovial cells and villous hypertrophy, and, later, some chronic inflammatory cell infiltration. Treatment consists of the immediate replacement of the missing plasma factor. In the case of haemophilia this involves the administration of 'cryoprecipitate' while for Christmas disease fresh plasma or special concentrates are given. The place of joint aspiration is controversial. If the haemarthrosis is under tension it is probably wise to aspirate the blood immediately following replacement therapy.

Pain relief in the acute phase is essential and should be achieved by adequate administration of analgesics, and occasionally with ice packs applied to the affected joints. Early mobilisation is essential.

Chronic Arthritis. Prevention of chronic arthritis is the main aim of treatment. Permanent joint damage depends on the frequency of haemorrhage into the joint together with the length of time that blood remains in the joint, producing damage to the articular cartilage. *Thus, early treatment of acute haemarthrosis is essential.* The rapid muscle wasting that occurs adjacent to affected joints must also be corrected, and splinting may be required to prevent deformity.

Permanent joint changes are degenerative, secondary to repeated haemarthroses, with destruction of joint surfaces, loss of joint space, and subsequent osteophyte formation. Repeated haemarthroses also cause both hyperaemia of epiphyseal plates with resultant irregular overgrowth, and periarticular fibrosis, both of which further contribute to the deformity and loss of function.

HYPERCHOLESTEROLAEMIC ARTHROPATHY

The metabolic inherited disorder, familial hypercholesterolaemia (Type II hyperlipoproteinaemia) may be associated with a migratory arthritis affecting small peripheral joints.

This condition is characterised by the development of widespread cutaneous xanthomata (which may also occur within tendons and attached to periosteum), arcus senilis, and premature atherosclerosis. There is a great increase in plasma cholesterol, β-lipoproteins, and phospholipids, with normal levels of plasma triglycerides and chylomicrons.

HYPERMOBILITY SYNDROMES

Joint or ligamentous laxity permitting hyperextension of the fingers and knees, and a tendency to dislocation of the shoulders and patellae, is not uncommon in otherwise normal individuals. This tendency is frequently familial. However, identical hypermobility of joints is also a part of certain inherited connective tissue disorders such as the *Ehlers-Danlos* and *Marfan's* syndromes.

Arthropathy results either from recurrent dislocations or, more commonly, as a result of repeated minor traumata. Joint pain and swelling are the usual manifestations, which may be prevented by the studied avoidance of trauma, and the maintenance of muscular strength, especially the quadriceps group if the knees are affected. Permanent joint changes are due to secondary osteoarthrosis.

HYPERPARATHYROIDISM

Hyperparathyroidism may lead to joint disease in one of three ways:

1. By leading to secondary (renal) hyperuricaemia (p. 159) which may be complicated by clinical gout.
2. By leading to chondrocalcinosis and pyrophosphate arthropathy (p. 178).
3. By producing metabolic bone disease with subchondral bony trabecular fractures, collapse of cysts, and what amounts to a traumatic synovitis. This may be widespread and mimic rheumatoid arthritis.

HYPERTROPHIC PULMONARY OSTEOARTHROPATHY

Clubbing of the fingers may be associated with many conditions, the most common being chronic pulmonary suppuration, bronchial carcinoma, and cyanotic heart disease. Less commonly this is seen in Laennec's or biliary cirrhosis, ulcerative colitis, and malabsorption syndromes. It may also be congenital, occurring in the absence of any other diseases.

Hypertrophic pulmonary osteoarthropathy is an extension of the more familiar clubbing of the fingers, and in a sense is a more complete expression of this reaction. By far the commonest cause is bronchial carcinoma. The patient presents with pain, swelling, and stiffness of peripheral joints. Apart from clubbing, the diagnosis rests on the characteristic radiological appearance of periosteal reaction with new bone formation (Fig. 17.2) adjacent to involved joints. The most common site is the distal end of the radius and ulna.

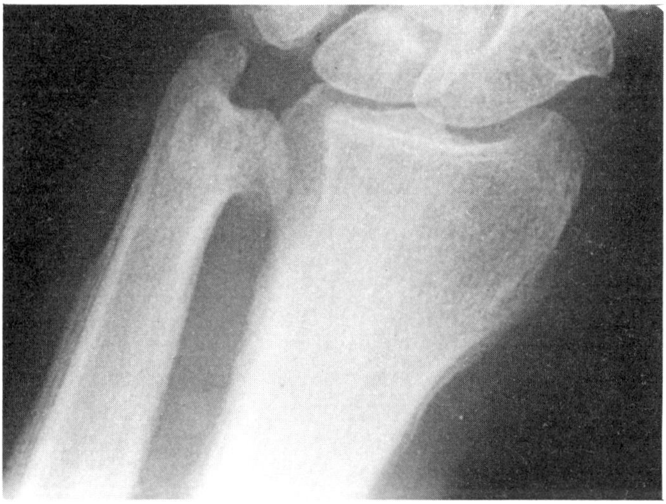

FIGURE 17.2 Hypertrophic pulmonary osteoarthropathy. Radiograph of a wrist showing periosteal reaction on the radius and ulna

For reasons not understood, resection of the carcinoma, or simply section of the vagus nerves supplying the affected lung, produces dramatic relief of the symptoms.

It is worth noting that the clinical development of hypertrophic pulmonary osteoarthropathy may be the first manifestation of a bronchial neoplasm.

HYPOGAMMAGLOBULINAEMIA

Congenital or acquired hypogammaglobulinaemia is characteristically associated with an increased susceptibility to infection, which may be overwhelming. Such patients are liable, of course, to septic arthritis but occasionally a true inflammatory arthropathy occurs. While this may have a striking resemblance to rheumatoid arthritis, it is non-erosive and tends to remit spontaneously, without residua. Tests for rheumatoid factor are regularly negative. The relationship between this type of arthropathy and rheumatoid arthritis is a matter for intriguing speculation; interestingly, subcutaneous nodules have been reported but histologically these lack the usual plasma cells.

NEUROPATHIC (CHARCOT'S) JOINTS

Although Charcot first described the prototype of the arthropathy which bears his name, in relation to tabes dorsalis, it is clear that any loss of joint sensation may cause a similar condition. Thus, any of the following may be responsible—

1 Tabes dorsalis
1 Syringomyelia
3 Diabetes mellitus
4 Leprosy
5 Paraplegia
6 Myelomeningocoele
7 Congenital indifference to pain
8 Charcot-Marie-Tooth disease

In ordinary practice only the first three are likely to be encountered.

The joint disturbance is characterised by gross destructive changes, joint instability and florid new bone formation (Fig. 17.3). Coarse grating crepitus is typical. Occasionally, there is a secondary inflammatory reaction within the joint producing effusion. It is often said that the Charcot joint is painless. There is, however, one exception—the diabetic tarsal neuropathic joint may be painful and present a clinical and radiological appearance suggesting a septic lesion.

OCHRONOSIS

Alkaptonuria is an inherited disorder of metabolism transmitted by a simple, recessive, autosomal gene. The liver enzyme *homogentisic acid oxidase*, responsible for the conversion of homogentisic acid to malelyl-aceto-acetic acid during the degradation of tyrosine, is absent. Homogentisic acid thus appears in the urine, which turns a dark colour on oxidation. The clinical manifestations, known as *ochronosis*, similarly

(a)

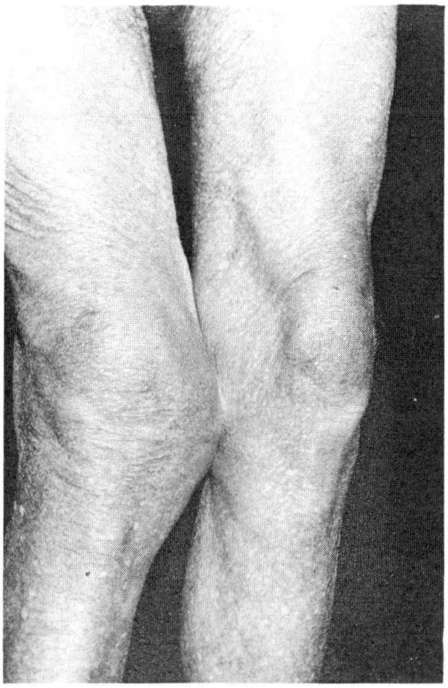

(b)

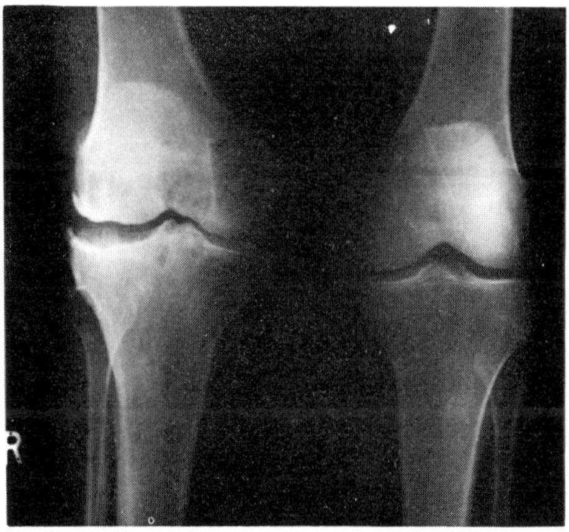

FIGURE 17.3 Syphilitic neuropathic arthropathy of the right knee

depend on its deposition in connective tissue, especially cartilage. Thus, the ears become discoloured, developing a slate blue appearance, and wax in the ears is also coloured. Pigmentation occurs of the skin of the axillae and groin, and over the nose.

The affected cartilage becomes hard and stiff so that the ears become thick and rigid: this disease is, therefore, more correctly classified under the heading of Metabolic Deposition Diseases.

The locomotor manifestations are usually confined to the spine, giving rise to backache and stiffness leading to complete spinal rigidity.

Radiologically, the intervertebral disc spaces are narrowed and the discs themselves calcified (Fig. 17.4). Secondary degenerative changes with osteophyte formation subsequently develop.

Rarely, a peripheral arthropathy develops due to deposition of the pigment in articular cartilage. The features are essentially those of degenerative joint disease. Particles of affected cartilage may break off and form loose bodies within the joint.

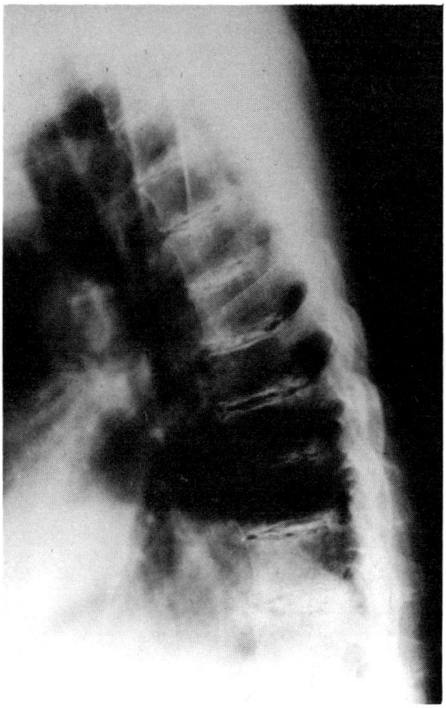

FIGURE 17.4 Calcification of the intervertebral discs in ochronosis (Courtesy Dr W. G. Wenley)

OSTEOCHONDRITIS DISSECANS

This is a common condition of unknown aetiology in which small and medium-sized flakes of articular cartilage become separated, to form loose bodies within the joint. The cartilage, since it is nourished by synovial fluid, remains viable and frequently ossifies.

This usually occurs in the second and third decades of life, affecting most commonly one knee, to produce intermittent pain often with effusion and locking. X-rays may reveal a depression in the articular contour when the detached flake of cartilage is accompanied by a piece of the adjacent subchondral bone. Surgical removal of the loose body is the only effective treatment.

PIGMENTED VILLO-NODULAR SYNOVITIS

As the name suggests, this is essentially a pathological diagnosis. Synovial tissue of the joints, bursae and tendon sheaths may be affected by this inflammatory granulomatous condition. Thus, either villous or nodular lesions occur, by hypertrophy of synovium, which contain multinucleate giant cells and haemosiderin, from which the pigmented appearance is derived. The pathogenesis is entirely unknown.

Clinically, this presents as a monarticular arthropathy in a young adult, sometimes with involvement of bursae or tendon sheaths. The commonest joint to be affected is the knee. Effusion usually occurs and, if aspirated, is found to be heavily bloodstained. Narrowing of the joint space or erosion of juxta-articular bone develops in longstanding cases.

Synovectomy has been advocated as the treatment of choice. On opening the joint the synovium is seen to be thickened and brown, with large numbers of long trailing villi, among which are scattered pedunculated or sessile nodules. The former may become separated and cause locking of the joint by acting as loose bodies. Since most joints do not permit a complete removal of synovium to be performed, recurrence is not unusual, and surgical treatment is frequently followed by irradiation to try to prevent this.

RELAPSING POLYCHONDRITIS

Relapsing polychondritis is a primary inflammatory disease affecting cartilage throughout the body, and occuring in middle age. The course is intermittent, and episodes of active inflammation are usually accompanied by general malaise and fever, together with elevation of the ESR. The aetiology is unknown.

Pain, swelling, and tenderness of subcutaneous cartilaginous structures, particularly the nose and pinnae, are common clinical manifestations and lead to collapse of the nose (Fig. 17.5) and deformity of the ears. However, inflammation of the sclerae and tracheal rings also occurs, the latter being a common cause of death from tracheal collapse and airway obstruction.

Articular cartilage may also be involved so that the condition masquerades as an inflammatory arthropathy, when in fact there is no true synovitis. Many joints are affected, including both cartilaginous joints (symphysis pubis and manubrio-sternal joint) and synovial joints. The joint pain, swelling, effusion, tenderness, and limitation of movement may resemble rheumatoid arthritis. Although tests for serum rheumatoid factor are negative, radiographs of the hands and feet may easily be mistaken for those of rheumatoid arthritis, because of somewhat similar 'erosive' appearances and joint space narrowing.

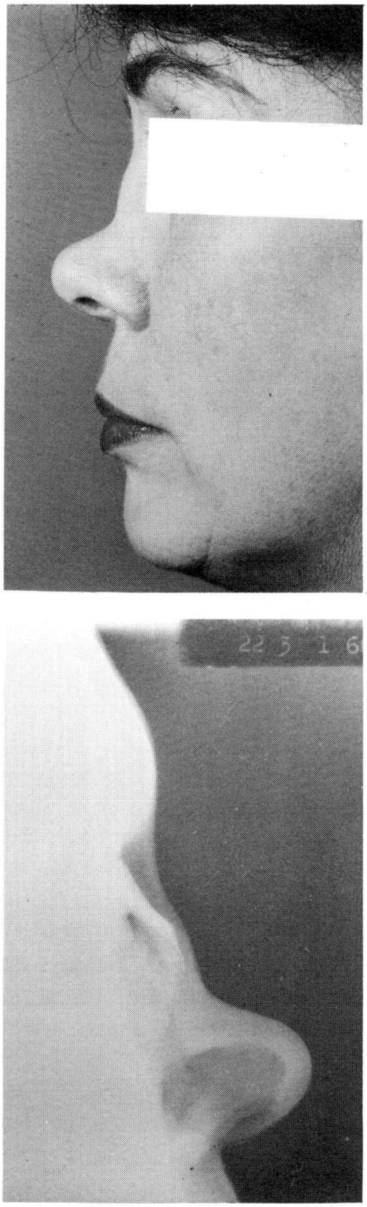

(a)

(b)

FIGURE 17.5 Loss of nasal cartilage in relapsing polychondritis

RUBELLA AND OTHER VIRUS INFECTIONS

Rubella, and occasionally other virus infections such as mumps, may be complicated by a distinct polyarthritis, especially when they occur in young adults. This can involve one, or many, joints and may present features suggestive either of mild rheumatic fever or rheumatoid arthritis. However it is self-limiting, lasting for 2 to 28 days. In rubella it may develop before, with, or after the rash, and is sometimes seen without a rash (presenting a difficult diagnostic problem). Carpal tunnel syndrome is not infrequent. The synovitis is histologically non-specific but the virus has been isolated from an involved joint. Treatment is symptomatic and a short course of corticosteroids is sometimes justified.

SARCOIDOSIS

Articular involvement during the course of sarcoidosis appears to fall into two distinct categories. First, there is the polyarthritis associated with erythema nodosum (*see* p. 277), usually occurring in the benign form of sarcoidosis which declares itself as hilar lymphadenopathy. This form of the disease usually occurs below the age of thirty years and is more common in women than in men. It is usually a self-limiting condition, the joints, glands, and skin lesions all subsiding spontaneously. This benign form of sarcoidosis is often referred to as Loefgren's syndrome. It may be aborted by steroid therapy.

In the second form of arthritis actual sarcoid granulomata occur in the synovium, in association with a more widespread form of the disease. The clinical appearance of the joints may resemble rheumatoid arthritis although fewer joints are usually involved.

Granulomata in the bones produce cystic lesions visible radiologically; but where the phalanges are affected there is diffuse swelling which may be mistaken for a small joint polyarthritis such as rheumatoid arthritis. Corticosteroids tend to produce only temporary remissions in this form of sarcoidosis and the long-term prognosis is poor. All types of sarcoidosis are more common among the negro races.

SERUM SICKNESS

This is a disease in which circulating immune complexes produce widespread vascular damage leading to pathological changes in many organs, including the joints. It characteristically follows an injection of foreign (horse) serum given for therapeutic purposes. Following the injection there is a latent period (4 to 10 days) during which it is assumed that the recipient is mounting a humoral antibody response against the foreign protein. When this humoral antibody enters the circulation it combines with any remaining foreign protein to form an immune antigen-antibody complex. The presence of this complex in the circulation is thought to be the immediate cause of the vascular damage. At this stage serum complement levels fall. The pattern of clinical response will depend on which vessels are most affected. The clinical picture consists of an urticarial eruption, generalised lymph node enlargement, angio-neurotic oedema and fever. Occasionally, non-thrombocytopenic purpura, proteinuria, oliguria, abdominal pain, and arthralgia also occur.

SYNOVIAL CHONDROMATOSIS

Synovial chondromatosis may cause pain and swelling of a joint usually with either limitation or locking during movement. Single joint involvement is usual, the knee being most commonly affected.

The joint manifestations are due to the presence of single or multiple cartilaginous loose bodies which become calcified or ossified. These are formed by metaplasia in the synovium, and subsequently separate. Any synovial tissue may be affected.

The synovium appears thickened with plaques of cartilaginous material visible on the surface, some of which become pedunculated. The condition is benign. Radiologically, multiple rounded opacities are seen in relation to the affected joint and its capsule when the cartilaginous deposits have become calcified.

Surgical removal of loose bodies, and, occasionally, synovectomy may be indicated.

SYNOVIAL RUPTURE

The presence of an effusion in a large weight-bearing joint such as the knee results in very high intra-articular pressures developing during normal exercise. This may lead to rupture of the synovial sac and escape of the fluid between the tissue planes of the calf. The clinical features are almost indistinguishable from those of a deep vein thrombosis, with calf pain, tenderness, and swelling, oedema around the ankle, and a positive Homans' sign. The fluid may become encapsulated, forming a visible and palpable calf cyst.

Because of the difference in treatment it is essential to distinguish this from a deep vein thrombosis. The history may indicate the likelihood of a synovial rupture if the patient noted a swollen knee, or the pain developed suddenly during exertion. The observant patient may have noticed that the swelling of the knee decreased as another developed in the calf.

An anthrogram performed within a few days of the rupture will show the typical appearance of the injected radio-opaque material tracking down into soft tissues of the calf.

While synovial rupture is recognised most frequently in the rheumatoid knee it also occurs in the elbow, and may occur with synovial effusions from other causes.

Treatment is seldom required. The rupture seals spontaneously and the fluid outside the joint is absorbed. Very rarely, excision of a calf cyst is required.

SYNOVIAL TUMOURS

Malignant synovioma is fortunately a very rare tumour. It is extremely malignant, and is derived from synovial cells.

Young males are most commonly affected, the lesion developing usually in a lower-limb joint although any joint may be involved. The tumour presents as a painless swelling adjacent to the joint, or rarely tendon. Radiologically, it appears as a soft tissue mass with adjacent periosteal reaction. Dissemination occurs directly by lymph vessels to the regional nodes, lung, and bony skeleton, where osteolytic lesions are the rule.

Histologically the tumour is a sarcoma with anaplastic spindle cells and epithelioid cells.

Treatment consists of wide excision, usually involving amputation of the affected limb, followed by irradiation. The prognosis is poor, five-year survival rates being between 30 and 50 per cent.

WHIPPLE'S DISEASE

Fatty diarrhoea, abdominal pain, weight loss, skin pigmentation, and chylous ascites occurring exclusively in males are the manifestations of this rare condition. Histologically, it is characterised by an infiltration of the submucosa of the ileum, and of the regional lymph nodes draining the ileum, with large foamy macrophages which stain positively by the Periodic Acid Schiff technique.

Whipple's disease may also be associated with an inflammatory, non-erosive, intermittent arthropathy, usually affecting the knees and, occasionally, other lower-limb joints. Serum rheumatoid factor is absent and X-rays of affected joints do not reveal erosive changes but may show peri-articular osteoporosis.

Information is not available as to whether the antibiotic therapy which has recently been shown to improve the bowel condition (and suggests a bacterial aetiology) has any effect on the joints.

Appendix A

Clinical Examination of the Locomotor System

H L F Currey

A number of excellent accounts of the systematic examination of the joints are available to the student, but most of these are primarily relevant to orthopaedic surgery. This section is therefore somewhat selective, with emphasis placed on those aspects of the examination that are particularly relevant to the diagnosis of rheumatic diseases. The student must realise that such an examination requires the acquisition of a skill, and we have therefore paid special attention to those joints which, in our experience, prove most difficult to examine properly.

Sound clinical assessment of the articular system in rheumatology requires no more than an extension of the basic methods of the clinician (inspection, palpation etc.) *plus* the application of simple mechanical principles based on the anatomical arrangement of the joint in question. Accurate measurements must be made wherever possible, and it is essential that they are recorded in a standardised manner so that they are intelligible to others.

METHOD OF EXAMINING A JOINT

It is a great convenience that the majority of joints are paired, and the most informative technique is one in which each method of examination is applied alternately to the two sides.

Assessment of a joint requires observation concerning the following:

Swelling
Pain
Skin changes
Muscle wasting
Movements
Deformity

Swelling

In osteoarthrosis this is typically *bony*, with osteophytes and new bone formation producing a firm gnarled feel. In inflammatory joint disease, swelling may be due either to *soft tissue swelling* or to *fluid*. The proliferated, oedematous synovium of the rheumatoid joint produces a boggy swelling, which needs to be distinguished from an effusion. An excess of fluid in the synovial cavity may occur in arthropathy from any cause (or, rarely, without arthropathy; for example, in a joint situated within an area of gross oedema from other causes, or in a joint close to a focus of acute inflammation – a 'sympathetic effusion'). The contour of a joint is altered in a characteristic way by the presence of an effusion, and careful comparison with the opposite side may reveal its presence. Proof of the fluid nature of a joint swelling may be obtained by 'cross fluctuation' across the synovial cavity. Localised cystic swellings near joints may represent distended bursae or cysts. Either may communicate with the main joint cavity to give, again, 'cross fluctuation'.

Pitting *oedema* of tissues overlying a joint is an indication of the acuteness of the inflammatory process. It is commonly seen, for example, in crystal synovitis. Exceptionally, it may be a feature of early rheumatoid arthritis (p. 20). However, apparent swelling of a joint may be produced by overlying oedema due to conditions outside the articulation. A common error, for example, is to regard acute pre- or infra-patellar bursitis as arthritis of the knee joint. Careful observation, in this instance, will show that the extent of the swelling does not correspond with the anatomical arrangement of the articular synovial cavity.

Pain

Apart from the spontaneous pain which may be present when an arthritic joint is at rest, physical examination must determine whether discomfort is produced by moving a joint or by pressure over it. Care may be necessary, however, in interpreting positive signs as evidence of arthritis. In the example quoted, that of acute pre-patellar bursitis, putting the knee through a full range of movement will certainly produce pain (by distorting inflamed tissues outside the joint), but a limited range of painless passive movement will also be demonstrable. Similarly, exquisite tenderness may be present over a localised area anteriorly, but no tenderness will be found over other areas where the joint cavity is accessible to examination. Thus, in an acutely inflamed joint, passive movement typically produces pain throughout the whole range, and tenderness can be elicited over all exposed aspects of the articulation. When these criteria are not fulfilled it is necessary to consider whether the inflammation may lie outside the joint. Well-known diagnostic pitfalls in this regard are the erroneous diagnosis of arthritis in children with juxta-articular inflammation due to acute osteomyelitis or acute leukaemia. Similarly, adults with de Quervain's syndrome (*see* p. 232) may mistakenly be diagnosed as suffering from arthritis of the wrist joint.

In the routine examination of the articular system, simultaneous movement and compression provide a useful rapid screening test for inflammation in hand and foot joints. Thus, the earliest physical sign of rheumatoid arthritis may be the discomfort produced (for example) in the metatarsophalangeal joint of the little toe by moving this articulation while compressing it between finger and thumb (*see* Fig. A21).

In degenerative joint disease, localised tender areas may be discovered in relationship to ligaments and other structures round the joint. These may be significant in indicating the site of local lesions responsible for symptoms.

It is convenient to classify joint tenderness into four grades by the following procedure. The examiner attempts to apply firm pressure to the joint by squeezing it (where practicable) between finger and thumb. If the joint is tender there will be one of four responses –

Grade I The patient complains of pain.
Grade II The patient complains of pain and winces.
Grade III The patient winces and withdraws the joint.
Grade IV The patient will not allow palpation of the joint.

The Overlying Skin

Redness of the skin indicates an acute inflammatory reaction within the joint. It is common in septic arthritis, crystal synovitis, and rheumatic fever. It is rare in rheumatoid arthritis. For reasons not understood, the skin overlying an acute gouty joint tends to be dry, while that overlying a rheumatic fever or septic joint is moist.

Increased warmth of the skin overlying an inflamed joint is a surprisingly definite and useful sign, and a sensitive indication of inflammation within the joint. It is usually positive when an effusion of any size is present. The test is performed by applying the same part of the observer's hand to the joint on each side of the body. When the hand is carried backwards and forwards in this way, any difference in temperature is readily appreciated. Only a difference is significant, and the test is obviously invalidated if one or other joint has been selectively warmed or cooled before the test, for example by the presence of dressings.

Muscle Wasting

Painful and inflamed joints characteristically produce a reduction in the bulk of nearby muscles. In a limb this can be documented as the circumference at a level defined with reference to a bony landmark.

Movement

Joint movements may be *active* or *passive*. In general, testing of passive movements is more informative about the state of an actual articulation, for active movements may be impaired by muscle weakness or lesions of tendons. In many situations it is wise to test both.

Full examination of a joint requires measurement of the range of normal movements and, also, testing for the presence of any abnormal motion. The observer notes whether the movements are painful and whether palpable *crepitus* is produced in the joint. Pain on movement has been mentioned above. Crepitus is an important indication of joint pathology. It is elicited by placing a palpating hand over the joint while the other hand moves the articulation passively. Crepitus is also audible with a stethoscope. Soft, fine crepitus may be felt in rheumatoid joints. This presumably indicates that the moving surfaces are no longer smooth cartilage, but fine granulations. Predictably, the development of osteoarthrosis is associated with more coarse crepitus, and in the badly damaged joint there may be gross grating. In the hip joint this may be so loud as to be audible as the patient walks into the consulting room. The extreme example of this is Charcot's arthropathy. Crepitus may also arise from tendon sheaths, and a creaking leathery crepitus is characteristic of tendon sheath involvement in progressive systemic sclerosis (p. 112). The familiar 'cracking' of joints, for example the loud snapping noises arising from knees during flexion while weight-bearing, or from hyper-extended finger joints, are of significance only in the situation where they form a prominent complaint by the patient, when they indicate hypochondriasis.

MEASUREMENT AND RECORDING OF JOINT MOVEMENTS

The American Academy of Orthopaedic Surgeons in 1965 published a booklet: *Joint Motion, Method of Measuring and Recording*. It was reprinted by the British Orthopaedic Association in 1966. This small volume describes a simple system of recording the range of joint movements, applicable to the whole body, which it is hoped will soon be universally adopted.

The system is based on the *neutral zero method*, in which all movements of a joint are measured from defined *zero starting positions*. Thus, the extended 'anatomical position' of an extremity (e.g. a straight knee) is regarded as being at zero degrees (rather than 180 degrees of some previous systems). From the zero starting position, movement is therefore recorded as the number of degrees of flexion, or (in the opposite direction) the number of degrees of extension. The range of flexion in a knee joint with limited motion might thus be recorded as '20–40 degrees'.

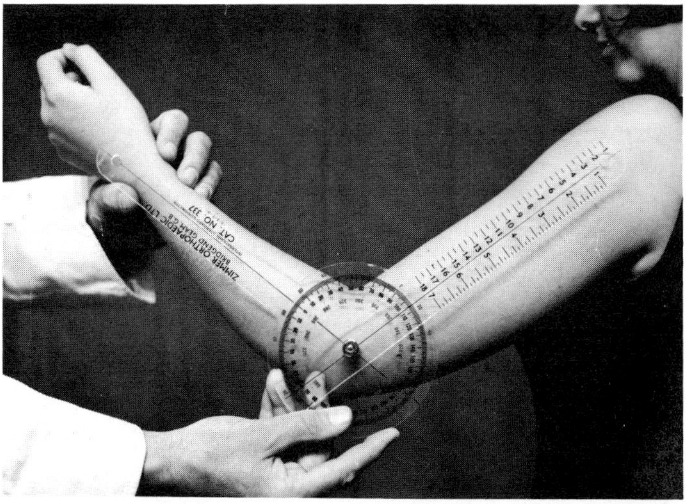

FIGURE A1 Accurate measurement of joint movement requires a *goniometer*

This would indicate 20 degrees of fixed flexion deformity, and an inability to flex beyond 40 degrees. A distinction is made between 'extension' and 'hyperextension'. When the movement opposite to flexion is a natural motion (e.g. at the wrist and shoulder joints) this is referred to as extension. When such a movement is unnatural (e.g. at the elbow and knee joints) it is referred to as hyperextension.

Clearly, the most meaningful assessment of movement in a paired joint is usually a comparison with the opposite side. Hence, all paired joints must be measured on both sides. In the following account of the method of examining various joints, the approximate normal range of movements are indicated and, where necessary, the zero starting position is defined.

For reasonably accurate (and reproducible as between one observer and another) recording of many joint movements a measuring device, or *goniometer*, is absolutely essential. This instrument consists of two arms hinged at one end, with a scale showing the angle formed between them. A suitable instrument for large joints should have arms about 12 inches long and a large, clear scale, which registers zero when the arms are extended to form a straight line (Fig. A1).

For really accurate recording of small joint movements, a strip of ordinary soldering metal can be moulded to the extensor surface of the adjacent bones and then used to trace the angle on to paper.

Standard nomenclature must be used to describe joints. The toes are named 'first' to fifth', but to avoid confusion, fingers are 'index, middle, ring, and little'.

THE CERVICAL SPINE

The patient stands or sits upright.

Rotation	(60°)*	'Look behind you to the right (or left)'.
Flexion	(45°)	'Look down'.
Extension	(45°)	'Look up'.
Lateral bending	(45°)	'Bend your head sideways, ear towards the shoulder'.

THE THORACO-LUMBAR SPINE

The major part of the spine is examined as a unit. Functionally there is variation; rotation taking place mainly in the dorsal region, bending movements in the lumbar area. However, it is difficult to test the different zones separately, apart from estimating differences by eye.

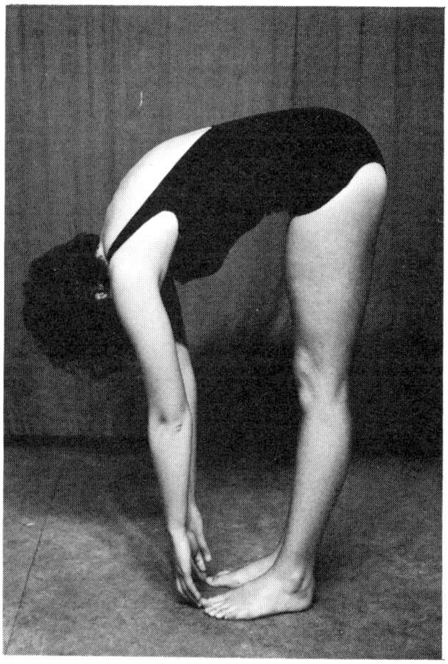

FIGURE A2 Estimation of forward flexion of the lumbar spine requires careful observation of this area during the manoeuvre 'touch your toes'

Adequate exposure is essential, and the ideal is a Bikini-type of garment. Inspection will show whether there is any abnormality of *posture*. The normal curvatures may be altered (*kyphosis* and *lordosis* signify curvatures concave forwards and backwards respectively), or there may be lateral curvature (*scoliosis*). Measurements are difficult to apply to altered spinal posture, and the only accurate recording is a clinical photograph. However, a useful measure in the fixed flexed spine of ankylosing spondylitis is the wall to tragus measurement, the patient standing upright

*Figures in parenthesis indicate approximate normal range.

with his back to the wall, with the heels against the wall. Particularly significant is a localised angulation (*gibbus*) indicating collapse of a vertebra, which may be traumatic, neoplastic, or infective. Firm pressure over the spinous processes may reveal localised tenderness.

Flexion. The standing patient attempts to touch his toes, keeping his knees straight. The observer views from the side (Fig. A2). The actual ability to touch the toes is unimportant (sufficiently mobile hips enable it to be done despite a rigid spine). The range of motion is judged by very careful observation of the movement of the lumbar region. This movement may be confirmed by placing the fingers over the lumbar spinous processes, the separation of these prominences during flexion will then be appreciated (using bony landmarks this separation can also be recorded by tape measure).

Extension. The standing patient bends over backwards, supported behind by the examiner's hand (Fig. A3). The range of motion is estimated by eye.

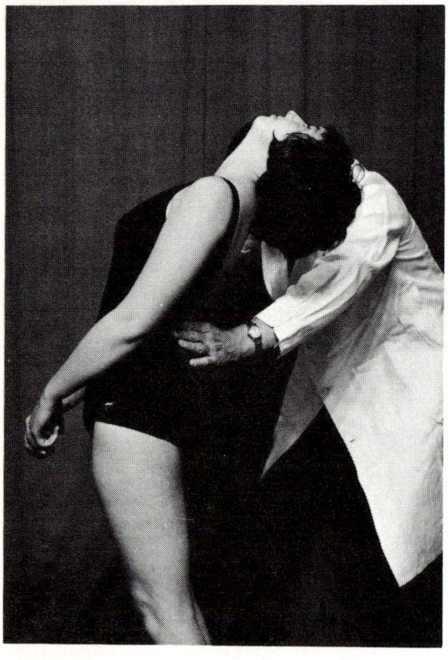

FIGURE A3 Lumbar spine extension

Lateral Bending. The standing patient slides first one hand, then the other, towards the floor, without allowing the trunk to bend forwards. The observer views from behind (Fig. A4). This much-neglected test may be of great value in distinguishing a disc lesion from early ankylosing spondylitis (in both, flexion tends to be restricted, but lateral bending is more limited in the latter condition).

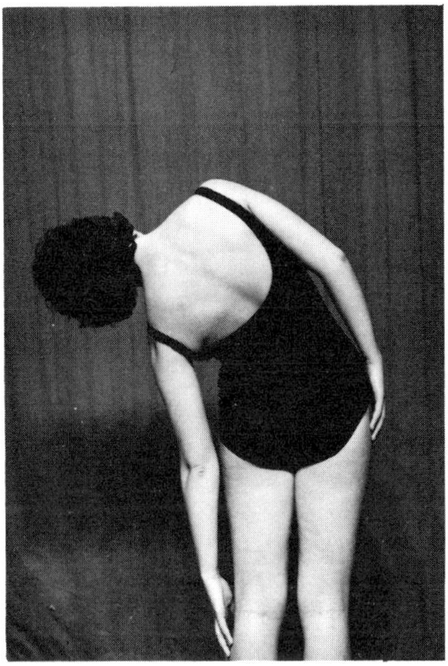

FIGURE A4 Lateral bending of the lumbar spine: 'Slide your left (or right) hand down your leg'

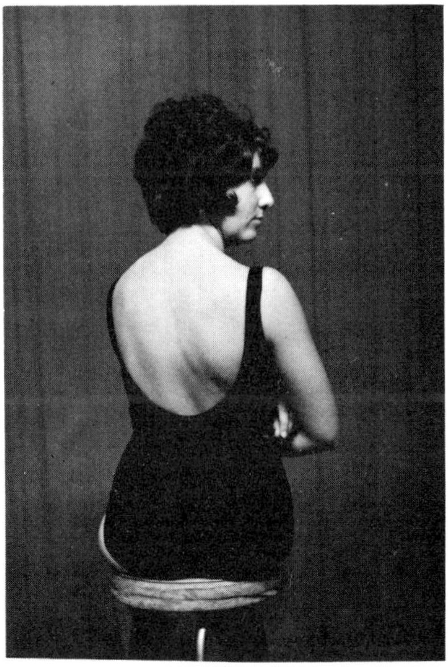

FIGURE A5 Thoracic spine rotation; tested in the sitting position to anchor the pelvis

Rotation. The patient sits on a stool (to fix the pelvis) and rotates the head and shoulders as far round as possible to each side. The observer views from behind (Fig. A5).

Chest Expansion. This is a useful index of costo-vertebral joint motion. The normal varies with build, the lower limit being about 5 cm. A significant reduction may occur early in the course of ankylosing spondylitis.

SACROILIAC JOINTS

The surface marking of these joints is the pair of dimples low in the lumbar area. Pain on pressure over these points is suggestive of sacroiliac irritability. The two joints are part of the rigid bony ring of the pelvis, and most manoeuvres designed to produce movement at these articulations depend on distortion of the pelvis as a whole. This is difficult to achieve, particularly in a powerfully built subject. The method of testing illustrated in Fig. A6 has proved effective. With the patient prone, firm

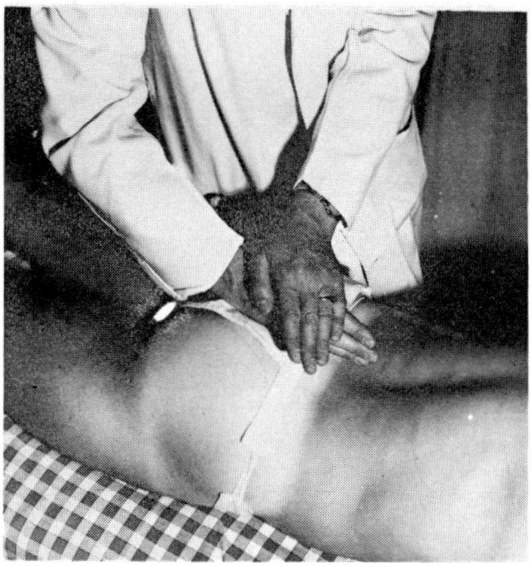

FIGURE A6 Testing for irritability of the sacroiliac joints by downward pressure on the lower sacrum. (*From* Mason, R. M. in *Textbook of Rheumatic Diseases*, 1969. Ed. Copeman, W. S. C. Edinburgh: Livingstone)

downward pressure is exerted over the lower one-third of the sacrum. This provides sufficient leverage for the sacrum to rotate fractionally between the pelvic bones, producing a sharp pain in the presence of active sacroiliitis.

THE MANDIBULAR JOINTS

This joint is located just anterior to the tragus of the ear. A palpating finger placed at this point will feel the head of the mandible sliding forwards as the jaw is opened. Pain and tenderness during this manoeuvre may occur when this joint is involved in an inflammatory arthropathy. More commonly, pathology in this articulation is due to an internal derangement secondary to such conditions as dental malocclusion. In this case the palpating finger may detect clicking and grating. The range of movement is documented as the distance to which the upper and lower incisors can be separated.

THE UPPER ARM

The Shoulder

Effusions of this joint may be difficult to detect, unless gross, when they produce a characteristic swelling which may involve the (often communicating) subacromial bursa.

Most movements of the shoulder are a combination of motion in the glenohumeral (ball and socket) articulation, and motion between the scapula and thorax. In order to test pure glenohumeral motion it is necessary to anchor the scapula with a hand placed across the clavicle and spine of the scapula (Fig. A7). Movements must thus be defined as *glenohumeral*

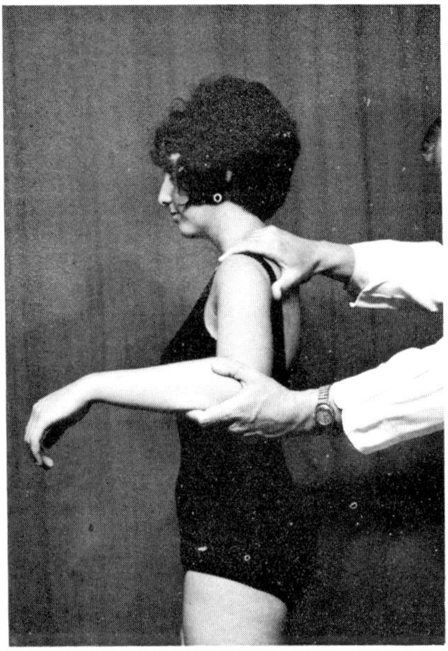

FIGURE A7 Shoulder abduction; the examiner's right hand is anchoring the scapula so that pure glenohumeral movement is tested

or *total shoulder*. Being a 'ball and socket' joint, very complex movements are possible at the shoulder. Analysis is simplified if the zero starting position is taken to be that in which the arm hangs by the side of the body with the palm facing forwards.

Special care is necessary in examination of the shoulder joint because of the frequency with which this articulation is affected by a number of ill-understood and, probably, not primarily arthritic conditions (tendinitis, bursitis, and capsulitis—*see* Chapter 15). In this group of disorders, pain may be provoked when particular movements are attempted against resistance, suggesting inflammation in the tendon(s) mediating the movement in question. With generalised capsulitis all glenohumeral movements are restricted and painful. In the common *supraspinatus tendinitis*, pain is typically produced through the middle one-third (60° to 120°) of active abduction, often abolished if the arm is in full external rotation.

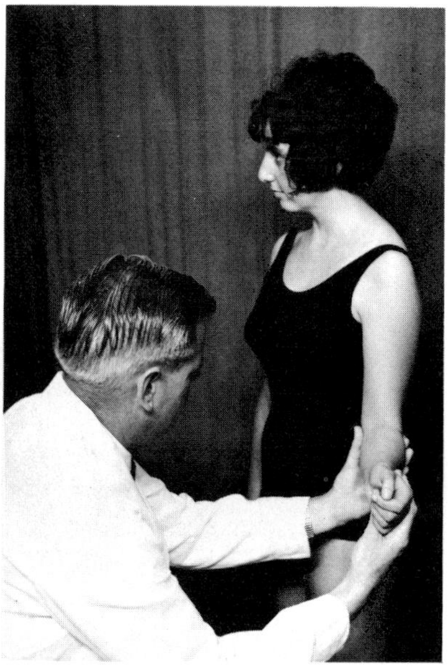

FIGURE A8 External rotation of the shoulder; a pure glenohumeral movement

Crepitus may not infrequently be elicited by movements of the shoulders in elderly subjects. As an isolated finding this usually does not signify osteoarthrosis (primary degenerative disease of the shoulder joint is anyhow rare).

Abduction (glenohumeral 90°, total 180°) Passive abduction is used to assess glenohumeral movement (Fig. A7). Attempted active abduction may reveal rupture or inflammation of the supraspinatus tendon.

Adduction (50°) Pure adduction is impossible because the thorax obstructs this movement. In practice, the arm is carried across the front of the chest (i.e. in partial flexion).

External rotation (60°) Fig. A8. This is the one shoulder movement to which scapulothoracic motion cannot contribute.

Internal rotation (90°) Except where very limited, this is conveniently documented as the height to which the thumb can reach in 'scratching the back' (Fig. A9).

Both internal and external rotation may also be tested with the shoulder joint in positions of flexion or abduction.

Flexion (glenohumeral 90°, total 180°) The arm is swung forward, as in marching.

Extension (65°) The arm is swung backwards, as in marching.

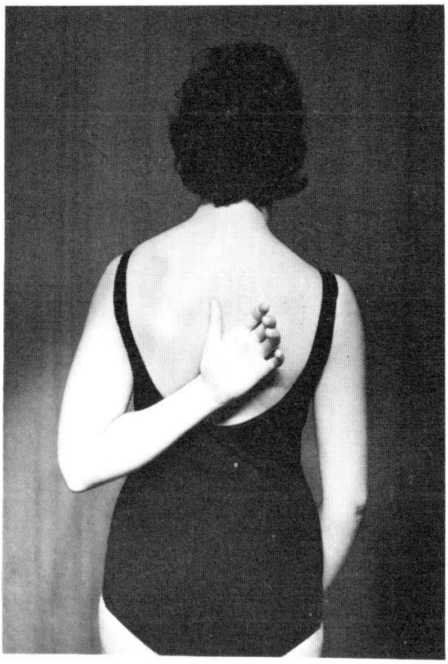

FIGURE A9 Internal rotation of the shoulder; a combined glenohumeral and scapula movement

Other Joints of the Shoulder Girdle and Thorax

Both the *acromio-clavicular* and *sterno-clavicular* joints are frequently the site of degenerative changes, but rarely give rise to symptoms. Placed superficially, they are readily accessible to inspection and palpation, and their movements can be studied by getting the subject to 'shrug shoulders'. The *sterno-manubrial* articulation may become painful in ankylosing spondylitis. In Tietze's disease (p. 237) there is painful swelling over the upper *costal cartilages*.

The Elbow

Effusions of this joint appear as bulging of the synovial cavity on either side of the olecranon posteriorly. Pain on pressure over the medial and lateral humeral epicondyles may indicate, respectively, *golfer's elbow* or *tennis elbow* (pp. 232 and 231). In passing, the examining thumb, slid down the olecranon and proximal subcutaneous border of the ulna, may encounter *rheumatoid nodules*, *gouty tophi*, or an enlarged *olecranon bursa*. The zero starting position is that in which the arm is in a straight line.

Flexion (150°)
Hyperextension (0°)

The Forearm

The zero starting position is that in which the elbow is beside the body and flexed to 90° with the thumb uppermost.

Pronation (80°)
Supination (90°)

The Wrist

This compound joint is frequently involved in rheumatoid arthritis; very rarely in primary osteoarthrosis. Local painful conditions, which have to be excluded before arthritis of the wrist is diagnosed, include recent or old *fractures of the scaphoid bone* and *de Quervain's tenosynovitis* (Chapter 15). The main movements are flexion and extension. Some lateral deviation is possible too. The zero starting position is that in which the hand is straight in line with the pronated forearm.

Extension (dorsi-flexion, 70°)
Flexion (palmar flexion, 70°)
Radial Deviation (20°)
Ulnar Deviation (30°)

The Hand

Careful examination of the hand is often as valuable in the differential diagnosis of polyarthritis as the examination of the whole of the rest of the patient. Uniquely, it provides the opportunity to study the distribution as well as the quality of arthritis, and it may also reveal characteristic changes in the skin, nails, and tendon sheaths. Function of the hand is peculiarly vulnerable to interference by lesions of tendons and their sheaths, and other associated soft tissues in addition to involvement of the joints as such; lesions at one point may produce important disturbance of more distal joints. Rheumatic disorders in the hands may thus produce serious interference with normal activities, and assessment of this involves examining the extremity as a functional unit. Finally, rheumatic disorders may interfere with peripheral nerve function in a number of ways, and examination of the hand must exclude, *inter alia*, compression of the median nerve in the carpal tunnel (p. 233). No assessment of an arthritic hand is complete without a neurological examination.

In seeking evidence of arthritis in a relatively normal hand, the two most helpful steps are the careful visual inspection of the outstretched fingers for the slight 'spindling' of the digits produced by early rheumatoid involvement of the proximal interphalangeal joints (*see* Fig. 3.7), and testing each of the small joints, in turn, for discomfort on pressure while the joint is moved passively (Fig. A10). This is a sensitive test for early arthritis.

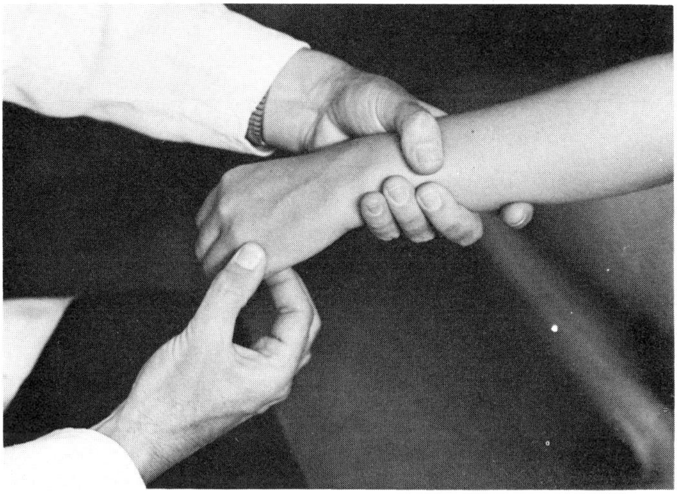

FIGURE A10 Testing for irritability of finger joints; compression and passive movement are applied simultaneously

It is worth remembering that the *flexor tendon sheaths* have linings similar to those of synovial joints, and are thus liable to be involved in the same pathological process. Effusions into these sheaths may be visible as sausage-shaped swellings along the flexor surface of the digits, or in the palm. Palpable nodules may be detected within the sheath, and in the condition *trigger finger* the area of stenosis can usually be located by careful palpation along the course of the tendon during movement of the digit. *Ruptured tendons* are revealed by loss of the active movement they serve.

Functional assessment of a hand involves consideration of the power and dexterity available for executing certain fundamental manoeuvres. As an example, four basic types of grip are illustrated in Fig. A11.

When the hand is involved in a well-developed arthritic process, the pattern of joint deformity and other local changes are often highly characteristic of the disease in question. These various patterns have been described under the relevant chapter headings, and only a few of the more 'classical' hands will be mentioned here. *Nodal multiple osteoarthrosis* produces a 'square hand' (*see* Fig. 14.1), with a firm bony swelling of the first carpo-metacarpal joint and wasting of the nearby thenar muscles. *Heberden's nodes* (firm pea-like swellings at the base of the distal phalanges) complete the picture. *Rheumatoid arthritis* in the early stages typically produces fusiform fingers from interphalangeal joint involvement (*see* Fig. 3.7). Later, the boggy swelling of wrist and

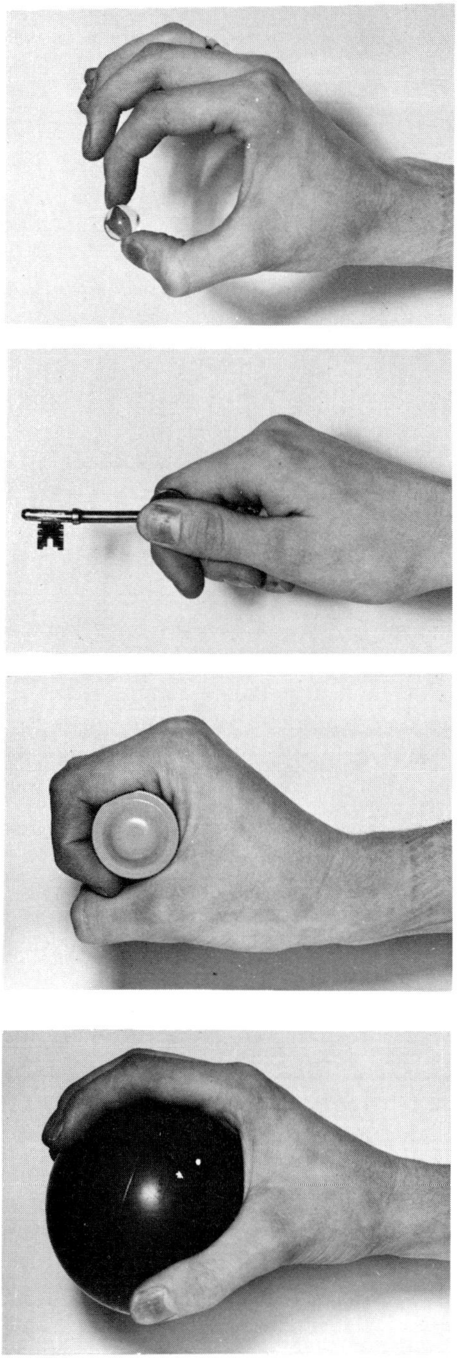

FIGURE A11 Four basic hand grips

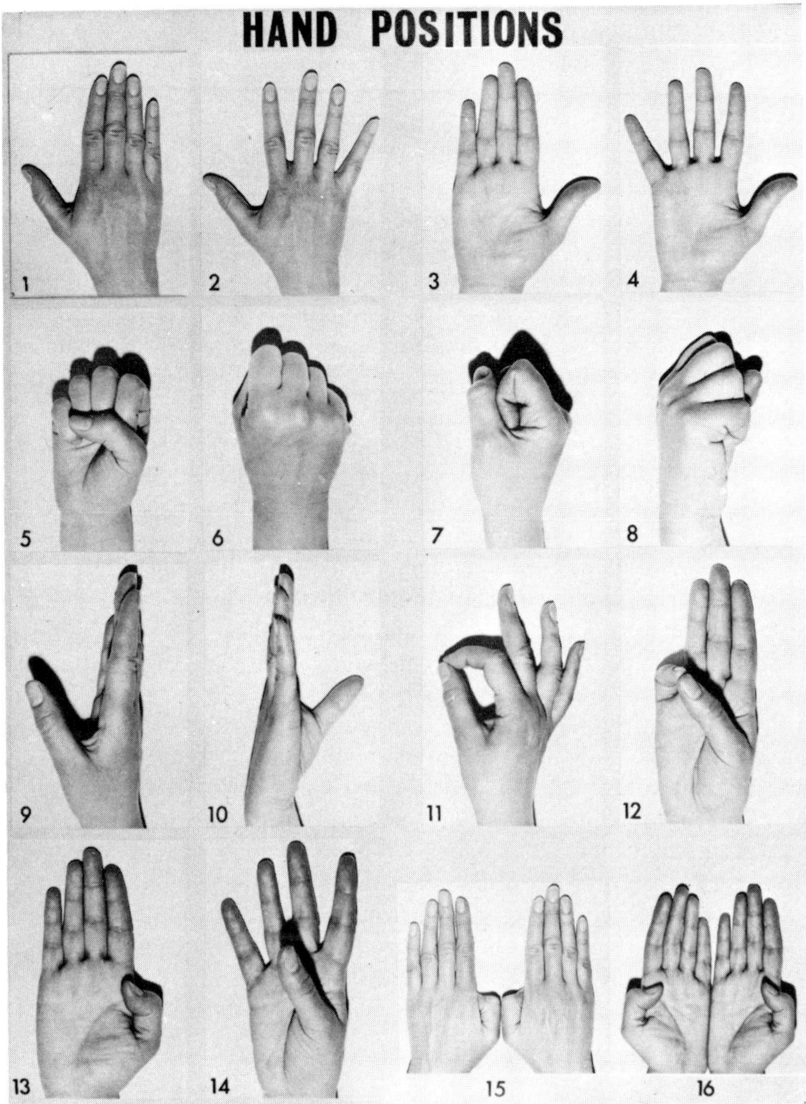

FIGURE A12 Chart used in ordering hand photographs (after one designed by Mr Adrian Flatt)

metacarpo-phalangeal joints, with wasted intrinsic muscles in between, present a characteristic picture (*see* Fig. 16.1). With advance of the disease in the hand, more gross deformities, due to joint destruction and tendon dysfunction, may lead to *ulnar deviation* of the fingers (often with palmar *subluxation* of the proximal phalanges (*see* Fig. 3.9) and, in the fingers themselves, *boutonniére* (Fig. 3.11) or *swan-neck* (Fig. 3.10) deformities. In the rheumatoid hand also, examination of the flexor tendon system may reveal effusions, ruptures, nodules, or stenosis; other features may be thin or transparent skin, and the nail-fold lesions indicative of digital arteritis.

Psoriatic arthropathy typically involves terminal interphalangeal joints, and the bulbous swelling of these articulations in association with psoriatic nail changes is characteristic (*see* Fig. 5.7). *Progressive systemic sclerosis* (p. 112), *systemic lupus erythematosus* (p. 134), and *dermatomyositis* (p. 122) may all produce mild symmetrical polyarthritis affecting the small joints of the hand, with the emphasis usually on the proximal interphalangeal joints. Each of these three conditions is also likely to produce characteristic skin changes in the hands. These are described in the relevant sections.

Measurement and recording of hand joint function presents considerable difficulty. Joint deformities can best be recorded by clinical photographs, for which purpose it is an advantage to have a set of standard views (such as the one adapted from Mr Adrian Flatt and illustrated in Fig. A12) to which the clinician refers when ordering photographs.

The actual range of movement of individual hand joints can be measured with a small goniometer, or by moulding a malleable strip of metal on to the dorsal surface of the adjacent bones, then using this to trace the angle on to paper. Changes in the size of proximal and distal interphalangeal joints can be recorded by using a set of jewellers' rings, while rather elaborate fluid displacement methods can be employed to measure changes in the size of a digit or the hand as a whole. Such measurements are of value mainly in the conduct of drug trials, where the influence of different therapeutic agents on the activity of inflammatory joint disease is being compared. Such trials have been the stimulus to develop various tests of hand function as a whole. Of these, the most useful is grip strength, in which a rolled-up, paediatric-sized sphygmomanometer cuff, inflated to 20 mm Hg, is gripped in the hand of the subject. The pressure he is able to exert on the bag is recorded in millimetres of mercury.

THE LOWER LIMB

The Hip

Accurate examination of the hip joint is one of the most important requirements for investigation of the locomotor system, and often the most neglected. Failure may be due to the inadequate circumstances in which the examination is carried out. Thus, a 'bathing trunk' type of garment provides the only satisfactory covering for the patient, and adequate assistance is essential if the subject is elderly or disabled.

Observation of the *gait* (with and without any walking aid used) may be informative and, while the patient is still standing, the *Trendelenberg test* can be performed by observing the relative heights of the two anterior-superior iliac spines while the patient stands first on one leg then on the other. Normally, the pelvis tilts upwards on the non-weightbearing side. Weight-bearing on a diseased hip may produce the opposite effect.

The remainder of the examination is carried out on a couch which must have two essential features: (*a*) it must be firm and non-sagging, (*b*) it must be away from the wall since, if fixed, it will never be possible to examine the left hip joint properly. The depth of the joint from the surface means that joint effusions, swelling, and local tenderness are much less often apparent than in superficial joints. Nevertheless, careful inspection, and deep palpation over, and just distal to, the middle of the inguinal ligament (i.e. over the front of the joint) may be informative. In suspected hip joint disease, abdominal examination is mandatory, and rectal examination is often indicated.

Measurements of leg length should also be made when hip joint pathology is suspected. True leg length is measured from the anterior-superior iliac spine to the medial malleolus (or other bony landmark), while apparent leg length is measured from umbilicus to the same lower point. Differences between the true lengths of the legs often indicate pathology in or near the hip joint on the shorter side, while differences between the apparent lengths (not reflected in true length differences) indicate lateral tilting of the pelvis, often due to an adduction deformity in a diseased hip joint.

The hip is another 'ball and socket' joint. Due to its deeper socket, the range of movement is less than in the shoulder joint, but the same problem arises in measurement; that of establishing whether movement is occurring at the acetabulo-femoral articulation itself, or whether the pelvis is being tilted. This requires careful observation and is made easier by the presence of an assistant to indicate the position of bony landmarks in the pelvis (Fig. A13). Unless otherwise specified, the zero starting position is that in which the leg is in line with the body, toes pointing anteriorly.

Flexion (115°). With the patient supine, the flexed knee is brought towards the abdomen (Fig. A14). The knee must be flexed to avoid a 'sciatic stretch' effect, and the angle recorded is that at which further flexion produces pelvic tilting. It is important to remember that a flexion deformity of the hip can be masked by pelvic tilting. Such a compensatory lumbar lordosis can be abolished by fully flexing the opposite hip joint (confirmed by a hand under the small of the back), and this will make apparent any fixed flexion deformity (Fig. A15).

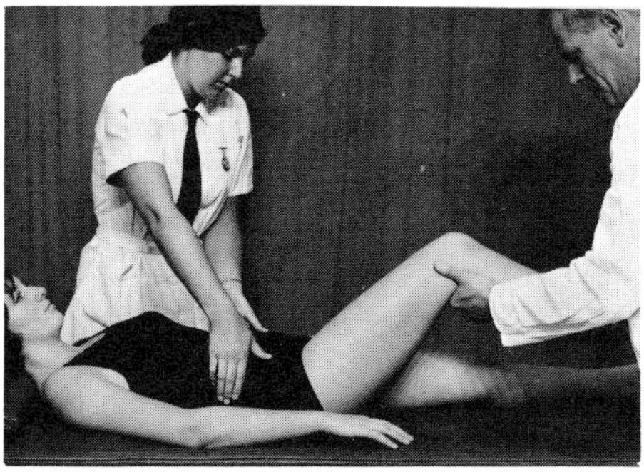

FIGURE A13 Hip movements can be mimicked by tilting the pelvis. Assessment of true hip movements may require the presence of an assistant to indicate the position of pelvic bony landmarks

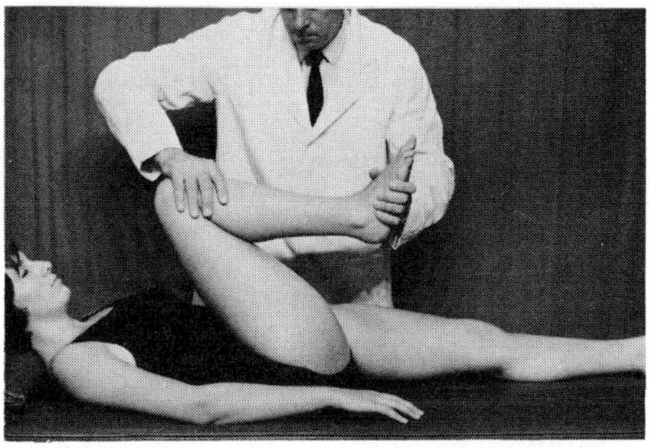

FIGURE A14 Hip flexion

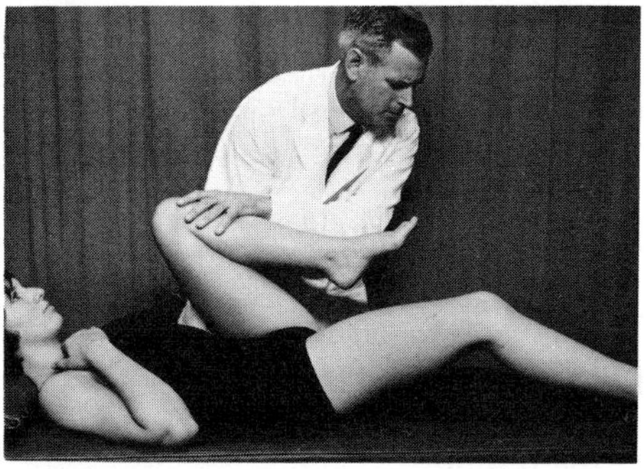

FIGURE A15 Flexion deformity of a hip joint may be concealed if there is compensating lumbar lordosis and pelvic tilting. Full flexion of the opposite hip will abolish the lumbar lordosis and reveal the flexion deformity

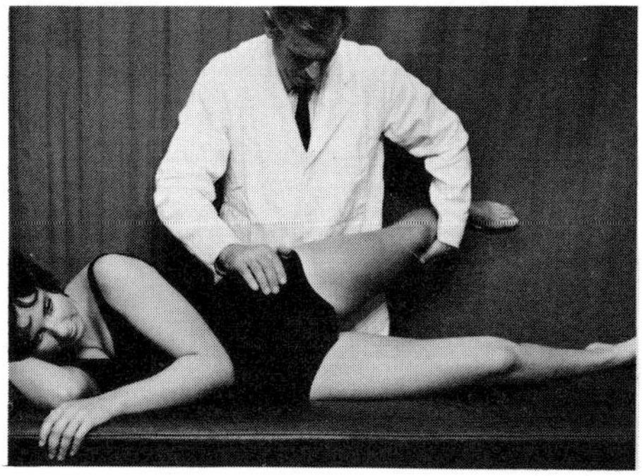

FIGURE A16 Extension of the hip joint. The examiner uses one hand to detect pelvic tilting

Extension (30°). With the patient lying on the opposite side, the observer, from behind, draws the leg backwards (Fig. A16). The angle recorded is that at which any further movement is achieved by pelvic tilting. An assistant is essential for this test if the subject is disabled.

Abduction (50°). With the patient supine, the leg is carried outwards. For serial measurements, the 'total straddle' can be recorded as the distance between the medial malleoli when both hips are abducted.

Adduction (45°). Similar to abduction, except that the leg is carried medially in front of the opposite limb.

Rotation (Internal 45°, External 45°). This may be tested with the leg in the standard zero starting position (which amounts to rolling the leg from

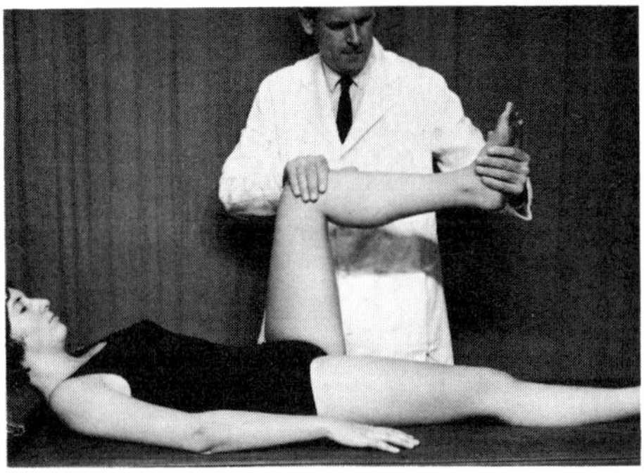

FIGURE A17 Internal and external rotation of the hip are here being tested with the hip joint in 90° of flexion

the side on the couch), or with the hip flxed to 45° or 90°. In practice, there is not much difference in the results obtained, and many clinicians find the 90° position most convenient (Fig. A17).

The Knee

Being superficial, the knee joint lends itself to much more precise examination than the hip. This requires familiarity with the surface markings of the joint, particularly the synovial cavity (with its supra-patellar extension), the line of the main joint space (level with the middle of the patellar ligament), and the collateral ligaments.

In a sense, there are two 'compartments' in this joint: the main articulation, and the patello-femoral. Physical examination may reveal that one or other compartment bears the brunt of any particular pathological process. *Patello-femoral lesions* tend to produce sharp pain on *active* extension of the knee, which is aggravated by backward pressure on the patellar during the movement. Patello-femoral discomfort and crepitus may also be elicited by sliding the patella sideways across the underlying femoral condyles. And at the extremes of medial and lateral displacement it may be possible to palpate part of the articular surface of the patella.

The complete investigation of a knee joint involves examination of all aspects of the joint (including posterior) both in the standing and lying positions.

Inspection (and comparison with the opposite knee) will reveal the presence of any swelling. This may be obviously due to distension of the joint with fluid, in which case a horseshoe-shaped swelling extends from the large supra-patellar pouch above, down the two borders of the patella, to fill in the depressions on either side of the patellar ligament. More often it requires palpation to identify the nature of any swelling. In osteoarthrosis, the bony hard, gnarled feeling is due to osteophytes. In inflammatory arthropathy there may be boggy, oedematous swelling of the synovium (soft tissue swelling) with or without fluid. A diagnosis of synovial effusion is made only when this can be demonstrated positively. Any soft swelling not accounted for by fluid is regarded as synovial. While gross effusions may be obvious, with cross-fluctuation from one part of the joint to another, smaller effusions may require meticulous technique for demonstration. The two most useful manoeuvres for this are illustrated in Fig. A18.

Inspection and palpation may also reveal localised tender areas (over sites of 'strain' in osteoarthrosis, or injured menisci) or swellings (such

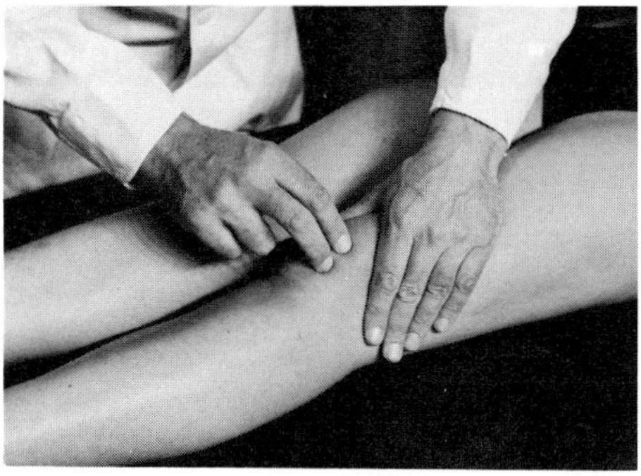

FIGURE A18 Two methods of testing for the presence of fluid in the knee joint

(*a*) The left hand forces fluid out of the suprapatellar pouch, while the thumb, index, and middle fingers of the right hand push the patella sharply downwards. A *patella tap* as the patella meets the femoral condyles is diagnostic of an effusion

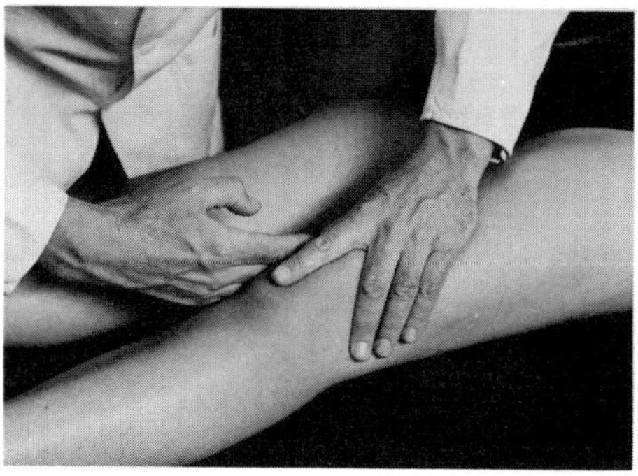

(*b*) The left hand forces fluid out of the suprapatellar pouch and also (with the index finger) anchors the patella. The right hand strokes downwards, first on one side of the patella then the other attempting to push fluid from side to side. If an effusion is present a characteristic outward bulging beside the patella is seen as the hand strokes the opposite side as meniscal cysts, or the cystic swellings in the popliteal space, so easily missed unless the back of the knee is carefully examined). Temperature differences are usually easily detected and provide a useful index of inflammation. Muscle wasting in the quadriceps, a sensitive index of knee-joint pathology, may be obvious on inspection. It can be recorded by comparing the circumference of the two thighs at a set distance (e.g. 15 cm) above the patella. Similarly, changes in actual joint swelling can be recorded as the circumference of the limb at the mid-point of the patellar ligament.

Apart from restricting the normal knee joint mobility, disease processes may interfere with function both by altering the alignment of the joint to produce *valgus* (knock-knee) or *varus* (bow-leg) deformities, and by increasing ligamentous laxity to the point where the articulation becomes unstable. Altered alignment should be recorded as an actual angle (ideally, both lying and weight-bearing). Tests for laxity are simply performed as part of the routine examination; lateral deviation of the knee is limited by the collateral ligaments, and antero-posterior gliding movements by the cruciates. Figure A19 illustrates two screening tests for instability.

FIGURE A19 Tests for instability of the knee:

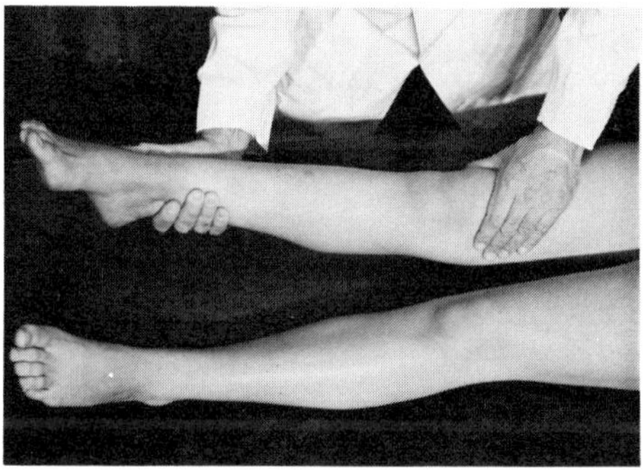

(*a*) Attempts to adduct and abduct the lower leg will reveal any lateral instability

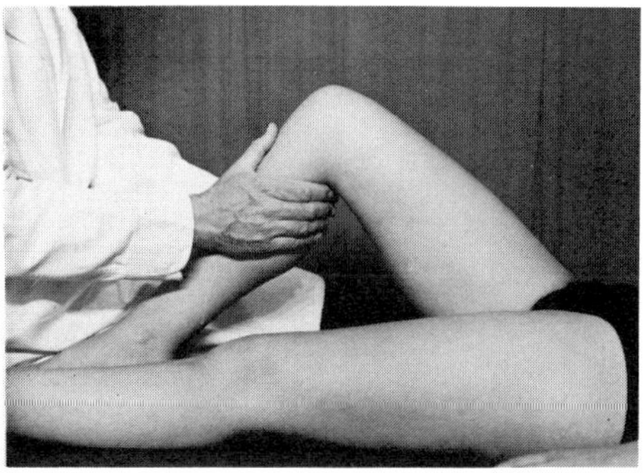

(*b*) Pulling and pushing reveals any antero-posterior laxity

Passive movement of the abnormal knee joint may produce pain and crepitus. In addition, when there is a tear of one or other meniscus, it may be possible to elicit a 'click' appreciated by a palpating finger over the meniscus in question. Various manoeuvres (such as alternating internal and external rotation applied to the foot during knee flexion and extension) may bring out this sign. Details of these will be found in orthopaedic texts.

The range of knee-joint motion is tested with the patient lying supine. The zero starting position is that in which the lower leg is in line with the thigh.

Flexion (135°)

Hyperextension (10°). This is variable, being an index of general ligamentous laxity. It is partly genetically determined, tending to be greater in coloured races.

The Ankle

Arthritis of the ankle joint has to be differentiated from ligamentous sprains. On the whole, sprains produce tenderness limited to one site, and pain particularly on movement in one direction, while active arthritis produces a joint that is tender along the whole joint line, and in which all movements are painful.

(a)

(b)

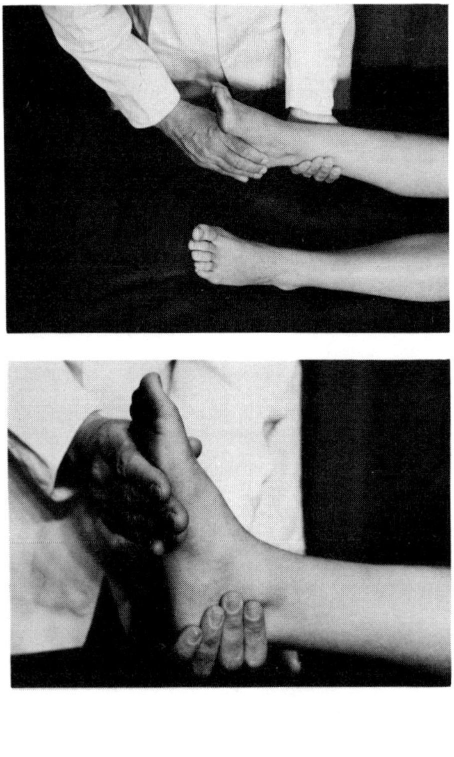

FIGURE A20 Testing passive movement in the foot. (*a*) The subtalar joint. (*b*) The midtarsal joint

The range of motion should be tested with the knee flexed. The zero starting position is that in which the sole of the foot is at right angles to the leg.

Flexion (plantar flexion, 50°)

Extension (dorsiflexion, 20°)

The Foot

The various articulations in the foot do not lend themselves to individual testing. It is customary to examine separately the subtalar joint and the midtarsal joints. The methods of testing passive movements at these two articulations are illustrated in Fig. A20. Approximately 5 degrees of both inversion and eversion is possible at the subtalar joint, and about 20 degrees of each of these movements at the midtarsal joints. But accurate measurements are difficult, and approximate comparisons between the two sides are often the best that can be achieved.

In patients with rheumatic disorders it is worth testing for *heel tenderness* both on the plantar surface and posteriorly at the point of insertion of the Achilles tendon (*see* p. 235). The Achilles tendon is also a relatively common site for detecting rheumatoid nodules.

Pedal complaints may result from a variety of abnormalities of the anatomy, posture, and tone of the foot. Such conditions are generally regarded as falling within the province of the orthopaedic surgeon rather than the rheumatologist, and the techniques employed in examining such feet will be found in orthopaedic textbooks.

The Toes

Most of the pathological appearances described as occurring in the fingers may be observed also in the toes. However, examination of the latter is generally much less rewarding. Routine locomotor examination should always include 'pinching' each metatarsophalangeal joint between forefinger and thumb while simultaneously flexing and extending it (Fig. A21). These joints are frequently involved early in rheumatoid arthritis,

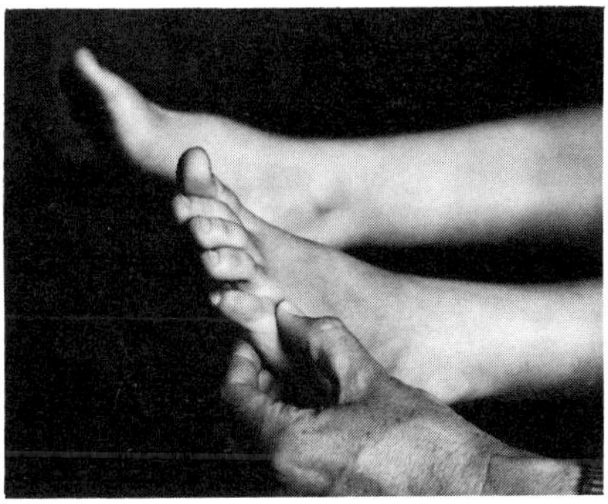

FIGURE A21 Simultaneous compression and passive movement of a metatarsophalangeal joint to detect irritability; an early sign of inflammatory arthropathy

and pain on this manoeuvre may be the first positive physical sign. Later in the course of an inflammatory arthropathy this test may reveal the thickened and subluxed joints that make walking so painful. Particularly in Reiter's disease (which affects mainly the lower limbs) these chronic changes may result in gross 'clawing' of the toes.

As in the hands, arthritis of terminal interphalangeal joints, with psoriatic involvement of the nail on the same toe, is characteristic of psoriatic arthropathy. Equally characteristic is the 'podagra' of acute gouty arthritis, in which the first metatarsophalangeal joint is swollen and exquisitely painful, with warm, red, and dry overlying skin.

Appendix B

Laboratory Investigations

Graham R V Hughes

RHEUMATOID FACTORS

Rheumatoid factors should more correctly be called 'antiglobulins', for they are antibodies (mainly of the IgM class) developed against altered gamma globulin (IgG immunoglobulin). The alteration that renders the subject's own globulin antigenic is thought to be the spatial distortion which this globulin molecule undergoes when it combines with antigen (*see* p. 9).

Rheumatoid factors are not specific for rheumatoid arthritis (Table B1). They are commonly present, for example, in the serum of patients with bacterial endocarditis. In the latter condition, bacteria coated with gamma globulin travel freely in the circulation, and are thought to provide the antigenic stimulus for the production of antiglobulins. In other conditions associated with the presence of antiglobulins, such as rheumatoid arthritis and liver disease, the mechanism is not clear.

Rheumatoid factors are heterogeneous and have a range of specificities; this is reflected in their varying reactivity with the human and rabbit gamma globulins used in the various tests. The range of specificities in any particular 'seropositive' subject will thus determine whether that serum will give a positive result with tests employing rabbit globulin, with those employing human globulin, or with both.

In practice, either human or rabbit gamma globulin (IgG) is attached to either sheep red blood cells or inert particles such as polystyrene (Latex), which then act as simple indicators of agglutination when the test serum is added.

LATEX FLOCCULATION TEST

Human gamma globulin is coated on to particles of polystyrene, and a small volume of this suspension is added to 'doubling dilutions' of the test serum. The highest dilution in which agglutination occurs is recorded as the titre. Sensitivity varies, but usually 1/80 is 'doubtful', and 1/160 or

TABLE B1

Causes of Positive Rheumatoid Factor Tests

Condition	Comments
RA	Especially those with nodules, erosions, or Sjögren's or Caplan's syndromes.
Normal persons	Approximately 4% of the population.
Relatives of RA patients	Slightly higher incidence, but low titres. For the most part these people escape the disease.
SLE	Up to 40%
Progressive systemic sclerosis	Up to 40%
Subacute bacterial endocarditis	Up to 25% positive. Reverts to negative with adequate antibiotic therapy.
Liver disease	Particularly infective hepatitis, chronic active hepatitis and cirrhosis.
Pulmonary fibrosis	Not necessarily associated with RA.
Leprosy	Up to 50%—usually in those with mutilating and osteoarticular disease.
Chronic pulmonary tuberculosis	5–20%
Conditions with raised gamma globulin levels	Positive tests may be found in sarcoidosis, multiple myeloma, macroglobulinaemia.
Sicca syndrome (Chapter 10)	Approaches 100%

over is 'positive'. This is the 'tube latex test'. A cruder 'slide test' gives a more rapid but less reliable answer. Similar tests can be performed using *bentonite* in place of polystyrene.

SHEEP CELL TEST (Rose-Waaler test)
A variety of tests employ sheep red blood cells coated with rabbit gamma globulin as the test system (Fig. B1). The source of the globulin is the serum of a rabbit that has been immunised against sheep red cells. Sheep red

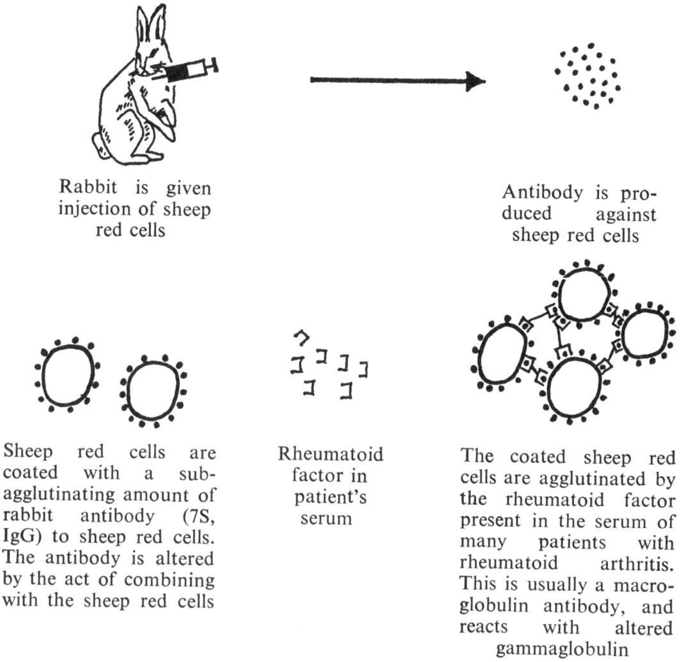

FIGURE B1 Mechanism of the Rose-Waaler reaction for rheumatoid factor (*From* Asherson, G. L., *Brit. med. J.*, 1967, **ii**, 417)

ells are then exposed to this serum (so-called 'amboceptor') diluted suffiiently so that the cells become coated with the rabbit IgG antibody, but re not quite agglutinated by it (a subagglutinating dilution). These sheep ells, now coated with rabbit IgG, are then added to doubling dilutions of ne patient's serum, and the most dilute (or highest titre) serum producing ed cell agglutination is noted. The specific reaction is the immune comination of rheumatoid factor and rabbit IgG. The red cells act merely s inert markers of the reaction.

A complication arises because the serum of certain subjects contains *eterophile antibody*, which will agglutinate normal sheep red cells and nus give false positive results. This difficulty is overcome in one of two ays: in one, the test sera are absorbed with sheep cells to remove any eterophile antibody before the test is performed. (This is the *sheep ell agglutination test* or *SCAT*.) Alternatively, the patient's serum is ested against both sensitised (coated) and unsensitised sheep cells, and ne ratio between the two titres is taken as the result. Thus, if a particular erum agglutinates sensitised cells at 1/128 and unsensitised cells at 1/4, ne result is recorded as $1/128 \div 1/4 = 1/32$. This is the *differential gglutination test* or *DAT*.

In practice, both the SCAT and the DAT are often recorded as th reciprocal of the titre, so that the example given above would be reporte simply as 32. The two tests are comparable. The lowest result regarde as positive is usually 16.

To some extent the latex and the sheep cell tests are complementary The former, because it employs human gamma globulin, is more sensitiv but less specific for rheumatoid arthritis. Thus, the (tube) latex test find its main usefulness as a relatively simple screening test for routine use while the more elaborate sheep cell methods are reserved for the mor precise testing of subjects with positive latex tests. The slide latex tes provides a very simple and rapid method for use when laboratory facili ties are not available.

THE LE-CELL TEST

The LE-cell is a phagocyte that has ingested altered nuclear material* The LE-cell phenomenon occurs in two stages. First, the nucleoprotei

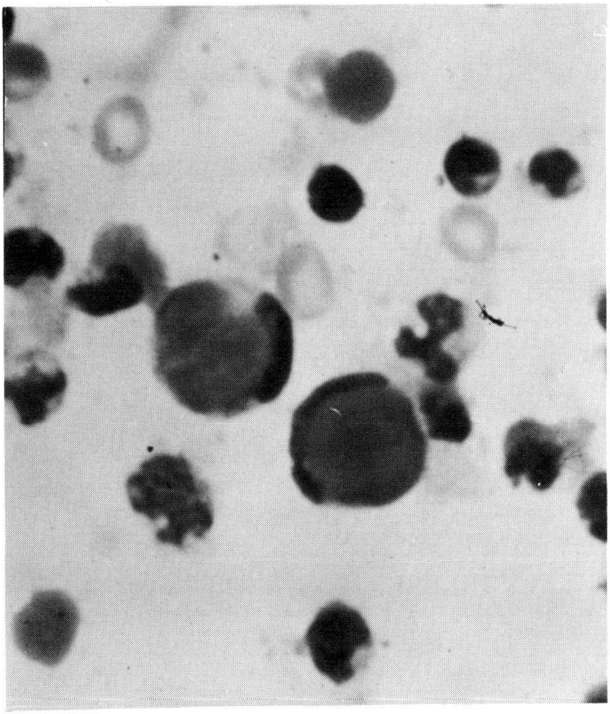

FIGURE B2 Two LE cells (Courtesy Dr D. M. Canning)

*The so-called 'tart cell' which may mimic the LE-cell, usually represents an ingeste lymphocyte, its nucleus staining blue, retaining its membrane and chromatin network, and not being obviously damaged.

of the cell nucleus is altered by antinuclear factor (IgG). Phagocytosis of the damaged or dead cell then occurs (Fig. B2).

This phenomenon may occur in bone marrow (where it was originally described) or in synovial fluid or pericardial fluid. The common laboratory test, however, makes use of peripheral blood where the phagocyte is a polymorphonuclear leucocyte.

Method. Peripheral blood is withdrawn and allowed to clot. The clot is then fragmented, thereby damaging some of the nucleated cells (the intact cell membrane largely protects the nucleus against antinuclear factor). The fragments of clot are sieved off, and the remaining fluid incubated before being centrifuged. The 'buffy coat' layer, containing the leucocytes, is then stained and carefully examined for LE-cells.

Significance of LE-cells. Depending on the care with which the test is performed, LE-cells are found in approximately 80 per cent of patients with SLE. They are also found in up to 10 per cent of patients with rheumatoid arthritis and, occasionally, in chronic active hepatitis (*see* p. 140), drug hypersensitivity, progressive systemic sclerosis, polyarteritis nodosa, and dermatomyositis.

ANTINUCLEAR FACTOR

The disadvantage of the LE-cell test is that it requires a careful and prolonged search and, even so, LE-cells may be missed.

With the introduction of immunofluorescent techniques more direct methods of demonstrating antinuclear activity became available. Antinuclear factor (ANF) is present in the serum of almost 100 per cent of cases of active SLE. It is, therefore, the best screening test for this disease. The disadvantage of this sensitive test is that it is less specific than the LE-cell test, and the list of diseases in which a positive ANF may occur is lengthy (*see* p. 140).

Method (Fig. B.3). Frozen sections of normal tissue (e.g. rat liver or thyroid) or peripheral blood smears, are incubated with the patient's serum. The cells are then washed, the antinuclear factor, if present, adhering to the cell nuclei.

The second stage of this 'sandwich' technique involves the incubation of the section with fluorescent antiserum to human gamma globulin (obtained from a goat immunised with human gamma globulin, the serum then conjugated to fluorescein). This antiserum adheres to the patient's globulin at sites where it is attached to the nuclei. After further washing, inspection by ultraviolet light microscopy reveals the distribution of fluorescein (and, hence, antinuclear activity) as brilliant apple-green fluorescence.

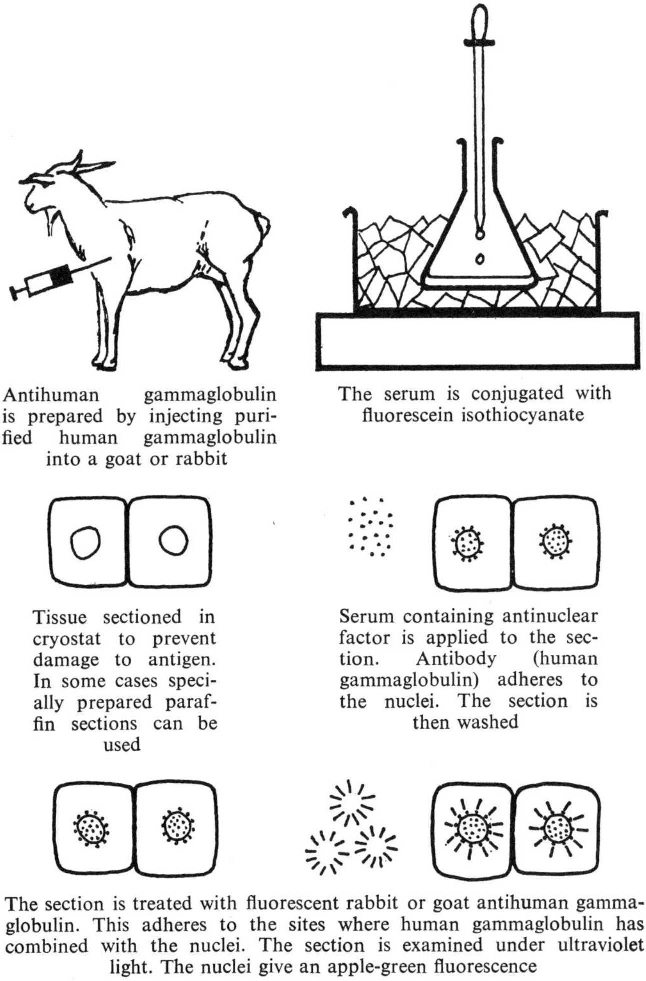

FIGURE B3 Immunofluorescent method for detecting antinuclear factor (*From* Asherson, G. L., *Brit. med. J.*, 1967, **ii**, 417)

URIC ACID

Plasma Uric Acid. Uric acid diffuses freely throughout the body fluids and plasma and blood uric acid estimations give similar results. The method commonly used is a colorimetric one, uric acid reducing Folin's phosphotungstic acid reagent to produce a blue colour. Most centres now use a modification of this method adapted for the autoanalyser.

The method has the slight disadvantage of giving readings up to 1 mg/ 100 ml too high, largely due to non-urate chromogens, but these disappear when the serum is stored for three weeks, or when heated to 60 degrees.

A second method makes use of the enzyme uricase which splits uric acid. This method, though more exact, is too time-consuming for general use.

In most centres the arbitrary upper limit of normal for serum uric acid is regarded as 7 mg/100 ml in males and 6 mg/100 ml in females.

Urine Uric Acid. For the estimation of urine uric acid, the same Folin's phosphotungstic acid method is used, at a dilution of 1 in 10.

Murexide Test. This method of staining for uric acid in suspected tophaceous material is less often used now that crystallographic methods are available. It remains, however, a simple and practical test. The tophaceous material is heated with 5 drops of nitric acid. After cooling, a few drops of ammonia solution are added, producing a purple colour (ammonium murexide).

HOMOGENTISIC ACIDURIA

In *alkaptonuria* (ochronosis) the alkalinised urine darkens on standing. The urine will also give a positive test for a 'reducing substance' (Benedict's test or Clinitest), but a negative result with enzyme tests for glucose such as Clinistix or Testape.

ANTISTREPTOLYSIN 'O' (ASO) TITRE

The streptococcus produces two distinct haemolysins – streptolysins 'O' and 'S'. The ability of streptolysin 'O' to haemolyse sheep red cells is depressed if serum containing ASO is added.

Using standardised streptolysin 'O' and sheep red cells, therefore, the dilution of the test serum necessary to produce inhibition can be assessed and recorded as a titre.

A positive ASO titre indicates recent infection with a streptococcus. The test is, therefore, non-specific, being positive following any streptococcal sore throat. However, in a suspected case of rheumatic fever, a high titre (over 1 in 800), or a rising titre, provides additional evidence for the diagnosis. (By convention this test is also reported as the reciprocal of the titre, i.e. 1/800 becomes '800'.)

EXAMINATION OF SYNOVIAL FLUID

Aspiration. Fluid from any synovial joint is suitable for examination. In practice, the most common site for aspiration of synovial fluid is the knee joint. Thorough antiseptic precautions are essential, the knee being cleaned over a wide area, and the remainder of the leg covered with sterile towelling.

A variety of sites can be used for aspiration, perhaps the most satisfactory being at a point between the upper and lower ends of the patella, on the medial border. Using a sterile swab, the groove between the patella and femur is palpated. At this site, local infiltration with 1 per cent lignocaine is performed. The aspiration needle (a 20 gauge needle may be necessary for more turbid fluid) is inserted at right angles to the skin, behind the posterior surface of the patella, and fluid is aspirated.

Appearance. Normal joint fluid is straw-coloured, clear, and viscous (and is present only in minute quantities). Inflammatory changes are associated with a greater volume of a more opaque fluid which is less viscous, and which will clot on standing if the fibrinogen content is sufficiently high. *Bloodstaining* is rarely due to the needle. It may occur in haemophilia, trauma, pigmented villo-nodular synovitis or, rarely, in synovitis of any cause, if sufficiently acute. Septic arthritis characteristically produces a grey, turbid fluid, but this is not invariable and no diagnostic reliance can be placed on naked-eye appearances.

Viscosity. The viscosity of joint fluid depends both on the concentration and the degree of polymerisation of its *hyaluronic acid* content. Inflammatory changes affect viscosity both by diluting the hyaluronic acid and by causing depolymerisation. The viscosity of the fluid is apparent as its 'stringiness' during transfer from syringe to container. Normal fluid is highly viscous; in rheumatoid arthritis, by contrast, the fluid may be quite watery.

Mucin Test. Addition of acetic acid (to a final concentration of 1 per cent) to normal or near-normal synovial fluid produces a firm mucin clot. Fluid from acutely inflamed joints gives a scanty and flocculent mucin clot. This test is usually not regarded as worth performing routinely.

Protein Content. As in other body fluids, the protein content of the synovial fluid is a measure of permeability changes in the lining and hence is a reflection of the acuteness of a synovitis. In degenerative joint disease a figure of 2 to 3 G/100 ml is common. In rheumatoid arthritis or crystal synovitis the figure is usually about 4 to 7 G/100 ml. A rough guide to the protein content is the speed of appearance and texture of any clot that forms.

Leucocytes. In order to perform cell counts, synovial fluid must immediately be mixed with EDTA (Versine) anticoagulant, and acetic acid should be omitted from any diluting fluid used. The viscosity of the fluid makes this examination rather inaccurate, and it is seldom done routinely. The degree of turbidity of a fluid provides a rough index of its cell content. In practice, degenerative joint disease may produce synovial leucocyte counts of 0 to 5,000 cells/mm^3, rheumatoid arthritis counts of the order of 5,000 to 50,000 cells/mm^3.

The morphology of the synovial fluid leucocytes can be studied, and differential counts carried out either on dry smears using Wright's stain, or on wet preparations (preferably using phase contrast microscopy). Again, this is seldom worth doing routinely. In general, rheumatoid effusions usually contain about 90 per cent neutrophil leucocytes, the remainder being mononuclear cells. In degenerative joint disease the percentage of mononuclear cells may be somewhat higher, while in septic arthritis and crystal synovitis almost every cell may be a polymorphonuclear. Rubella arthritis may yield a relatively high mononuclear count. Very large (40μ) cells with cellular inclusions (Pekin cells) may be seen in Reiter's disease. Multiple small, dark inclusions may be seen in the cytoplasm of polymorphonuclear leucocytes in a wide variety of circumstances. These 'ragocytes' are most common in rheumatoid arthritis, but are not diagnostic of this condition (*see* p. 12).

Rheumatoid Factor. Though infrequently looked for, this may occasionally be found in synovial fluid before it becomes positive in the blood, and may prove helpful in diagnosis.

Crystals. See Chapter 11.

Bacteriology. See Chapter 12.

SYNOVIAL BIOPSY

'Open' biopsy involves the surgical exploration of the joint (arthrotomy) with removal of a piece of synovium under direct vision. For 'closed' biopsy the technique is essentially that of needle aspiration. A variety of biopsy needles is available, the choice depending on individual preference. This method of biopsy is safe and, generally, gives a satisfactory piece of synovium for histology.

ARTHROSCOPY

Endoscopic examination of the knee joint under local anaesthetic is now practicable, and is being tested. It is a relatively safe and simple procedure that permits inspection, photography, and biopsy of certain areas of the joint. Unlike ordinary (blind) biopsy, it enables the site to be selected.

The usefulness of both arthroscopy and closed biopsy is limited, of course, by the fact that open arthrotomy is also a relatively safe and simple operation, and it clearly offers advantages in the information it can provide.

Appendix C

(Extract from the report by The Royal College of Physicians of London on the training of consultants)*

Schedule of Training

Rheumatology and/or Physical Medicine

A. *The Pre-registration Year* (at present 12 months: 6 months Medicine, 6 months Surgery)

B. *General Professional Training*
For 3 years:
Hospitals posts, that is, House Physician, House Surgeon or resident in a special hospital or a special department of the general hospital. The post of House Surgeon in an Orthopaedic department and House Physician in a Neurology department will be of advantage.
Or laboratory posts in sciences basic to medicine.
Experience should be obtained of general clinical medicine at Registrar or equivalent academic level.

C. *Vocational (Specialist) Training*
For 4 Years:
General medicine at Registrar (or equivalent academic) level with at least two years of Senior Registrar (or equivalent appointment) in Rheumatology or in a post combining general medicine with Rheumatology. During this period experience should be acquired in Physical Medicine and rehabilitation.

D. A number of posts in hospitals have been recommended by the College as suitable for Consultant training and it is advisable that, as far as possible, time in training should be spent only in such posts. Rotation between 'university/teaching' and other hospitals at some stage during the training years is an advantage.

*We are grateful to the Registrar, The Royal College of Physicians of London, for permission to publish this Schedule. A new report on Consultant Training is in preparation at the time of going to press, but we are informed that, although the form in which the Schedules are presented may be altered, there will be no essential changes.

Editors

E. A year can with advantage be spent in research or other special experience at home or abroad at some stage, and no strict sequence of posts need be observed before appointment to a Senior Registrarship or its equivalent. Research may be pursued contemporaneous with Registrar experience. Preferably, a research fellowship should be obtained for a period of one or two years; in this case one year may be deducted from the period of Senior Registrarship.

F. Time spent in general practice or working overseas in a relevant appointment or in the medical branch of one of the Services may be recognised as making up part of the training.

Index